**Books are to be returned on or before
the last date below.**

(555)

Fundamentals of Clinical Ophthalmology

Glaucoma

Fundamentals of Clinical Ophthalmology

Glaucoma

Edited by

Roger Alan Hitchings
Professor of Glaucoma and Allied Studies
Institute of Ophthalmology and
Moorfields Eye Hospital, London

Series Editor
Susan Lightman
Professor of Clinical Ophthalmology
Institute of Ophthalmology and
Moorfields Eye Hospital, London

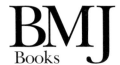

BMJ
Books

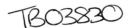

First published in 2000
by the BMJ Publishing Group, BMA House, Tavistock Square,
London WC1H 9JR

www.bmjbooks.com

British Library Cataloguing in Publication Data

A catalogue record for this book is available from the British Library

ISBN 0-7279-1448-0

Typeset by J&L Composition Ltd, Filey, North Yorkshire
Colour Origination by Tenon & Polert Colour Scanning, Hong Kong
Printed and bound in Italy

Contents

Contributors

K Barton
Consultant Ophthalmic Surgeon, Moorfields Eye Hospital, London, UK.

A Béchetoille
Professor of Ophthamology, Centre Hospitalier Universitaire, Angers, France.

P T K Chew
Associate Professor, Department of Ophthalmology, National University Hospital, Singapore.

A H Child
Honorary Senior Lecturer, Glaucoma Research Unit, Moorfields Eye Hospital, London, UK.

P J Foster
Research Fellow, Moorfields Eye Hospital and Institute of Ophthalmology, University College London, UK.

S G Fraser
Friends of Moorfields Glaucoma Research Fellow, Moorfields Eye Hospital, London, UK.

T Garway-Heath
Consultant Ophthalmic Surgeon, Moorfields Eye Hospital, London, UK

A Heijl
Professor and Chairman, Department of Ophthalmology, Malmö University Hospital, Malmö, Sweden.

R A Hitchings
Professor of Glaucoma and Allied Studies, Institute of Ophthalmology, University College London and Moorfields Eye Hospital, London, UK.

G J Johnson
Rothes Professor of Preventive Ophthalmology, Department of Epidemiology and International Eye Health, Institute of Ophthalmology, University College London, UK.

J Jonas
Associate Professor of Ophthalmology, Friedrich–Alexander–University Erlangen–Nürnberg, Erlangen, Denmark.

P T Khaw
Professor of Glaucoma Studies and Wound Healing and Consultant Ophthalmic Surgeon, Moorfields Eye Hospital and Institute of Ophthalmology, University College, London, UK.

G Kobelt
Managing Director, Health Dynamics International, France.

G K Krieglstein
Professor and Chairman, University Eye Hospital, Cologne, Germany.

C Migdal
Consultant Ophthalmologist, Western Eye Hospital, London, UK.

I E Murdoch
Consultant Ophthalmic Surgeon, Moorfields Eye Hospital, London, UK.

M Papadopoulos
Glaucoma Fellow, Moorfields Eye Hospital and Institute of Ophthalmology, University College, London, UK.

P Shah
Consultant, Birmingham and Midlands Eye Centre, Birmingham, UK (Formerly Galucoma Fellow, Moorfields Eye Hospital and Institute of Ophthalmology, University College London, UK).

G L Spaeth
Director, William and Anna Goldberg Glaucoma Service and Research Laboratory, Wills Eye Hospital, Philadelphia, USA and Professor of Ophthalmology, Jefferson Medical College, Philadelphia, USA.

J C Tsai
Assistant Professor of Ophthalmology, Vanderbilt Univerity School of Medicine, Nashville, Tennessee, USA.

A C Viswanathan
Specialist Registrar, Moorfields Eye Hospital, London and Honorary Research Fellow, Laboratory of Physiological Optics, Institute of Ophthalmology, University College London, UK.

A Wells
Glaucoma Fellow, Moorfields Eye Hospital and Institute of Ophthalmology, University College, London, UK.

R P L Wormald
Consultant Ophthalmologist and Head of Clinical Epidemiology, Moorfields Eye Hospital, and Institute of Ophthalmology, University College, London, UK.

Preface to the *Fundamentals of Clinical Ophthalmology* series

This book is part of a series of ophthalmic monographs, written for ophthalmologists in training and general ophthalmologists wishing to update their knowledge in specialised areas. The emphasis of each is to combine clinical experience with the current knowledge of the underlying disease processes.

Each monograph provides an up to date, very clinical and practical approach to the subject so that the reader can readily use the information in everyday clinical practice. There are excellent illustrations throughout each text in order to make it easier to relate the subject matter to the patient.

The inspiration for the series came from the growth in communication and training opportunities for ophthalmologists all over the world and a desire to provide clinical books that we can all use. This aim is well reflected in the international panels of contributors who have so generously contributed their time and expertise.

Susan Lightman

Preface

This single volume guide to one of the more common eye diseases sets out to highlight the importance of the subject within ophthalmology. To achieve this it has not only to define, develop treatment strategies, and assess the outcome of treatment for the glaucomas, but also to assess their impact both on the patient, as well as on society as a whole.

To accomplish these aims the book first defines glaucoma, looking at the differentiation of the different types and the changing perception of what is primary open angle glaucoma. Chapters discuss the features of primary open angle glaucoma, concentrating on optic disc, visual field and intraocular pressure signs. Knowing these signs, the book looks at methods of population screening and the results of population studies. Although a large part of the book focuses on open angle glaucoma, for this variety has received most attention from ophthalmologists, major chapters on angle closure glaucoma recognise the importance of this subset of the primary glaucomas world-wide. Individual chapters address the important subjects of both congenital and secondary glaucomas.

Treatments for the glaucomas are discussed in detail. This discussion includes both the principles behind treatment, as well as the efforts to establish an evidence base for the effectiveness of different treatments. All treatments have a price tag; the costs are investigated both for different treatments and in different countries. It is appropriate therefore to consider the cost to the patient as well as the cost of the therapy. As different treatments can have similar outcomes but different price tags, the cost effectiveness of different treatments can be used to decide between them.

Treatment for glaucoma is no longer a matter of reducing intraocular pressure. The outcome should relate to preserving visual function, as well as change, or lack of it, in the optic nerve head. All treatments can bring their own problems or side effects and a knowledge of these allows the practising physician to make valued judgements between alternatives, as well as advise the patients on risks as well as benefits.

The glaucomas form a heterogeneous group of eye diseases, each with the potential to severely affect the lifestyle of the sufferer. This book sets out to make it easier for the general ophthalmologist to reduce the likelihood of that occurring.

Roger Hitchings

1 What is primary open angle glaucoma?

R A HITCHINGS

This chapter looks at primary open angle glaucoma, defines it and sees what sets it apart both from other glaucomas and from other diseases of the optic nerve. It then sets out broad principles of management. Early references not readily available have been cited in the text, the remainder have been placed in the bibliography.

Primary open angle glaucoma: development of a disease

The development of our concept of glaucoma has followed the development of methods of examination of the eye. When this was limited to external inspection and later with a magnifying glass or loupe, the identification of ocular disease was restricted to those physical signs externally visible. Patients with progressive and painless visual loss often had no external sign of abnormality and may only have shown some evidence for cataract. Early writings often failed to distinguish between cataract and glaucoma. Recognition that the eye felt hard to the touch was noted by Bannister in his book "A worthy treatise of the eyes" where he described "alteration of the colour of the crystalline humour, with a durosity or hardness of the whole eye . . .". Elsewhere he describes the "Eie be grown more solid and hard . . . than it should be". (Bannister R. A worthy Treatise of the eyes. London 1622). In 1745 Johann Platner described absolute glaucoma "with hardness of the eye, a sea green colour to the pupil and a dilated pupil" (Platner JZ.

Institutiones Chirugiae rationales cum medical cum manualis. Lipsiae 1745; 889). Mackensie[1] described the signs and symptoms of glaucoma and suggested surgical puncture of the coats of the eyes as treatment.

The ophthalmoscope allowed examination of the ocular contents and soon recognition of glaucomatous cupping (Weber A. Ein Fall von parteiller Hyperamie der chorioidea bei einem Kaninchen. *Arch f Ophthalmol* Berlin 2. 1855; 133) and Heinrich Muller ascribed glaucomatous cupping to increased intraocular pressure (Mueller H. Beschreibung einiger von Prof von Graefe exsterpierter Augaepfel. *Arch f Ophthalmol* Berlin 4.1858; 363). Separation of glaucomatous from normal optic disc appearance was first performed by Elschnig (Elschnig A. Ueber physiologische, atrophischeund glaukomatoese Exkavation. *Ber Disch Ophthalmol* 1907; **34**: 2).

The central field defects now accepted as typical for chronic glaucoma were first identified with the use of the campimeter or tangent screen. Von Graefe is credited with being the first to recognise their use in this way. It was the introduction by Bjerrum of the Tangent screen that popularised the routine use of perimetry for identifying visual field defects. The arcuate or Bjerrum scotoma was first described by this technique (Bjerrum. 1890 *Nordisk Ophthal* Tidskrift, vol 2, p3) and further elaborated by Sinclair (Sinclair AHH. *Trans Ophth Soc UK* 1905; 384).

The development of instruments that gave accurate measurements of intraocular pressure

(IOP) was followed by surveys to assess the range of IOPs in the population. The results from these surveys led to the definition of a "normal" intraocular pressure together with a concept of an "abnormal pressure" (taken to be exceeding 2 or 3 SD [standard deviation] above the mean).[2,3] It was suggested that individuals with a high IOP would inevitably develop glaucomatous cupping and visual field loss, for the condition of the eye was already abnormal.[1] These eyes with elevated IOP were labelled "ocular hypertension".[4–6] This term tended to become synonymous with preglaucoma, or early open angle glaucoma without damage[6] and in many countries was considered sufficient indication to begin IOP lowering treatment. It was only with the long-term follow-up of groups of ocular hypertensives that the relative risk of developing glaucoma (in the absence of other risk factors) only rose dramatically when the IOP exceeded 30 mm Hg.[8–10] The association between ocular hypertension (OHT) and the development of glaucoma was considered multifactorial and complex.[11]

Concurrent development of methods of quantifying visual loss revealed characteristic patterns of loss seen with optic disc excavation. Cup sizes were expressed as a total of the whole disc. Pickard noted that small cups could exit in glaucomatous eyes and large cups in normal eyes.[12] Armaly introduced the concept of the cup: disc ratio[13] finding that less than 10% of the population had a cup: disc ratio exceeding 0.5, subsequently confirmed on the Framingham study.[14] Glaucomatous visual field defects could be correlated with changes at the neuroretinal rim (so called disc-field correlation)[15–17] and helped produce the triad of signs that made up chronic glaucoma: raised IOP, glaucomatous cupping and visual loss. This triad so imprinted itself upon the collective ophthalmological awareness that at the end of the 20th century the diagnosis of chronic glaucoma still rests on this trio of signs.[18]

The cause of the elevated IOP remained a mystery. The ophthalmoscope allowed recognition of intraocular signs associated with hardness of the eye. The cause of the elevated pressure was variously ascribed to hypersecretion of aqueous, excessive retention of aqueous, vascular disturbances within the eye and neurological disturbances outside the eye.

The development of gonioscopy, and the association of angle closure with acute and congestive glaucoma provided one mechanism. Salzmann was the first to use gonioscopy in the study of glaucoma. He found partial closure in these cases of congestive glaucoma (Salzmann M. Die Ophthalmoskopie der Kammerbucht. Klin Monatbl. F. Augenheikl. 1914; 52: 561). The concept of pupil block and its relief was first promulgated by Curran (Curran EJ. A new operation for glaucoma involving a new principle in the aetiology and treatment of Primary Glaucoma. *Arch Ophthalmol* 1920; 49: 131). Tronscosco studied 87 cases and found angle closure in 72% with acute or subacute glaucoma. He suggested that in these glaucomas an initially open angle closed later in the attack. (Troncosco M. Closure of the Chamber Angle in Glaucoma. *Arch Ophthalmol* 1935; 14: 557). Sugar concluded that the anterior chamber angle is open but narrow before an attack, but closed during an attack of congestive glaucoma (Sugar HS. The Mechanical factors in the etiology of acute glaucoma. *Am J Ophthalmol* 1941; 24: 851). Interestingly this approach was contested by Duke Elder who maintained that the narrowness of the angle was caused by the congestion and followed the acute attack (Duke Elder S, Baranay HE, Goldmann H, *et al.* Glaucoma a Symposium. C Thomas Springfield 1955). It was only the development of the concept of pupil block and cure of the condition by iridectomy that the argument was concluded (Haas J, Scheie HG. Peripheral iridectomy in narrow-angle glaucoma. *Trans Amer Acad Ophth* 1952; 56: 589). Subsequent studies differentiated these eyes from those with wide anterior chamber angles for which an alternative cause for the elevated IOP had to be found.

The possible causes for increased IOP in primary open angle glaucoma were considered to be either trabecular sclerosis, interference with aqueous drainage via Schlemm's Canal, obstruction to venous drainage from the eye, or overproduction of aqueous. Barkan attributed the raised IOP to trabecular sclerosis (Barkan O. Glaucoma: classification, causes and surgical control. *Am J Ophthalmol* 1938; **21**: 1099). Most experimental studies favoured trabecular sclerosis, placing the site of maximum resistance on either side of the Canal of Schlemm. Baranay and Scotchbrook showed that hyaluronidase reduced outflow resistance (Baranay E, Scotchbrook A. The effect of testicular hyaluronidase on the resistance to flow through the angle of the anterior chamber. *Acta Physiol Scand* 1954; **30**: 2408) and Barkan showed that an internal trabeculotomy dramatically reduced the resistance to aqueous outflow (Barkan O. Primary Glaucoma: Pathogenesis and classification. *Am J Ophthalmol* 1954; **37**: 724). Linner measured the pressure drop between the anterior chamber and the Canal of Schlemm localising the site of outflow resistance to the trabecular meshwork (TM) (Linner E. The outflow pressure in normal and glaucomatous eyes *Acta Ophthamol* 1955; **33**: 101). These views were substantiated by a series of experiments by Grant on enucleated human eyes.[19,20]

These changes seemed to be the result of a degenerative process causing loss of IOP control. An increase in outflow resistance led to the need for a higher intraocular pressure to maintain fluid flow through the anterior chamber. This process was associated with increased stress around the optic nerve head, causing mechanical distortion and reduced blood supply. The morphometric changes that followed became recognised as characteristic for glaucoma, and the disease was termed "primary open angle glaucoma" (POAG). This separated it from various secondary glaucomas, closed angle glaucomas and the deformed eyes seen in congenital glaucoma.

From this plateau of understanding, doubts on pathogenesis and mechanisms arose. As has been noticed the relationship between raised IOP and visual loss was not as simple as originally proposed.[21] Additional factors such as age, a positive family history of POAG and cup: disc ratio had to be implicated, and so the disease became multifactorial in nature. The IOP alone was considered sufficient cause only when the level was spectacularly high. (See Wilson for review.[22]) Total population studies revealed that a significant proportion of eyes with glaucomatous optic neuropathy had an IOP within the normal range (22–25 mm Hg).[3] When this concept of "normal pressure glaucoma" (initially "low tension" or "normal tension" glaucoma) was accepted, it cast doubts upon the validity of the triad of signs needed for diagnosis. This concern became particularly acute when it became known that these patients had normal aqueous humour dynamics.[27] The role of "pressure" in pathogenesis was becoming less secure and only maintained by the idea that the IOP in eyes with normal pressure glaucoma (NPG), although within the normal range, was "too high for the eye". It became downgraded to the level of a risk factor. Having noted this, there remains considerable variation in the definition of POAG as a recent review reveals.[28]

The late 20th century saw a considerable drive towards rationalising the visible changes at the optic disc and in the visual field. The retinotopic distribution of fibres and the characteristic nature of visual loss recognised in glaucoma meant that specific types of visual loss had characteristic changes visible at the optic nerve head.[15–17] The morphometric disc changes seen were typified and later typed, first to allow pattern recognition in this disease, and then to give possible indications as to pathogenesis (see also Chapter 5). That sequential changes occurred at the optic nerve head, was first recorded half a century ago by Ransome Pickard (Pickard R. Alteration in the size of the normal optic disc cup *Br J Ophthalmol* 1948; **32**: 955). Analysis of sequential optic disc photographs showed changes occurring in eyes with ocular hypertension suggesting conversion to glaucoma, before demonstrable visual field defects could be seen.[29,30] Similarly, retinal nerve fibre layer loss was seen to precede detectable visual field defects.[31] The view that early glaucoma could have normal visual function was given impetus with the demonstration of significant neuronal loss in the optic nerves of eyes known to have ocular hypertension but without visual field loss.[30,32] Again doubts were being cast on the triad of signs needed for diagnosis. It was not doubted that retinal nerve fibres and hence visual function, were being lost, just our ability to recognise it was insufficiently well developed.

Improved methods of examination of visual function lead to better pattern recognition, both in visual performance (where a move away from white-on-white perimetry, suggested by the theory of parallel processing and selective loss of visual function[33]) and in preferential large fibre loss in early glaucoma,[34] giving the promise of earlier detection of visual loss in glaucoma. Threshold perimetry associated with age derived from normal performance data allowed the development of standard criteria for visual loss[35] (see Chapter 6). Optic disc photographs allowed the recognition of signs for glaucoma with varying sensitivity and specificity figures to match. The development of measurement data, both with optic disc imaging and retinal nerve fibre layer measurements (particularly when matched against a normal data base), allowed the move towards the separation of the glaucomatous from the normal optic disc with increasing confidence.[36-38] The confidence that flowed from these examinations still allowed recognition of abnormality and the diagnosis of glaucoma before reproducible defects in visual function are recognised.

How can we define primary open angle glaucoma today? From the above discussion it can be seen that it is an optic neuropathy, with characteristic morphometric changes at the optic nerve head, that may or may not be associated with detectable loss of visual function and may have an intraocular pressure above the normal range. It has no obvious cause.

Primary open angle glaucoma: varieties

Primary open angle glaucoma occurs in such a wide variety of forms that it can be hard to see how the same causative process existed for all. It is appropriate therefore to look at different descriptive types. These have been subdivided by age at presentation, associated refractive errors and by the presence of an IOP within the normal range.

Simple primary open angle glaucoma

Population screening has characterised in western countries the typical patient to be a middle aged or elderly individual, having a slowly developing optic neuropathy with progressive visual loss. These characteristics have been described fully by Wormold (see Chapter 3).

Afro-Caribbeans

Population studies from Barbados[39] and from London[40] have shown that at diagnosis the typical Afro-Caribbean patient is younger, has a higher presenting IOP and more severe optic disc disease than their Caucasian counterpart. The eye is more resistant to treatment and carries a worse prognosis.[41] There has been the suggestion that Afro-Caribbeans in the USA are even more at risk than those on Barbados, perhaps because of as yet unrecognised environmental factors, and this may hold true for urban dwellers in the UK too.

Juvenile onset primary open angle glaucoma

These patients often have a strongly positive family history,[42] and present with or without some evidence of underdevelopment of the anterior iris stroma, (giving a characteristic flat featureless and usually dark brown appearance). These eyes usually present with an IOP in the high 30s and show marked resistance to topically applied hypotensive treatment. Left untreated progressive optic disc cupping develops. Filtration surgery is usually needed at an early stage in their management.

Primary open angle glaucoma with high myopia

These patients are at risk from developing glaucoma at any age. A recurring tragedy is the schoolchild who eventually presents because the optometrist can no longer provide normal vision with spectacle or contact lenses. Alternatively they are referred by the neurologist having presented as a case of optic atrophy of unknown cause. The glaucoma in the elderly myopic individual may go undiagnosed because of difficulties in examining the optic disc and visualising the "shallow" cupping typical in these eyes.[43] Even though there is peripapillary atrophy the optic disc should remain pink in colour, and if not, whatever the IOP, glaucoma should be considered.

Normal pressure glaucoma

This is a large subdivision of the POAG family, outside Japan it is present in up to 30%+ of newly diagnosed cases, and is the commonest variety of POAG within Japan. The condition is underdiagnosed in Western countries because the main trigger for case finding is elevated IOP. Without it the index of suspicion falls and in consequence glaucomatous cupping may be overlooked. In many instances aqueous dynamics are normal,[27] with normal diurnal curves for IOP and normal values for aqueous outflow. Despite this finding recent studies have confirmed a role in management for reducing IOP[44-46] although it remains uncertain as to whether this approach can cure the condition or just buy time before the optic neuropathy progresses. Although there have been a number of studies to suggest that there are morphometric differences between the optic disc appearances in high tension and normal tension glaucoma, the overlap between the two subdivisions is too great for these differences to be of value in clinical practice. That there is a primary defect at the optic disc seems likely however, for recurring optic disc haemorrhages are more characteristic of this type of primary glaucoma than the high tension variety.

Glaucoma as a progressive disease

Clinicians know intuitively that glaucoma is a progressive disease. It is known from cross-sectional analyses of patients presenting with glaucoma which show that the extent of the visual field loss is greater in the older patient, suggesting progression with time.[47] It is also known from untreated ocular hypertension or poorly controlled high tension glaucoma that there is progressive loss of visual function. What is not known is the rate at which it occurs. We assume that this will be at a higher rate in those eyes with higher IOPs. We also assume that the rate may well be linear (in Normal Pressure Glaucoma at least).[48] We like to think that lowering IOP will reduce if not halt the rate of deterioration, but again, outside normal pressure glaucoma there is little evidence (from an inability to measure rate of change) that we have achieved this. Our treatment is based on the assumption that lowering IOP does modify rate of change. Knowledge of the rate of change before a therapeutic intervention would greatly enhance our ability to show that this had been altered as a result of treatment.[44,49]

Patients rarely recognise progression of their disease until the late stages. The earliest stages occur without demonstrable visual loss as tested with white-on-white perimetry. Early visual field defects are overlooked within the binocular field. Loss of function is noticed by the patient as difficulties in adjusting to the light in darkened rooms, difficulties when driving the car at night or in the rain, difficulties from glare, and in terminal stages of the disease, difficulties with the visual field. Progression is noted by the patient as a hazy recognition that some or all of these symptoms are getting worse. A recent study of symptoms associated with demonstrated progression showed reasonable correlation between these symptoms and worsening of the disease.[50]

What do we treat when managing glaucoma?

The eye

Treatment for glaucoma is all too often directed towards the eye in question, to the exclusion of the rest of the patient. It has to be remembered that a significant proportion of glaucoma patients has no symptoms up until the time of diagnosis. Our treatment may well create symptoms and we have to keep the level of these below the gain from treatment as perceived by the patient. Accordingly, easily tolerated topically applied medicines and techniques of glaucoma and laser surgery least likely to produce discomfort are all to be preferred.

The amount of treatment to be given will depend upon the amount of IOP lowering required and what is a target end point IOP. This will depend in part on a simple actuarial analysis of the patient's life expectancy together with an assessment of the rate of visual loss and an estimate of how (any) further visual loss will impede upon the patient's lifestyle. For example, even a slow rate of visual deterioration will have a harmful effect over decades in the young patient, but little effect on the elderly. By contrast an eye with a threat to fixation will become symptomatic with any further loss, particularly if the corresponding retinal location has already been lost in the first eye. Therefore the elderly, the eye without fixation threat and the eye with a known slow rate of change, need not have the same stringent low target pressure set if giving further treatment would cause additional symptoms and side effects.

The patient

As noted above, many patients are asymptomatic at presentation. They are more prepared to accept treatment, which at the least will cause an interference in their lifestyle, if they can understand the process behind it. An informed decision will imply agreement in their treatment, which in turn will help them to comply with it. The systemic as well as the ocular side effects need to be fully explained before starting treatment, rather than explain them afterwards.

The doctor

All doctors try to treat disease. Treatment considered inadequate to control the disease process is seen as a reason to increase the treatment even if the potential for side effects is greater, e.g. whether to recommend glaucoma surgery for a patient with uncontrolled ocular hypertension. The ophthalmologist has to be able to "cry halt" at each incremental treatment stage before rushing on to the next. On occasion masterly inactivity and a wait and see approach is a safer one for the patient. At each stage the patient needs to be kept fully informed as to the thoughts behind any management decisions.

The family

Many glaucoma patients are elderly, and may have difficulty complying with a treatment regime. Family support is essential under these circumstances, so that all may have an understanding for the need for compliance and on occasion assist in management decisions as to the best approach to maintain it.

References

1 Mackensie W. A practical treatise on diseases of the eye. London, Longman, Rees, Orm, Brown and Green, 1830.
2 Leydhecker W, Akiyama K, Neumann HG. Der intra-okulare Druck gesunder menschlicher Augen. *Klin Monatsbl Augenheikl* 1958; **133**: 662.
3 Hollows FC, Graham PA. IOP, Glaucoma and Glaucoma suspects in a defined population. *Br J Ophthalmol* 1966; **50**: 570–86.
4 Pohjanpelto PEJ, Plava J. Ocular hypertension and glaucomatous optic nerve damage. *Acta Ophthalmol* 1974; **52**: 194–201.

5 Kolker AE, Becker B. "Ocular Hypertension" vs open-angle glaucoma: a different view. *Arch Ophthalmol* 1977; 586.

6 Phelps CD. Ocular hypertension: to treat or not to treat? *Arch Ophthalmol* 1977; **95**: 588.

7 Chandler D, Grant WM. "Ocular Hypertension" vs open-angle glaucoma. *Arch Ophthalmol* 1977; **95**: 585.

8 David R, Livingston DG, Luntz MH. Ocular Hypertension a long-term follow-up of treated and untreated patients. *Br J Ophthalmol* 1977; **61**: 668–74.

9 Hovding G, Aasved H. Prognostic factors in the development of manifest open angle glaucoma. A long-term follow-up study of hypertensive and normotensive eyes. *Acta Ophthalmol Copenh* 1986; **64**: 601–8.

10 Armaly MF, Krueger ED, Maunder LE, *et al.* Biostatistical Analysis of the Collaborative Glaucoma Study. *Arch Ophthalmol* 1980; **98**: 216–373.

11 Quigley HA, Enger C, Katz J, Sommer A, Scott R, Gilbert D. Risk factors for the development of glaucomatous visual field loss in ocular hypertension. *Arch Ophthalmol* 1994; **112**: 644–9.

12 Pickard R. A method of recording disc alterations and a study of the growth of normal and abnormal disc cups. *Br J Ophthalmol* 1923; 7: 81–91.

13 Armaly MF. The optic cup in the normal and glaucomatous eye. *Invest Ophthalmol Vis Sci* 1970; **9**: 42–59.

14 Leibowitz HM, Krueger DE, Maunder LR, *et al.* The Framingham Eye Study monograph: An ophthalmological and epidemiological study of cataract, glaucoma, diabetic retinopathy, macular degeneration, and visual acuity in a general population of 2631 adults, 1973–5. *Surv Ophthalmol* 1980; **24**: 335–610.

15 Read B, Spaeth GL. The practical and clinical appraisal of the optic disc in glaucoma. *Trans Am Acad Ophth Otolaryngol* 1974; **78**: 255–67.

16 Spaeth GL, Hitchings RA, Sivalingam E. The optic disc in glaucoma: Pathogenetic correlation of five patterns of cupping in chronic open-angle glaucoma. *Trans Am Acad Ophth Otolaryngol* 1976; **81**: 217.

17 Hitchings RA, Spaeth GL. The optic disc in glaucoma 11: Correlation of the appearance of the optic disc with the visual field. *Br J Ophthalmol* 1977; **61**: 107–13.

18 Shields MB. Primary Open-Angle Glaucoma. In: Anonymous Textbook of Glaucoma. Baltimore: Williams and Wilkins 1993: 172–97.

19 Grant WM. Experimental aqueous perfusion in enucleated human eyes. *Arch Ophthalmol* 1963; **69**: 783–801.

20 Grant WM. Further studies of facility of flow through trabecular meshwork. *Arch Ophthalmol* 1958; **60**: 523–33.

21 Quigley HA. Reappraisal of the mechanisms of glaucomatous optic nerve damage. *Eye* 1987; **1**: 318–22.

22 Wilson MR, Martone J. Epidemiology of chronic open angle glaucoma. In: Ritch, Shields MB, Krupin T (eds). The Glaucomas. 1st edn. St Louis: Mosby 1996: 753–68.

23 Tielsch JM, Sommer A, Witt K, Katz J, Royall RM. Blindness and Visual Impairment in an American Urban Population. *The Baltimore Eye Survey* 1990; **108**: 286–90.

24 Klein BE, Klein R, Sponsel WE, *et al.* Prevalence of glaucoma. The Beaver Dam Eye Study. *Ophthalmology* 1992; **99**: 1499–504.

25 Dielemans I, Vingerling JR, Wolfs RCW, Hofman A, Grobbes DE. The Prevalence of Primary Open Angle Glaucoma in a population based study in The Netherlands. The Rotterdam Study. *Ophthalmology* 1994; **101**: 1851–5.

26 Coffey M, Reidy A, Wormald RPL, Wu XJ, Wight LA, Courtney P. Prevalence of glaucoma in the west of Ireland. *Br J Ophthalmol* 1993; **77**: 17–21.

27 Larsson LI, Rettig ES, Sheridan PT, Brubaker RF. Aqueous humor dynamics in low-tension glaucoma. *Am J Ophthalmol* 1993; **116**: 590–3.

28 Bathija R, Gupta N, Zangwill L, Weinreb RN, *et al.* Changing definition of glaucoma. *J Glaucoma* 1998; 7: 165–9.

29 Pederson JE, Anderson DR. The Mode of Progressive Disc Cupping in Ocular Hypertension and Glaucoma. *Arch Ophthalmol* 1980; **98**: 490–95.

30 Quigley HA, Addicks EA, Green R, Maumanee AE. Optic nerve damage in human glaucoma: 2. The site of injury and susceptibility to damage. *Arch Ophthalmol* 1984; **99**: 635–49.

31 Sommer A, Katz J, Quigley HA, *et al.* Clinically detectable nerve fiber atrophy precedes the onset of glaucomatous field loss. *Arch Ophthalmol* 1991; **109**: 77–83.

32 Quigley HA, Dunkelberger GR, Green WR. Chronic human glaucoma causing selectively greater loss of large optic nerve fibers. *Ophthalmology* 1988; **95**: 357–63.

33 Livingstone M, Hubel D. Segregation of form, color, movement and depth: Anatomy, physiology and perception. *Science* 1988; **240**: 740–9.

34 Quigley HA, Sanchez RM, Dunkelberger GR, L'Hernault NL, Baginski TA. Chronic glaucoma selectively damages large optic nerve fibers. *Invest Ophthalmol Vis Sci* 1987; **28**: 913–20.

35 Heijl A, Lindgren A, Olsson J. A package for the statistical analysis of computerised visual fields. *Doc Ophthalmol Proc Soc* 1987; 153–68.

36 Iester M, Mikelberg FS, Courtright P, Drance SM. Correlation between the visual field indices and Heidelberg retina tomograph parameters. *J Glaucoma* 1997; **6**: 78–82.

37 Iester M, Mikelberg FS, Drance SM. The effect of optic disc size on diagnostic precision with the Heidelberg retina tomograph. *Ophthalmology* 1997; **104**: 54–58.

38 Wollstein G, Garway-Heath D, Hitchings RA. Identification of early glaucoma cases with the scanning laser ophthalmoscope. *Ophthalmology* 1998; **105**: 1557–63.

39 Leske MC, Connell AM, Schachat AP, Hyman L. The Barbados Eye Study. Prevalence of open angle glaucoma. *Arch Ophthalmol* 1994; **112**: 821–9.

40 Wormald RP, Basauri E, Wright LA, Evans JR. The African Caribbean Eye Survey: risk factors for glaucoma in a sample of African Caribbean people living in London. *Eye* 1994; **8**: 315–20.

41 The Advanced Glaucoma Intervention Study (AGIS): 3. Baseline characteristics of black and white patients (see comments). *Ophthalmology* 1998; **105**: 1137–45.

42 Morissette J, Cote G, Anctil JL, *et al.* A common gene for juvenile and adult-onset primary open-angle glaucomas confined on chromosome 1q. *Am J Hum Genet* 1995; **56**: 1431–42.

43 Jonas JB, Dichtl A. Optic disc morphology in myopic primary open-angle glaucoma. *Graefe's Arch Clin Exp Ophthalmol* 1997; **235**: 627–33.

44 Bhandari A, Crabb DP, Poinoosawmy D, Fitzke FW, Hitchings RA, Noureddin BN. Effect of surgery on visual field progression in normal-tension glaucoma. *Ophthalmology* 1997; **104**: 113–17.

45 Collaborative normal tension glaucoma study group. Comparison between glaucomatous progression between untreated patients with normal-tension glaucoma and

patients with therapeutically reduced intraocular pressures. *Am J Ophthalmol* 1998; **126**: 487–97.

46 Collaborative normal tension glaucoma study group. The effectiveness of intraocular pressure reduction in the treatment of normal-tension glaucoma. *Am J Ophthalmol* 1998; **126**: 498–505.

47 Jay JL, Murdoch JR. The rate of visual field loss in untreated primary open angle glaucoma. *Br J Ophthalmol* 1993; **77**: 176–8.

48 Crabb DP, Fitzke FW, McNaught AI, Edgar DF, Hitchings RA. Improving the prediction of visual field progression in glaucoma using spatial processing. *Ophthalmology* 1997; **104**: 517–24.

49 Katz J, Gilbert D, Quigley HA, Sommer A. Estimating progression of visual field loss in glaucoma. *Ophthalmology* 1997; **104**: 1017–25.

50 Viswanathan AC, McNaught AI, Poinoosawmy D *et al*. Severity and stability of glaucoma: patient perception compared with objective measurement. *Arch Ophthalmol* 1999; **117** (4): 450–4.

2 Epidemiology of primary open angle glaucoma

S G FRASER

Primary open angle glaucoma (POAG) is a condition that lends itself well to epidemiological studies in that it is reasonably common but relatively little is known about its pathogenesis. This is mirrored in the fact that most of the major population based studies have taken place in Europe and North America, areas where POAG is the commonest form of glaucoma.

The aim of this chapter is to review the prevalence and incidence of POAG from the point of view of these studies and then to review current thinking regarding risk factors.

Prevalence

The prevalence of a disease is the proportion of a population with the disease at a point in time. It is obviously impossible to examine an entire population for glaucoma, but an estimate can be made from examining random samples of the population. The prevalence obtained will be an approximation of that of the total population, as long as the study is large enough and the subjects are chosen in a truly random fashion.

Over the last 10–15 years there have been a number of population based studies that have, by adopting strict diagnostic criteria to the diagnosis of glaucoma and choosing their subjects in a random fashion, given an invaluable insight into the epidemiology of POAG. The important concepts required for population based studies are summarised in Table 2.1.

Table 2.1 The important elements to look for in a population based study

1. A reasonably large sample size
2. Whether the random sample is truly random
3. What efforts were made to find out if those subjects who declined to take part in the study were broadly representative of the study population
4. Careful consideration of diagnostic criteria for the disease
5. Preferably a number of observers agreeing on a subject being labelled as having or not having the disease in question

The area of the study, the sample size and the prevalence figures of some of these recent studies are detailed in Table 2.2.

In summary, these studies indicate a prevalence for POAG of 1.5–2% for Caucasians and 6–8% for Afro-Caribbeans. It is however, important to remember that quoting an overall prevalence figure for glaucoma is of limited value as race, age and possibly gender have such a profound effect that prevalence rates are best stated in relation to these variables. These factors are discussed in the relevant sections later in the chapter.

Incidence

The incidence of a disease is the rate at which new cases occur in a population during a specified period. Studies of POAG incidence are plagued by difficulties in diagnosing early disease and the need for prolonged follow-up of subjects. Thus, there are few rigorous studies of glaucoma incidence to date. This situation

Table 2.2   Prevalence of POAG in some recent studies

Name/locality of study	Sample size	Age range (years)	Racial distribution	Prevalence POAG
Baltimore[1] (USA)	5308	> 40	Mixed	White 1.29%
				Black 4.74%
Beaver Dam[2] (USA)	4926	43–84	Caucasian	2.1%
Roscommon[3] (Eire)	2186	> 50	Caucasian	1.87%
Blue Mountains[4] (Australia)	3654	> 49	Caucasian	3%
BARBADOS[5] (WI)	4709	40–84	Mixed (Mainly black)	Black 7%
Rotterdam[6] (Netherlands)	10 000	> 55	Caucasian	1.1%
St Lucia (WI)[7]	1679	> 30	Black	8.8%

should alter in the future as some of the large-scale population studies re-examine their initial cohorts to see the proportion of normal patients who have gone on to develop glaucoma.

Most incidence figures at present are calculated from the prevalence of the disease in different age ranges. This method was used to calculate incidences in white patients from around 20 cases of POAG per 100 000 persons per year at the age of 50, to around 200 cases per 100 000 for those who are 80.[8] Similar calculations for black patients indicate a higher incidence at all age groups from 200 cases per 100 000 persons per year at age 50, to 600 cases per 100 000 per year at age 80.

Of the available studies the Bedford survey found an overall annual incidence of 0.048 – this is not separated for age groups and relates only to Caucasian patients.[9]

Risk factors

There is a wealth of literature regarding risk factors for POAG and it is important when reading of the findings of these studies, to think how the studies were conducted.

Hospital based studies can be subject to selection bias in which certain patients are over represented in the hospital setting. Good examples of this are myopes and diabetics, in which regular eye examinations are likely, so increasing the likelihood for glaucoma being detected and for the patient to be referred to a clinic. Thus hospital based studies tend to over-estimate the proportion of glaucoma patients with myopia and diabetes which then implicates them as risk factors for the disease.

Population based studies are generally more useful than hospital based, but this advantage is lost if the study subjects are not selected randomly. If, for example, a study asks for volunteers, it is those who have greater concerns regarding glaucoma, e.g. those with a family history of glaucoma, who are more likely to present for examination. If the sample is not truly random, the influence of such factors as family history of glaucoma will be overestimated.

Local risk factors for primary open angle glaucoma

Intraocular pressure (IOP)

Although there is little doubt that raised IOP is a major risk factor for glaucoma, it is not the *sine qua non* it was once thought to be. There is strong evidence that IOP is intimately associated with glaucoma. This is summarised in Table 2.3.

Figure 2.1, from the Baltimore Eye Study,[10] is a plot showing that the relative risk of glaucoma rises with IOP. It is also important to note that this risk begins to rise, i.e. is greater than one, from about 16mm Hg. The commonly used cut-off between "normal tension" glaucoma (≤21 mm Hg) and "high tension" glaucoma (> over 21 mm Hg) is therefore meaningless. Although the use of the terms normal/low tension glaucoma can be helpful, to think of them

Table 2.3   Evidence that IOP is a risk factor for POAG

- The prevalence of POAG rises with increasing IOP[10] (see also Figure 2.1)
- Patients who have their IOP lowered (by whatever means) usually have their visual field loss slowed
- The eye with the higher IOP tends to lose field more quickly and this occurs even if both IOP's are below 21 mm Hg
- In studies where IOP is excluded from the definition of glaucoma it is strongly related to the risk of glaucoma

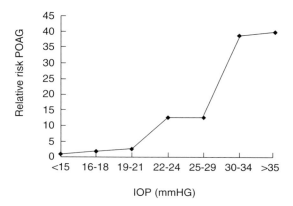

Figure 2.1   The risk of Primary Open Angle Glaucoma at varying levels of intra ocular pressure (from Sommer et al.)[10]

as a different disease to POAG, is not. A more realistic concept is to consider that an individual's optic nerve has a level of IOP that it can or cannot withstand. At a clinical level this is manifest by the presence or absence of visual field decline. If field loss is occurring, individuals need their IOP reduced to a level that stops (or more realistically, slows) this decline.

The concept of IOP as the major risk factor for glaucoma, rather than a diagnostic requisite, does mean that there must be some other factor or factors that act with the particular pressure in an eye to produce characteristic glaucomatous changes.

The optic nerve head

As well as being an important marker of the presence and advancement of glaucoma, the structure of the optic nerve head may play a role in the pathogenesis of glaucoma.

There are two main theories regarding the mechanism of optic nerve damage in glaucoma.[11] The mechanical theory (IOP related) suggests that the pressure head acts directly on the lamina cribrosa. This structure is less well supported superiorly and inferiorly at the disc margin, and it is here that the initial damage occurs, producing the characteristic arcuate defects. Variations in ganglion cell support at the disc may explain the variations between IOP susceptibilities between individuals with similar IOPs.

The alternative theory is the vascular mechanism of damage in which changes within the microcirculation of the disc capillaries are responsible for glaucomatous changes. Whether this is primarily vascular or secondary to IOP has not been elucidated.

Epidemiological studies have also implicated disc variation as a risk factor for glaucoma with both vertical and horizontal cup: disc ratio correlated positively with subsequent field loss. The Collaborative Glaucoma study[12] indicated that a high ratio was a risk factor for developing field defects.

One of the proposed reasons that black people have a greater prevalence of POAG than white people, despite having no differences in their IOPs, is that black people have been noted to have larger discs and larger cup: disc ratios than white people. Larger discs and discs with large cup: disc ratios have been found to be more susceptible to glaucomatous damage.[11]

Myopia

A number of studies have found a strong association between myopia and POAG. One study found a twofold excess prevalence of POAG in myopes,[13] while another found a fivefold risk.[14] Like diabetes the effect of myopia is overestimated in hospital based studies and it is likely that large scale population studies will find that the association is much smaller than once thought.

Systemic risk factors for primary open angle glaucoma

Age

Population studies have shown that one of the most important risk factors for developing POAG is increasing age. All the population based studies shown in Table 2.2 found an increased prevalence of POAG with increasing age. As well as being consistent across various studies, the magnitude is uniformly large with prevalence rates four to ten times higher in the oldest age group compared to the baseline (usually subjects in their forties).

Genetic

There is little doubt that a positive family history of glaucoma puts an individual at increased risk of glaucoma. Estimates have varied from 13–47% of POAG cases being familial. There is a 5–20 times prevalence rate in those with a positive family history. A number of new genes and loci have been found in the last two to three years and as it is probable that POAG is polygenic, this is likely to be a fruitful area in the future.

From an epidemiological perspective, studies of family history and glaucoma are prone to bias, which probably explains the widely differing prevalence rates in different studies. Patients who know a member of their family has glaucoma are more likely to present to a clinic and are more likely to attend for surveys. Family history data is provided by the patient and can therefore be subject to recall bias.

Probably the most accurate estimate of the association of family history and risk of developing glaucoma is from unbiased population studies with a high response rate such as the Baltimore Eye Study.[15] This did find that family history was a significant risk factor for POAG, but less so than in most other published studies. They found that the odds ratio of having POAG for those with siblings with the disease was 3.69, parents with the disease

2.17 and for those with children with the disease 1.12.

Gender

The Baltimore,[1] Beaver Dam,[2] Roscommon[3] and Blue Mountains[4] studies did not find males or females to be at significantly greater risk of glaucoma. However, the Barbados eye study[5] did find that males had an age adjusted risk of 1.4 compared with females while the Rotterdam study[6] found a three times increased risk for males. Conversely, the Dalby study[16] indicated a higher risk for females. Overall, it seems unlikely that gender is a major risk factor for developing glaucoma.

Diabetes

Diabetes has long been implicated as a risk factor for POAG, and the relative risk is calculated at 2.8 for having POAG if the patient was diabetic.[17] Wilson et al. had similar findings.[6] These were both hospital based studies and as described above are likely to overestimate the association. Population based studies of glaucoma have mostly found no association of glaucoma and diabetes (Baltimore, Barbados) or a small association (Beaver Dam).

The Rotterdam and Blue Mountains Eye studies did find an increased risk of POAG in diabetics therefore it seems that although the risk for diabetics is less than previously thought it is not possible to fully exclude a link.

Systemic hypertension

Studies of the role of blood pressure (BP) in the pathogenesis of glaucoma are, like diabetes, bedevilled by hospital bias. A number of studies have found a direct relationship between rise in BP and rise in IOP,[18] but it has been harder to find a similar association between BP and POAG.

The Baltimore Eye study investigators realising that simply comparing the BP of individuals with and without glaucoma was unlikely to provide a definitive answer, looked at the vascular perfusion pressure of their subjects.[18] The perfusion pressure is the BP (systolic, diastolic or mean) minus the IOP and when it was calculated for the subjects in the study, showed a strong association between the prevalence of POAG and *low* diastolic perfusion pressure (Figure 2.2). The graph indicates that those subjects with diastolic perfusion pressures below 30mm Hg had an age adjusted risk of POAG six times higher than those with pressures of 50mm Hg or greater.

The hypothesis is that optic nerve damage may be occurring in these subjects because of poor optic nerve perfusion. This theory is further enhanced by the results of 24 hours BP monitoring which shows that patients with profound falls in their BP overnight ("nocturnal dippers") have an increased risk of POAG.[19]

A further refinement of the hypothesis also comes from the Baltimore workers, who found that younger subjects (less than 60 years) with raised BPs, had a lower risk of POAG than the age matched normal population. Conversely, older subjects (over 70 years) had a higher risk than their aged matched controls. The authors suggest the reason for this may be that hypertension actually improves optic nerve head flow initially, but once secondary vascular changes

occur with prolonged hypertension resistance to blood flow increases.

The two findings of the Baltimore Eye Study may be related in that the vascular changes of prolonged hypertension, result in loss of blood vessel autoregulation, reducing the ability of the nerve head vessels to respond to a reduction in diastolic perfusion. It is important to stress that this theory, although elegant, still requires far more evidence.

Racial risk factors for primary open angle glaucoma

Over the last decade large scale population studies have shown that individuals of African, African American and African Caribbean origin are at higher risk of POAG compared to Caucasians. The prevalence values (Table 2.2) are illustrative of this. Overall, the studies indicate around a fourfold excess prevalence in black as compared to white subjects and this difference persists in all age groups.

The Barbados study[5] found a gradient in prevalence by racial group with the highest risk being in those subjects describing themselves as black. A lower prevalence was found in those who classified themselves as of mixed race and the lowest prevalence was for those who were white. Interestingly, the London Afro-Caribbean study[20] showed a statistically significant association between IOP and skin colour, but not between skin colour and glaucoma.

Not only is there a higher prevalence of POAG amongst black people but there is evidence that the onset of the disease is at a younger age.[1] In one study the average age of glaucoma patients in Jamaica was found to be 10 years less than the American average,[1] with the average age at presentation for black patients being 49.5 years while for whites it was 59.8 years.[21]

At the present time there is little data regarding POAG risk in other racial groups such as those from the Indian sub-continent, Hispanics, Eastern Europeans or Polynesians.

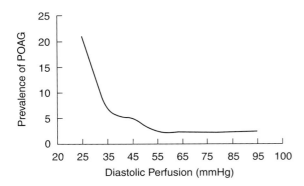

Figure 2.2 The relationship between the prevalence of POAG and diastolic perfusion pressure of subjects from the Baltimore Eye Survey (from Tielsch *et al*[18])

Environmental risk factors for primary open angle glaucoma

Socioeconomic factors

There has been little work done on socioeconomic status and POAG. One study found a higher prevalence of glaucoma in outdoor manual workers than in indoor workers (the latter having the higher income). A similar study found a higher rate of glaucoma in manual labourers compared to clerical workers, although this was not controlled for race.[22]

It would seem likely that those factors which influence access to adequate medical care such as income, educational level and socioeconomic status, would have an effect on the occurrence of glaucoma.[23] Whether this is true or not has yet to be proved, but there is evidence that lower socioeconomic status is related to later presentation of POAG and therefore carries an increased likelihood of subsequent blindness.[24]

Cigarette smoking

Although studied fairly well, smoking has not been shown to be a risk factor for glaucoma in most studies. One hospital based case control study could find no association between smoking and glaucoma,[17] nor could the Beaver Dam study[25] show a relationship between smoking and POAG.

Alcohol intake

A link has been found between alcohol consumption and the risk of glaucoma.[17] Once again it seems likely that non-population based studies will be biased, with heavy drinkers having more contact with health services and therefore increasing their opportunity of having their glaucoma diagnosed. Thus when alcohol intake is looked at on a population basis, as in the Beaver Dam study[25] there is no suggestion of a relationship between alcohol and glaucoma.

References

1 Tielsch JM, Sommer A, Katz J, Quigley HA, Royall RM, Javitt J. Racial variations in the prevalence of primary open angle glaucoma. *JAMA* 1991; **266**: 369–74.

2 Klein BEK, Klein R, Sponsel WE, *et al*. Prevalence of glaucoma. *Ophthalmolgy* 1992; **99**: 1499–504.

3 Coffey M, Reidy A, Wormald R, Wu XJ, Wright L, Courtney P. Prevalence of glaucoma in the west of Ireland. *Br J Ophthalmol* 1993; **77**: 17–21.

4 Mitchell P, Smith W, Attebo K, Healey PR. Prevalence of Open-Angle Glaucoma in Australia. *Ophthalmology* 1996; **103**: 1661–9.

5 Leske MC, Connell AMS, Schachat AP, Hyman L. The Barbados Eye Study – Prevalence of Open Angle Glaucoma. *Arch Ophthalmol* 1994; **112**: 821–9.

6 Dielemans I, Vingerling JR, Wolfs RCW, Hofman A, Grobbe DE, de Jong PTVM. The Prevalence of Primary Open Angle Glaucoma in a Population based study in the Netherlands. *Ophthalmology* 1994; **101**: 1851–5.

7 Mason *et al*. National Survey of the Prevalence and Risk Factors of Glaucoma in St Lucia, West Indies. *Ophthalmology* 1989; **96**: 1363–8.

8 Quigley HA, Vitale S. Models of Open Angle Glaucoma Prevalence and Incidence in the United States. *Invest Ophthalmol Vis Sci* 1997; **38**: 83–91.

9 Perkins ES. The Bedford glaucoma survey: 1. Long term follow-up of borderline cases. *Br J Ophthalmol* 1973; **57**: 179–85.

10 Sommer A, Tielsch JM, Katz J, *et al*. Relationship between intraocular pressure and primary open angle glaucoma among White and Black Americans. *Arch Ophthalmol* 1991; **109**: 1090–5.

11 Sommer A. Glaucoma: Facts and Fancies. *Eye* 1996; **10**: 295–30.

12 Armaly MF, Krueger DE, Maunder L, *et al*. Biostatistical analysis of the collaborative glaucoma study. 1. Summary of report of the risk factors for glaucomatous visual field defects. *Arch Ophthalmol* 1980; **98**: 2163–71.

13 Wilson MR, Hertzmark E, Walker AM, Childs K, Epstein DL. A Case-Control Study of risk factors in open angle glaucoma. *Arch Ophthalmol* 1987; **105**: 1066–71.

14 Perkins ES, Phelps CD. Open angle glaucoma, ocular hypertension, low tension glaucoma and refraction. *Arch Ophthalmol* 1982; **100**: 1464–7.

15 Tielsch JM, Katz J, Sommer A, Quigley HA, Javitt, JC. Family History and risk of primary open angle glaucoma. *Arch Ophthalmol* 1994; **112**: 69–73.

16 Bengtsson B. The prevalence of Glaucoma. *Br J Ophthalmol* 1981; **65**: 46–9.

17 Katz J, Sommer A. Risk factors for primary open angle glaucoma. *Am J Prev Med* 1988; **4**: 110–4.

18 Tielsch JM, Katz J, Sommer A, Quigley HA, Javitt JC. Hypertension, Perfusion Pressure and Primary Open-Angle Glaucoma. *Arch Ophthalmol* 1995; **113**: 216–21.

19 Meyer JH, Brandi-Dohan J, Funk J. Twenty four hour blood pressure monitoring in normal tension glaucoma. *Br J Ophthalmol* 1996; **80**: 864–7.

20 Wormald RPL, Basauri E, Wright LA, Evans JR. The African Carribean eye survey: risk factors for glaucoma in a sample of African Carribean people living in London. *Eye* 1994; **8**: 315–20.

21 Wilson R, Walker A, Dueker DK, Pitts-Crick R. Risk factors for rate of progression of glaucomatous visual field loss. *Arch Ophthalmol* 1982; **100**: 737.

22 Bjornssong. The primary glaucomas in Iceland: Epide-

miological studies. *Acta Ophthalmologica* suppl. 1967; **91**: 93–9.

23 Leske MC, Rosenthal J. Epidemiological aspects of open angle glaucoma. *Am J Epidemiol* 1979; **109**: 250–72.

24 Fraser SG, Bunce CV, Wormald RPL. Risk factors for late presentation of Chronic Glaucoma. *Inv Ophth Vis Science* 1999; **40**: 2251–7.

25 Klein BE, Klein R, Ritter LL. Relationship of drinking alcohol and smoking to prevalence of open angle glaucoma. *Ophthalmology* 1993; **100**: 1609–13.

3 Primary open angle glaucoma: screening

R P L WORMALD

The effects of glaucoma in its most severe form are totally disabling. Its insidious onset and prolonged asymptomatic phase have earned it the epithet "the thief of sight". For this reason, glaucoma was sometimes sited in textbooks of public health or screening as a typical example of a condition for which screening is appropriate.

However, a number of difficulties must be overcome if mass screening for the detection of early glaucoma is ever to become a reality. Here, it is important to be clear about the definitions of screening. Some might consider the opportunistic testing of intraocular pressure (IOP) and possibly other assessments during a routine sight test for spectacles as screening. Yet when compared to national programmes for breast cancer or cancer of the cervix, there is clearly a difference. Mass screening starts with a clear definition of the target population which must be enumerated and each individual provided with a unique identifier. This is essential so that the performance and organisation of the population screening can be monitored, in particular in terms of coverage of the population at risk. Such a notion never occurs in the context of glaucoma testing in any nation.

Screening is the presumptive identification of individuals within a defined population who might benefit from further assessment.[1] Recent recommendations in the UK for glaucoma "Case Finding" (a term now used for opportunistic testing) advise the use of all three traditional tests (discs, fields and pressures) which is no different to diagnostic testing. The American Academy of Ophthalmology in their Preferred Practice Guidelines recommend the "comprehensive adult eye evaluation" for all case finding.[2]

Proper screening requires not only the existence of a valid and reliable screening test, but also a clear and agreed definition of what the disease is and is not – in other words a clear case definition. Both these issues are problematic in glaucoma.

Consideration of existing tests for gaucoma

Because glaucoma is relatively rare in white populations, and its onset insidious, meaningful conclusions on the performance of various screening tests for the disease can be derived only from population-based studies.[3–5] Studies conducted in clinics with known proportions of cases, controls and suspects, can be misleading when it comes to anticipating the behaviour of a test in the population at large. This is because the prevalence of the condition is artificially inflated in the clinic study and the case mix is very different in the community.

The Baltimore Eye Study was used to look at the validity of various screening tests for the detection of glaucoma, in particular IOP and optic disc cupping.[6] Both perform very poorly individually and not much better in combination. This is because there appear to be numerous cases that have normal pressure and discs at the survey, but who have reproducible and typical glaucomatous visual field defects. The case definition for glaucoma was the presence of such a defect and the independent agreement of two ophthalmologists that there was a progressive problem requiring intervention.

Recently, evidence that many nerve fibres may be lost before a reproducible visual field defect can be demonstrated, has added further confusion. Some people who have raised IOP, abnormal discs and normal fields, may well be on their way to becoming frank glaucoma cases and therefore in pragmatic terms, should be treated as such. The evidence, based on postmortem examination of optic nerve specimens and the photographic demonstration of arcuate defects in the retinal nerve fibre layer, requires further validation.[7] Another study recently demonstrated that motion sensitivity abnormality precedes the appearance of frank visual field defects by a number of years.[8] Similarly, the appearance of an optic nerve head haemorrhage can precede field loss by many years.

Some argue that the cases that matter are those with high IOP because they are thought to be likely to progress rapidly and are likely to be influenced by IOP reduction. IOP fluctuates diurnally (more so in glaucoma), with each cardiac cycle and varies with the instrument used to measure it. A single normal or indeed high measurement means little. Disc appearance is more robust (it does not fluctuate), but many false negative and positive errors still occur. Not only are there many people whose discs appear grossly abnormal but whose fields are full but worse, there are many who have a normal appearance of their disc but definite and reproducible visual field defects. Fields too are associated with numerous false positives[9] which decrease with learning experience. There is the inevitable trade-off between sensitivity and false positive rate the more sensitive the test, the greater the number of false positive errors. Reducing the false positive rate by decreasing the sensitivity of the test means that more subtle and early cases will be missed and so the false negative rate increases.

Table 3.1 summarises the findings of the

Table 3.1 Detection rate, false positive rate and positive predictive value of the currently accepted tests for glaucoma screening, calculated from the published results of population-based epidemiological studies.

	1966[28] Florida	1966[29] Ferndale	1968[30] Bedford	1977[31] Framingham	1991[6] Baltimore	1992[32] Beaver	1993[5] Ireland	1994[9] Rotterdam
IOP cut off	25.9	21+	21+	>21	>21	>21	>21	>21
Disc cut off		GOND	GOND	0.5+	>0.5	0.5+	>0.5	0.5+
Sample size	67,193	4231	5941	2433	5308	4926	2186	3062
Glaucoma prevalence	1.4%	0.98%	0.93%	1.9%	2.5%	2.1%	1.88%	1.1%
IOP detection rate	100%	84%	89%	48%	47%	68.3%	51.2%	61.8%
IOP false-positive rate	1.4%	8.5%	6.5%	10.9%	7.6%	5%	5%	1.5%
IOP predictive value	48.5%	8%	11.3%	8.8%	13.7%	23.5%	17%	31%
C/D ratio detection rate	–	61.5%	38.2%	58%	48%	100%	98%	100%
C/D ratio false-positive rate	–	2%	1.2%	15.4%	10.6%	12%	2.8%	18.3%
C/D ratio predictive value	–	23.5%	23%	7.6%	–	15.2%	41%	5.8%
Gold standard	Dr	Dr	Dr	VF	Dr	Dr	VF	VF

Dr, Clinician; VF, Visual fields; IOP, Intraocular pressure; C/D ratio, Cup to disc ratio; GOND, Glaucomatous optic nerve damage as a clinical diagnosis.

This table should only be taken as an approximation as we have had to derive the values from the published literature. This has resulted in a number of assumptions being made such as:

- All published prevalence figures have been assumed as percentages of the whole study sample unless otherwise indicated in the published literature.
- Some of the studies (such as the Framingham) give more than one value for prevalence of glaucoma, here the most recently published figure has been used for calculation.
- Some of above studies did not give numbers with raised IOP or cup/disc ratios etc, therefore these numbers were derived from the percentages given in the text.

major population-based glaucoma surveys from which we could abstract estimates of detection (sensitivity) and false positive rates for IOP and optic disc cupping. These all show high false negative and false positive rates.

In the UK, work by the International Glaucoma Association[10] and others has shown that the highest proportion of appropriate referrals to the hospital eye service is made by optometrists via the general practitioner. The accuracy of their referrals improves with the number of investigations they routinely perform as they get closer to the "comprehensive adult eye examination", which is of course, not screening. Before the introduction of sight test charges,[11] optometrists were probably testing a high proportion of the population at risk in the UK, though clearly missing many cases. This was due to an excessive reliance on IOP as the primary screening test which also gave rise to a high false positive referral rate. It is estimated that only one in ten persons found at cross-section with an IOP > 21 mm Hg has glaucoma, and yet with this arbitrary statistical definition of the upper limit of normal, optometrists are legally bound to refer. This leads to gross wastage of scarce health care resources while half the glaucoma sufferers in the population remain undetected.

Current screening possibilities

There is a very long presymptomatic phase of the disease during which early identification and treatment would benefit the sufferer, at least in the opinion of most ophthalmologists, although this has never been proven in a randomised placebo controlled trial. There is no single test at present sufficiently valid for the efficient identification of sufferers at primary screening. Existing performance of current case finding practice is poor with a low sensitivity (around 50%), and a very poor positive predictive value (around 10%). The resource implications of the implementation of a national screening programme, which involves measuring IOP, optic disc cup: disc ratio and visual fields, in terms of societal costs and gains, has never been fully considered. Doubtlessly they would be very considerable bearing in mind that such a development would have to justify the opportunity cost of moving resources from another health sector. The screening tests currently available are acceptable to most patients and are neither dangerous nor invasive. However, there are problems in adequately funding a comprehensive eye exam approach in the NHS using optometrists in their current half business/half primary eye care mode.

Future developments

A fundamental problem in screening for glaucoma is the lack of a single, acceptable, cheap, robust and valid test for glaucoma. It needs to be able to reliably detect early stages of the disease and differentiate it from normals or other disturbances of visual function.

Several devices that are now under investigation may be able to do this, and in addition, detect optic nerve fibre damage before frank visual field loss is detectable. They are based on motion detection which is, it is thought, subserved by the larger class of ganglion cell, and those most vulnerable to damage in the early stages of the disease. Potentially, motion detection tests are cheap, simple, user friendly and possibly suitable for self-testing on standard PCs or videos. Hospital-based trials have shown good validity but community-based trials are awaited.[12]

This type of test might provide a primary screening test which could be offered at primary care centres, either GP surgeries or optometrists premises. The ideal properties of this test would be such that any person who performs the test normally has a very low probability of having glaucoma. However, 10–15% of persons doing the test will have results that are abnormal depending on various parameters, including cut off criteria and age of the sample. Those failing the test could then be advised to go on to more detailed case-finding assessment using the traditional three tests, preferably in the primary care setting, although facilities for glaucoma assessment could be provided at the local hospital. By eliminating the 85% or more of normal cases from the more detailed assessment, far fewer false positives should occur. The sensitivity should also be improved because the primary screening device should be very good at picking up true positives.

Other high-tech solutions may be offered with different approaches to imaging the retina and optic disc. Nerve fibre layer photography requires skilled photographers and dedicated camera and processing techniques. As long as the optical media are clear, excellent visualisation of the retinal nerve fibre layer is possible with grooves or defects clearly visible before frank functional loss is detectable.[13,14] However, the absence of grooves does not mean that there is no glaucoma.

The scanning laser ophthalmoscope can provide detailed information on the structure of the optic nerve head and detect changes in the area of neuroretinal rim thickness or cup volume.[15,16] But expense, lack of portability and the fragility of this equipment mean that this technique is not yet applicable to population screening. It is unlikely to become appropriate unless the cost of the technology dramatically falls or, indeed, society becomes a lot more affluent. In addition, the use of a scanning laser ophthalmoscope at present requires trained personnel for its operation as well as for interpretation of the results. The results are unlikely to be comparable in different ethnic groups as the thickness of the nerve fibre layer as well as the disc sizes and the cup:

disc ratios differ in different ethnic groups. There is little data on the use of this instrument in population-based studies, and normal values for different populations are not available at present.

Newer perimetric techniques such as short-wavelength automated perimetry are based on the theory that loss of blue-yellow sensitivity occurs early in glaucoma.[17] At present this remains experimental, not widely available and has not been used in large-scale studies.

"Oculokinetic" perimetry (OKP) is a deliberately "low-tech" device designed for use in primary care settings.[18] It consists of a printed card that is cheap to produce. Although it may miss many equivocal or early cases, it will detect most cases with dense scotomata of anything more than trivial dimensions.[19] Similarly, lower-tech suprathreshold visual field screening devices such as the Henson CFS 2000, the Takagi ATS and the Friedmann Mark II may offer the most practical solutions to the problem for the time being. Table 3.2 compares the detection and false positive rates for these devices. Most of these studies were clinic-based, however, with an inflated glaucoma prevalence so that the positive predictive value (PPV) is meaningless.[20–22]

In response to all the new modalities becoming available and being developed, Prevent Blindness America has issued very general criteria that could be used to judge suitable future devices for screening.[23] These include high sensitivity (85–95%), cheap to buy (US$5,000–10,000) and low running costs (about US$1 per patient screening), ease of use and short testing time, as well as good portability.

Table 3.2 Performance of suprathreshold visual field screening devices.[20–22]

Device	Detection rate	False positive rate	Gold standard
Takagi ATS	90%	25%	Octopus 2000 (G1)
Henson CFS2000	90.5%	11.6%	to itself (higher spec)
Humphrey 72	52%	10%	to its own threshold
Oculokinetic perimetry	90%	1.5%	Friedman Mark II

Cost

A seminal study of the cost of glaucoma screening based on IOP testing was undertaken in the USA.[24] Because of poor test validity, it concluded that it would be a prohibitively expensive and inefficient exercise. Hitchings using crude data has calculated the cost of glaucoma blindness in the UK.[25] Needless to say, purely in monetary terms leaving out quality of life considerations, the cost to society is high. There is little value in attempting to model cost of screening based on existing methods because of their known failings, but there may be value in developing a model based on using a motion testing strategy as a primary screening device. Tuck and Crick have carried out cost-effectiveness studies on testing for POAG. They conclude that this can only be justified if it forms either part of an overall eye examination, or case finding in high risk groups such as the Afro-Caribbean population over 40 years of age, or those with a strong family history of POAG.[26] This strategy of screening for high risk groups will have to await the results of community-based trials for realistic estimates of validity, and a trial of this type may take two or three years. The trial could also inform questions on the acceptability of introducing yet another screening responsibility on the primary care sector.

What this trial could not do was to provide information on the cost-effectiveness of screening. The principal outcome for such a trial would be the rates of glaucoma blindness in the screened versus unscreened population. Because this event is so rare in the population as a whole and because the course of the disease so indolent, the trial would have to be of huge dimensions to have any chance of picking up the effect of screening.

Probably the only way to assess the cost-effectiveness in a national setting such as the UK, would be to improve the reliability of blind registration statistics and then implement screening for, say, in Wales or Scotland. The registration statistics could then be monitored for a number of years and scrutinised for changes in the rate of registration for glaucoma over that time comparing the screened with the unscreened population. This would only work if registration statistics could be improved to a sufficient level of reliability.

It is clear from the above considerations that it would take considerable time to establish a national screening programme for glaucoma (none exists in any industrialised nation). With the results of the investigation of the new technology, modelling of cost can then be carried out. This would be followed by setting up the infrastructure for a large trial, while the validity of registration is improved. The trial itself would have to run for at least six years, which would mean 10–15 years before any useful answers could be expected.

In the mean time, much can be done to modify case-finding procedures in the light of new epidemiological evidence. The African Caribbean Eye Survey[27] in Haringey, North London, found a fourfold increase in glaucoma for Afro-Caribbeans which concurred with the findings of the Baltimore Eye Study[3] and the risk of glaucoma for Afro-Americans. Afro-Caribbeans and subjects from other races with a family history of glaucoma can be targeted with specific health awareness programmes and encouraged to seek testing for glaucoma at a dedicated local facility.

References

1 Peckham C, Dezateuxc, (eds). B Med Bulletin 1998.
2 American Academy of Ophthalmology. Preferred practice pattern Primary open angle glaucoma.1992.
3 Tielsch JM, Sommer A, Katz J. The Baltimore Eye Survey: Racial variations in the prevalence of primary open-angle glaucoma. JAMA 1991; 266: 369–74.
4 Leske MC, Connell AMS, Schachat AP. Hyman L. The Barbados Eye Study; prevalence of open angle glaucoma. Arch Ophthalmol 1994; 112: 821–9.
5 Coffey M, Reidy A, Wormald R, Wu X, Wright L, Courtney P. Prevalence of glaucoma in the West of Ireland. Br J Ophthalmol 1993; 77: 17–21.
6 Tielsch JM, Katz J, Singh K, et al. A population-based evaluation of glaucoma screening. Am J Epidemiol 1991; 134: 1102–10.
7 Quigley HA. Open angle glaucoma. Medical progress review article. N Engl J Med 1993; 328 (15): 1097–106.
8 Wu X, Reidy A, Coffey M and Wormald R. Impaired

motion sensitivity as a predictor of subsequent field loss: The Roscommon Glaucoma Survey. *Br J Ophthalmol* 1998; **82**: 534–7.

9 Dielmans I, Vingerling JR, Wolfs RCW, Hofman A, Grobbe DE, De Jong PTVM. The prevalence of POAG in a population-based study in the Netherlands. *Ophthalmology* 1994; **101**: 1851–5.

10 Tuck MW, Crick RP. Screening for glaucoma: age and sex of referrals and confirmed cases in England and Wales. *Ophthalmic Physiol Opt* 1992; **12**: 400–4.

11 Laidlaw DAH, Bloom PA, Hughes AO, Sparrow JM, Marmion VJ. The sight test fee Effect on ophthalmology referrals and rate of glaucoma definition. *Br J Med* 1994; **309**: 634–6.

12 Wu X, Wormald RPL, Fitzke F, Nagasubramanian S, Hitchings RA. Laptop computer perimetry for glaucoma screening. *Invest Ophthalmol Vis Sci* 1991; **32** (Suppl): 810.

13 Quigley HA, Katz J, Derick RJ, Gilbert D, Sommer A. An evaluation of optic disc and nerve fibre layer examinations in monitoring progression of early glaucoma damage. *Ophthalmology* 1992; **99**: 19–28.

14 Nicholl JE, Katz LH, Steinman WC, *et al.* Optic disc computerized analysis comparing three photographic techniques. *Invest Ophthalmol Vis Sci* 1989; **90** (Suppl): 174.

15 Cioffi GA, Robin AL, Eastman RD, *et al.* Confocal laser scanning ophthalmoscope. Reproducibility of nerve head topographic measurements with the confocal laser scanning ophthalmoscope. *Ophthalmology* 1993; **100**: 57–62.

16 Weinreb RN, Shakiba S, Zangwill L. Scanning laser polarimetry to measure the nerve fiber layer of normal and glaucoma eyes. *Am J Ophthalmol* 1995; **H9**: 627.

17 Johnson LA, Brandt JD, Khong AM, Adams AJ. Short-wavelength automated perimetry in low-, medium-, and high-risk ocular hypertensive eyes. *Arch Ophthalmol* 1995; **113**: 70.

18 Alvarez E, Damato BE, Jay JL, MacClare E. Comparative evaluation of oculokinetic perimetry and conventional perimetry in Glaucoma. *Br J Ophthalmol* 1988; **72**: 258–62.

19 Sponsel WE, Ritch R, Stamper R, *et al.* Prevent Blindness America visual field screening study. *Am J Ophthalmol* 1995; **120**: 699.

20 Greve M, Chisholm LA. Comparison of the oculokinetic perimetry glaucoma screener with two types of visual field analysis. *Cam J Ophthalmol* 1993; **28**: 201–6.

21 Cotagliola C, Russo V, Camera A, Scibelli G. The takagi automated tangent screen ATS85 for the detection of glaucomatous patients. *Ann Ophthalmol* 1991; **23**: 18–20.

22 Vernon SA, Henry DJ, Jones SJ. Calculating the predictive power of the Henson Field Screener in a population at risk of Glaucomatous field loss. *Br J Ophthalmol* 1990; **74**: 220–2.

23 Stamper RL. Glaucoma Screening. *J Glaucoma* 1998; **7**: 149–150.

24 Eddy DM, Sanders LE, Eddy JF. The value of screening for glaucoma with tonometry. *Surv Ophthalmol* 1983; **28**: 194–205.

25 Hitchings RA. Glaucoma Screening . *BNJ Ophthalmol* 1993; **77**: 326.

26 Tuck MW, Crick RP. The cost-effectiveness of various modes of screening for primary open angle glaucoma. *Ophthalmol Epidemiol* 1997; **4** (1): 3–17.

27 Wormald RPL, Basouri E, Wright LA, Evans JR. The Afro-Caribbean eye survey: risk factors for glaucoma in a sample of African-Caribbean people living in London. *Eye* 1994; **8**: 315–20.

28 Frydman JE, Clower JW, Fulghum JE, Hester MW. Glaucoma detection in Florida. *JAMA* 1966; **198** (12): 99–102.

29 Hollows FC, Graham PA. Intraocular pressure, glaucoma and glaucoma suspects in a defined population. *Br J Ophthalmol* 1966; **50**: 570–86.

30 Banks JLK, Perkins ES, Tsolakis S, Wright JE. Bedford Glaucoma Survey. *Br J Med* 1968; **1**: 791–96.

31 Kahn HA, Milton RC. Revised Framingham eye study prevalence of glaucoma and diabetic retinopathy. *Am J Epidemiol* 1980; **111**: 769–76.

32 Klein BEK, Klein R, Sponsel WE, *et al.* Prevalence of Glaucoma: The Beaver Dam Eye Study. *Ophthalmology* 1992; **99**: 1499–504.

4 Genetic Screening for glaucoma

A H CHILD

Recent advances in molecular genetics of glaucoma have made it possible to screen families for glaucoma where linkage to a proven locus, or demonstration of a causative gene mutation, is possible.[1] This has paved the way for the introduction of DNA screening in family glaucoma clinics which could lead to the concentration of scarce resources on preventive management in those demonstrated to be at increased risk. Those shown to be not carrying the familial gene can be reassured and advised to attend for glaucoma screening after the age of 40, as in the general population.

This advance in glaucoma prevention was built on evidence from surveys which indicated that on average 30% of juvenile and adult onset glaucoma subjects have at least one affected close relative (parent, sibling, offspring).[2] The inheritance pattern is autosomal dominant with reduced penetrance, with both sexes affected and direct vertical transmission from parent to child. Usually females are more often affected than males,[3] which indicates sex-influence on the expression of the causative gene. Other genetic disorders such as hypertension and diabetes, inherited independently, can potentiate the effects of the glaucoma gene, increasing the severity of visual loss. This is seen especially in black Afro-Caribbean populations where these overlapping disorders have been carefully studied.[4]

Congenital glaucoma is inherited in an autosomal recessive manner, both parents being unaffected carriers. The potential risk for each offspring is one in four, as is evident in large families.[5] However, in most western nations small families with, on average, two children, usually contain only one affected child. Genetic screening of subsequent children at birth using cord blood, or buccal samples, is possible in families where even one of the parental mutations has been detected. This is very reassuring, especially as the measurement of IOPs in infants and young children can be extremely difficult, often requiring general anaesthesia.

Selection of families for linkage studies

Families with glaucoma having a minimum of three living affected members in at least two generations, can be studied using candidate gene and random genome search techniques. In addition pooled linkage studies of families known to have the same subtype of glaucoma can be performed. All family members must have careful phenotyping. This will include age of onset (congenital, juvenile, early mid and late adult onset), IOP (normal or high pressure) and ocular appearance (optic disc size and morphometry, the presence of pseudoexfoliation, or pigment dispersion). It is reasonable to expect several different genes for each clinical subset amounting to an approximate total of 25 genes (Table 4.1).

GLC1A

The first locus for juvenile open angle glaucoma (JOAG) was discovered in 1993, mapped

Table 4.1 Table of loci described for glaucoma genes

Glaucoma Type	Locus (gene)	No. of families	Country of Origin	Clinical Features	Publication
Juvenile Onset (Dominant) also shown to cause adult onset in 3% of familial cases	GLC1A 1q24 (TIGR/MYOC*)	10	USA confirmed internationally	onset < 20 yrs. high pressure, surgery	*Nature Genet* 1993; **4**: 47–50 *Science* 1997; 275: 668–707
Adult Onset (Dominant)	GLC1B 2cen–q13	18 3	UK	low–moderate, moderate–high, tension 1OP < 30, onset 40/50	*Genomics* 1996; **36**: 142–50
	GLC1C 3q21–q24	1	USA	moderate–high pressure onset > 35 years	*Am J Hum Genet* 1997; **60**: 296–304
	GLC1D 8q23	1	USA	mixed normal and high pressure	*Am J Ophthalmol* 1998; **126**(1): 17–28
	GLC1E 10p14–p15	1	UK	typical normal pressure	*Am J Hum Genet* 1998; **62**(3): 641–52
	GLC1F 7q35–q36	1	USA	high pressure	*Arch Ophthalmol* 1999; **117**: 237–41
Congenital (Buphthalmos) Autosomal recessive	GLC3A 2p21 Cytochrome P4501B1(CYP1B1) over 20 new mutations from Turkey, France, U.K. (Pakistani), Gypsies of Slovakia, Saudi Arabia, etc.	20	Turkey, Canada	onset at birth or under 1 year requires surgery	*Genomics* 1995; **30**: 171–7 *Hum Mol Genet* 1997, **6**: 641–647
	GLC3B 1p36.2–36.1	4	Turkey, Canada		*Hum Mol Genet* 1996; 5(8) 1199–203

* TIGR/MYOC, <u>T</u>rabecular meshwork <u>I</u>nducible <u>G</u>lucocorticoid <u>R</u>esponse protein (myocilin)

to the 1q21–q31 region (long arm of chromosome 1) and assigned as GLC1A.[6] The use of GLC1 symbol for all types of primary open angle glaucoma (POAG) has been approved by the Hugo Nomenclature Committee; the letters A, B, C, etc. are assigned to each newly discovered locus. Mutations found in patients from Scotland, France, Japan, Germany and French Canada confirmed the gene TIGR/MYOC (**tr**abecular meshwork **i**nduced **g**lucocorticoid **r**esponse protein, also known as myocilin) as a cause of this glaucoma phenotype.[1] This gene is involved in the pathophysiology of glaucoma by causing obstruction of the aqueous outflow with its product, resulting in increased intraocular pressure (IOP). Some families linked to this locus have both JOAG and adult onset POAG.[7,8] In our Edinburgh family[9] we were able to offer buccal sample screening for two children, each at a 50/50 risk of inheriting the gene. Only one child carried the mutation, and the normal child was spared eye examinations from then on (Figure 4.1).

Neonatal cord blood or buccal sample screening could now be provided for any family large enough to demonstrate linkage to this region, or in which the family gene mutation is present in at least two affected members and not present in unaffected members.

Evidence for genetic heterogeneity has been reported.[10,11] Some clustering of mutations has been described. Most are missense mutations occurring in exon III. A predominantly reported mutation is the Gln368STOP observed in 25 familial, 15 sporadic cases, and 1 normal healthy subject.[12] Mutations in this region may involve the cell binding activity of this protein.[13] Interference with the uptake or metabolism of the protein may lead to its accumulation, obstruction of aqueous outflow and increased IOPs resulting in optic nerve damage, and leading to glaucomatous visual loss.

Adult onset chronic open angle glaucoma (COAG)

GLC1B

The onset of this form of glaucoma is usually after the age of 40 years. The first locus (GLC1B) has been assigned to the 2cen–q13 region.[14] An additional 12 families have been found to segregate.[1] The phenotype is less severe than that found in GLC1A linked families. The mean age of onset was 53 years and pressures ranged from normal to high, with most having moderate pressure glaucoma. Ocular surgery was necessary to control pressures in 42% of patients.

GLC1C

The second locus for adult onset POAG has been described in a single American family, mapping to the 3q21–24 region.[15] The 10 affected members shared a phenotype with onset after the age of 35 years, high IOPs, abnormal cup:disc ratios and visual loss. Three had surgical treatment to control pressures.

GLC1D

This locus for mixed normal and high pressure glaucoma has been found in one American family.[16] The phenotype in this family was variable with onset of visual field loss in middle age, followed by a modest elevation of IOP and progression of the disease in older individuals.

GLC1E

A specific locus for normal pressure glaucoma (NPG) has recently been assigned to 10p14–p15.[17] Unpublished heterogeneity tests in a further eight families indicate that other genes must also be responsible for NPG. The original family study provided a low score of 10.00 and demonstrated the potential for screening, with only 3 out of 18 at risk offspring in generation IV carrying the affected haplotype (Figure 4.2). Prevention of visual loss in these members through early presymptomatic

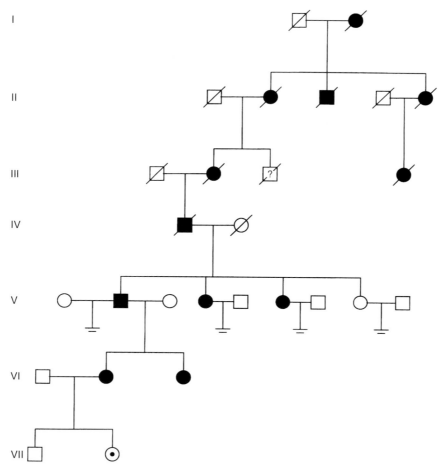

Figure 4.1 Seven generation Edinburgh family with juvenile onset primary open angle glaucoma.[9]
The mutation in the TIGR/MYOC gene was demonstrated in blood samples from living affected adults (closed squares, affected males; closed circles, affected females; open symbols, unaffected males and females). Two preschool children in generation VII were screened using buccal sample DNA. One was found affected and will continue with eye pressure checks. The other is not carrying the mutation and need not be checked in childhood.

identification is especially important in NPG where the usual indicator risk, elevated IOP, is absent.

Primary congenital glaucoma (PCG) or buphthalmos

GLC3A

This disorder manifests from birth up to 3 years of age and is inherited in an autosomal recessive manner (Figure 4.3). When an affected

parent marries an unaffected carrier the condition may present as a rare pseudo-dominant vertical transmission[18] (Figure 4.4). Genetic screening of an apparently unaffected partner prior to the first pregnancy can offer limited reassurance that no mutation is carried in this first gene on chromosome 2p21. It seems to be a major gene of importance worldwide in many racial groups. Mutations have been described in families from Turkey, French Canada, United Kingdom,[18] Saudi Arabia[19] and Slovakia.[20]

In one consanguineous Pakistani family

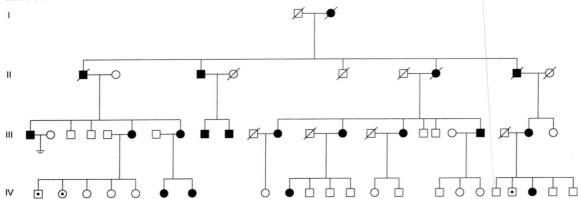

Figure 4.2 Four generation English family with normal pressure glaucoma.[17]
This family demonstrates the potential for screening. Closed figures denote affected status. In generation IV, only 3/18 presymptomatic at risk offspring carry the complete affected haplotype (carrier). Regular complete medical screening should permit early preventive treatment.

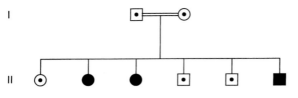

Figure 4.3 Primary Congenital Glaucoma (GLC3A).[18] Consanguineous Pakistani family with first cousin parents carrying identical mutations, and 3/6 children affected (closed symbols). Prenatal diagnosis is now available for any future pregnancy of the parents. Fiancée mutation screening is requested by the family, for any arranged marriage in generation II, in order to avoid the birth of affected offspring.

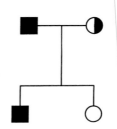

Figure 4.4 Primary congenital glaucoma (GLC3A).[18] Inherited in an autosomal recessive manner, this condition may present as a rare pseudo-dominant vertical transmission, when an affected person marries an unknown carrier.

residing in England, three out of six children were affected[18] (Figure 4.3). Both parents' mutations were identical as expected. The parents requested prenatal diagnosis for any future pregnancy, and screening of fiancées for their two eldest children of marriageable age, in order to avoid having affected offspring.

Causative mutations have been found in the cytochrome P4501B1 (CYP151) gene, clustered at the 5 prime end of the conserved exon III.[18] This fact will make it possible to screen the general population for detection of gene carriers.

The mode of action of CYP1B1 is, as yet, unclear. However, it belongs to a group of P450 super-family multigenes, monooxygenase genes responsible for phase I metabolism.

CYP1B1 participates in the metabolism of a molecule important for normal development and function of the anterior eye segment, perhaps a steroid,[21] or it may regulate corneal transparency and aqueous humour secretion[22, 23] leading to corneal clouding and increased IOP, as found in congenital glaucoma.

GLC3B (1p36)

Four families out of eight with PCG were found to be linked to this locus, suggesting that at least one further locus will be found.[24] A large number of genes have been reported in this band 1p36.2–36.1, but none can be directly attributed as a possible cause of congenital glaucoma.

Other glaucomas

A locus for pigment dispersion syndrome on the 7q35–q36 region has been described,[25] but further confirmation would be valuable. Loci for other types of glaucoma such as pseudo-exfoliative glaucoma are actively being sought.

Unusual inheritance patterns

Overlapping families

Where both parents are affected with dominantly inherited glaucoma a calculated risk of one in four for inheriting both causative genes is rarely observed in practice. Such families are not useful for studies to find glaucoma genes, but will be of great interest in studying the interaction of different genes – are they additive in effect? Is the age of onset that of the earliest type, or even earlier? Is the severity greater than that of either parent? Is the treatment response less?

Pseudodominance

Occasionally one finds a parent and child with congenital glaucoma, suggesting dominant inheritance (Figure 4.4). Mutation testing reveals that the "unaffected" partner is an unwitting carrier of a mutation for congenital glaucoma, so that the risk for offspring, instead of being 100% for unaffected carrier status (one affected parent), is actually 50% for affected status, a high risk.

Founding father effect

In the inbred Slovakian population which has the highest incidence of congenital glaucoma in the world (1:1250), every affected child studied has a double complement of the same mutation presumably all inherited from a single ancestor.[20] In this population, screening of every newborn would be easy, practical and very effective in terms of offering preventive treatment.

The insidious onset of glaucoma has always made it difficult to diagnose the disease at an early stage. Current case finding techniques are unwieldy and costly. The recent discovery of many genes believed to predispose to this disease could rapidly lead to DNA screening of at risk family members, permitting presymptomatic preventive therapy, or reassurance regarding unaffected status.

The genes discovered to date, namely TIGR/MYOC for juvenile glaucoma and CYP1B1 for congenital glaucoma, affect development of the trabecular meshwork, probably involving steroid metabolism. A better understanding of the processes involved could potentially lead to therapies which restore or replace an abnormal trabecular cell population, allowing correction of the process causing raised IOP rather than treating it as a complication.

References

1 Sarfarazi M. Recent advances in molecular genetics of glaucomas. *Hum Mol Genet* 1997; **6**: 1667–77.
2 Shin DH, Becker B, Kolker AE. Family history in primary open angle glaucoma. *Arch Ophthalmol* 1977; **95**: 598–600.
3 Johnson AT, Allward W, Sheffield V, Stone E. Genetics and glaucoma. In Ritch R, Shields BM, Krupin T (eds). Mosby, St Louis. *The Glaucomas* 2: 39–54.
4 Mason RP, Kosoko O, Wilson MR, *et al.* National survey of the prevalence and risk factors of glaucoma in St Lucia, West Indies. Part I. Prevalence findings. *Ophthalmology* 1989; **96** (9): 1363–8.
5 Sarfarazi M, Akarsu AN, Hossain A *et al.* Assignment of a locus (GLC3A) for primary congenital glaucoma (Buphthalmos) to 2p21 and evidence for genetic heterogeneity. *Genomics* 1995; **30**: 171–7.
6 Sheffield VC, Stone EM, Alward WL, *et al.* Genetic linkage of familial open angle glaucoma to chromosome 1q21–q31. *Nat Gen* 1993; **4**: 47–50.
7 Morissette J, Cote G, Anctil JL *et al.* A common gene for juvenile and adult onset primary open angle glaucomas confined on chromosome 1g. *Am J Hum Genet* 1995; **56**: 1431–42.
8 Meyer A, Bechetoille A, Valtot F, *et al.* Age dependent penetrance and mapping of the locus for juvenile and early-onset open angle glaucoma on chromosome 1q (GLC1A) in a French family. *Hum Genet* 1996; **98**: 567–71.
9 Stoilova D, Child A, Brice G, *et al.* Identification of a new "TIGR" mutation in a family with juvenile onset primary open angle glaucoma. *Ophthalmol Genet* 1997; **18:3**. 109–18.
10 Wiggs JL, DelBono EA, Schuman JS, Hutchinson BT, Walton DS. Clinical features of five pedigrees genetically linked to the juvenile glaucoma locus on chromosome 1q21–q31. *Ophthalmology* 1995; **2**: 1782–9.
11 Brezin AP, Bechetoille A, Hamard P, *et al.* Genetic heterogeneity of primary open angle glaucoma and

ocular hypertension: linkage to GLC1A associated with an increased risk of severe glaucomatous optic neuropathy. *J Med Genet* 1997; **34**: 51–8.

12 Allward WLM, Fingert JH, Coote MA, *et al.* Clinical features associated with mutations in the chromosome 1 open angle glaucoma gene (GLC1A) N Engl J Med 1998; **338** (15): 1022–7.

13 Polansky J, Fauss D, Chen P, *et al.* Cellular pharmacology and molecular biology of the trabecular meshwork inducible glucocorticoid response gene product. *Ophthalmologica* 1997; **211**: 126–39.

14 Stoilova D, Child A, Trifan OC, Crick RP, Coakes RL, Sarfarazi M. Localization of a locus (GLC1B) for adult-onset primary open angle glaucoma to the 2cen–q13 region. *Genomics* 1996; **36**: 142–50.

15 Wirtz MK, Samples JR, Kramer PL, *et al.* Mapping a gene for adult-onset primary open angle glaucoma to chromosome 3q. *Am J Hum Genet* 1997; **60**: 296–304.

16 Trifan OC, Traboulsi EI, Stoilova D, *et al.* The third locus (GLC1D) for adult-onset primary open angle glaucoma maps to the 8q23 region. *Am J Ophthalmol* 1998; **126** (1): 17–28.

17 Sarfarazi M, Child A, Stoilova D, *et al.* Localization of the 4th locus (GLC1E) for adult-onset primary open angle glaucoma on the 10p15–p14 region. *Am J Hum Genet* 1998; **62** (3): 641–52.

18 Stoilov I, Akarsu AN and Sarfarazi M. Identification of three truncating mutations in cytochrome P4501B1 (CYP1B1) as the principal cause of primary congenital glaucoma (buphthalmos) families linked to the GLC3A locus on 2p21. *Hum Mol Genet* 1997; **6**: 641–47.

19 Bejjani BA, Lewis RA, Tomey KF, *et al.* Mutations in CYP1B1, the gene for cytochrome P4501B1, are the predominant cause of primary congenital glaucoma in Saudi Arabia. *Am J Hum Genet* 1998; **62**: 325–33.

20 Plasilova M, Ferakova E, Kadasi L, *et al.* Linkage of autosomal recessive primary congenital glaucoma to the GLC3A locus in Roms (Gypsies) from Slovakia. *Human Heredity* 1998; **48** (1): 30–3.

21 Hayes CL, Spink DC, Spink BC, Cao JQ, Walker NJ, Sutter TR. 17beta-estradiol hydroxylation catalyzed by human cytochrome P4501B1. *Proc Nat Acad Sci USA* 1996; **93**: 9776–81.

22 Schwartzman ML, Masferrer J, Dunn MW, McGiff JC, Abracham NG. Cytochrome P450, drug metabolizing enzymes and arachidonic acid metabolism in bovine ocular tissues. *Curr Eye Res* 1987; **6**: 623–30.

23 Schwartzman ML, Balazy M, Masferrer J, Abraham NG, McGiff JC, Murphey RC. Schwartzman ML, Masferrer J, Dunn MW, McGiff JC, Abraham NG. Cytochrome P450, 12(R)–hydroxyicosatetraenoic acid; a cytochrome P450 dependent arachidonate metabolite that inhibits Na+, K+ATPase in the cornea. *Proc Nat Acad Sci USA* 1987; **84**: 8125–9.

24 Akarsu AN, Turacli ME, Aktan SG, *et al.* A second locus (GLC3B) for primary congenital glaucoma (Buphthalmos) maps to the 1p36 region. *Hum Mol Genet* 1996; **5**: 1199–203.

25 Anderson J, Pralea A, Del Bono EA, *et al.* A gene responsible for the pigment dispersion syndrome maps to chromosome 7q35–q36. *Arch Ophthalmol* 1997; **115**: 384–8.

5 Primary glaucomas: optic disc features

J JONAS, T GARWAY-HEATH

Glaucoma leads to morphologic changes in the intrapapillary and parapapillary region of the optic nerve head and in the retinal nerve fibre layer. The morphologic classification of the glaucomas thus depends on the differentiation between the physiologic variability of the appearance of the optic disc and retinal nerve fibre layer (RNFL) in normal eyes, and the changes seen in patients with glaucomatous and non-glaucomatous optic nerve damage.

For the ophthalmoscopic assessment of the optic nerve head and RNFL, variables can be used which are: size and shape of the optic disc, size and shape of the neuroretinal rim, optic cup size, disc haemorrhages, parapapillary atrophy, localised and diffuse diminution of the diameter of the retinal arterioles, and visibility of the RNFL.

Optic disc morphometry: features

Optic disc size

The optic disc area is not constant among individuals but shows an interindividual variability of about 1:7 in a normal Caucasian population (Figures 5.1, 5.2).[1,2] There are normal eyes with rather small optic discs and there are normal eyes with very large optic discs. The optic disc area is independent of age beyond an age of about 3–10 years. Within a range of minus 5 to plus 5 diopters of refractive error, optic disc size increases very slightly with increasing myopic refractive error. In eyes with high myopia, the optic disc is markedly larger,

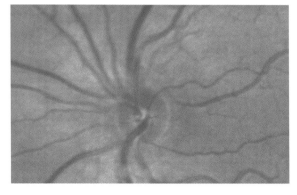

Figure 5.1 Abnormally small, otherwise normal optic disc.
Note: no cupping; good visibility of the retinal nerve fiber layer; no marked parapapillary atrophy.

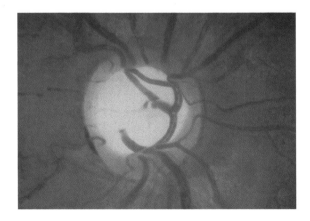

Figure 5.2 Abnormally large, otherwise normal optic disc with high cup:disc diameter ratios (Primary macrodisc with pseudoglaucomatous macrocupping). Note: normal shape of the neuroretinal rim: it is broadest in the inferior disc region, followed by the superior disc region. The rim is smallest in the temporal disc region ("ISNT'T rule").

and in eyes with marked hyperopia the optic disc is pronouncedly smaller than in emmetropic eyes. Size of the optic disc depends on race.[3] Caucasians have relatively small optic discs, followed by Mexicans, Asians, and Afro-Americans who have the largest optic discs. Susceptibility for glaucomatous optic nerve fibre loss may mainly be independent of optic disc size.

The optic disc can be measured using optic disc photographs, or with the help of computerised semiautomatic devices such as scanning laser ophthalmoscopes and laser polarimeters, or by ophthalmoscopy.[1] The horizontal and vertical disc diameters are measured ophthalmoscopically using a standard Goldmann three mirror contact lens and a commercial slit-lamp with adjustable length of the beam. Instead of the Goldmann contact lens, other ophthalmoscopic devices can be used such as the Zeiss four mirror contact lens,[4] a simple modified ophthalmoscope, or other ophthalmoscopic lenses.

Optic disc shape

The shape of the optic disc, which is usually slightly vertically oval, is not correlated with age, sex, right and left eye, and body weight and height.[2] An abnormal optic disc shape is significantly correlated with increased corneal astigmatism and amblyopia. Especially in young children, if an optic disc with abnormal shape is found in routine ophthalmoscopy, keratometry or skiascopy should therefore be performed to rule out corneal astigmatism and to prevent amblyopia.[2]

Neuroretinal rim size

As the intrapapillary equivalent of the retinal nerve fibres and optic nerve fibres, the neuroretinal rim is one of the main targets in the ophthalmoscopic evaluation of the optic nerve.[5,6] The neuroretinal rim size is not interindividually constant but shows, similar to the optic disc and cup, a considerably high inter-

individual variability.[1,2] It is correlated with the optic disc area – the larger is the disc, the larger is the rim.[2,7] The correlation between rim area and disc area corresponds with the positive correlation between optic disc size, optic nerve fibre count, and number and total area of the lamina cribrosa pores.[2]

In contrast to glaucomatous optic neuropathy, non-glaucomatous optic nerve damage is usually not associated with a pronounced loss of neuroretinal rim.

Neuroretinal rim shape

In normal eyes the neuroretinal rim shows a characteristic configuration. It is based on the vertically oval shape of the optic disc and the horizontally oval shape of the optic cup.[2] The neuroretinal rim is usually broadest in the Inferior disc region, followed by the Superior disc region, the Nasal disc area, and finally the Temporal disc region (ISN'T rule, as termed by Elliot Werner/Philadelphia) (Figure 5.2). The characteristic shape of the rim is of utmost importance in the diagnosis of early glaucomatous optic nerve damage.

In glaucoma neuroretinal rim is lost in all sectors of the optic disc with regional preferences depending on the stage of the disease.[2,5,6] In eyes with modest glaucomatous damage, rim loss is found predominantly at the inferotemporal and superotemporal disc regions. In eyes with moderately advanced glaucomatous atrophy the temporal horizontal disc region is the location with relatively the most marked rim loss. In very advanced glaucoma the rim remnants are located mainly in the nasal disc sector, with a larger rim portion in the upper nasal region than in the lower nasal region. This sequence of disc sectors (inferotemporal, superotemporal, temporal horizontal, nasal inferior and nasal superior) correlates with the progression of visual field defects with early perimetrical changes in the nasal upper quadrant of the visual field and a last island of vision in the temporal inferior part of the visual field in eyes with almost absolute glaucoma. It indicates that an early diagnosis of glaucoma, especially the temporal inferior and the temporal superior disc sectors, should be checked for glaucomatous changes.[2,8–10]

Optic cup size in relation to the optic disc size

Parallel to the optic disc and the neuroretinal rim, the optic cup also shows a high interindividual variability (Figures 5.1, 5.2). In normal eyes the areas of the optic disc and optic cup are correlated with each other – the larger the optic disc, the larger the optic cup.[1,2] In small optic discs cupping normally does not occur. Large optic discs usually have a large optic cup. Early or moderately advanced glaucomatous optic nerve damage may erroneously be overlooked in small optic discs with relatively low cup:disc ratios, if one does not take into account that small optic discs normally have no optic cup.[2] The glaucomatous eyes with small optic discs and pseudonormal but glaucomatous minicups often show glaucomatous abnormalities in the parapapillary region, such as a decreased visibility of the retinal nerve fiber layer, diffusely and/or focally diminished diameter of the retinal arterioles, and parapapillary chorioretinal atrophy. In contrast, a large optic cup in a large optic disc should not lead to the diagnosis of glaucoma if the other morphologic variables, especially the shape of the neuroretinal rim and the visibility of the RNFL, are normal.

Cup:disc ratios

Due to the vertically oval optic disc and the horizontally oval optic cup, the cup:disc ratios in normal eyes are larger horizontally than vertically. It is important for the diagnosis of glaucoma, which in the early to medium advanced stages, the vertical cup/disc diameter ratio increases faster than the horizontal one.[2,8–10]

As ratio of cup diameter to disc diameter, the cup:disc ratios depend on the size of the optic disc and cup (Figures 5.1, 5.2). The high inter-

individual variability of the optic disc and cup diameters explain that the cup:disc ratios range in a normal population between 0:0 and almost 0:9. Due to the correlation between disc area and cup area, the cup:disc ratios are low in small optic nerve heads and they are high in large optic discs. An unusually high cup:disc ratio, therefore, can be physiologic in eyes with large optic nerve heads, while an average cup:disc ratio is uncommon in normal eyes with small optic discs.[2] Eyes with physiologically high cup:disc ratios in macrodiscs should not be overdiagnosed to be glaucomatous, and eyes with low cup:disc ratios in small optic nerve heads in combination with increased intraocular pressure should not be underdiagnosed to be only "ocular hypertensive".

Optic disc haemorrhages

Splinter-shaped or flame-shaped haemorrhages at the border of the optic disc are a hallmark of glaucomatous optic nerve atrophy.[11] Rarely found in normal eyes, disc haemorrhages are detected in about 4–7% of eyes with glaucoma. Their frequency increases from an early stage of glaucoma to a medium advanced stage and decreases again towards a far advanced stage. Disc haemorrhages may not be found in disc regions or eyes without detectable neuroretinal rim. In early glaucoma they are usually located in the inferotemporal or superotemporal disc regions. They are associated with localised retinal nerve fiber layer defects, neuroretinal rim notches and circumscribed perimetrical loss.

The diagnostic importance of disc haemorrhages is based on their high specificity, since they are only rarely found in normal eyes; that they usually indicate the presence of glaucomatous optic nerve damage, even if the visual field, is unremarkable in that they suggest progression of glaucoma. Disc haemorrhages are, however, not pathognomonic for glaucoma, since they can also occur in other optic nerve diseases such as disc drusen.[12] Due to the low prevalence of disc haemorrhages in eyes with glaucoma, sensitivity of disc haemorrhages to differentiate between normal eyes and glaucomatous eyes is low. It also explains why disc haemorrhages are not a useful tool in screening examinations for glaucoma.

Parapapillary chorioretinal atrophy

Parapapillary chorioretinal atrophy can be divided into a central β zone characterised by visible sclera and visible large choroidal vessels, and a peripheral α zone with irregular hypopigmentation and hyperpigmentation (Figure 5.3).[2,13] Histologically, β zone correlates with a complete loss of retinal pigment epithelium cells and a markedly diminished count of retinal photoreceptors. Alpha zone is the equivalent of pigment irregularities in the retinal pigment epithelium. Correspondingly, β zone corresponds psychophysically to an absolute scotoma, and α zone to a relative scotoma.[2]

In normal eyes, both α zone and β zone are largest and most frequently located in the temporal horizontal sector, followed by the inferior temporal area and the superior temporal region. They are smallest and most rarely found in the nasal parapapillary area. Alpha zone is present in almost all normal eyes and is thus more common than β zone (mean frequency in normal eyes is about 15–20%). The myopic scleral

crescent present in highly myopic eyes differs histologically from the glaucomatous β zone in non-highly myopic eyes.[2] In the region of the myopic crescent, only the inner limiting membrane and underlying RNFL or its remnants cover the sclera, while in glaucomatous β zone, Bruch's membrane and the choroid is interposed between sclera and the remnants of the RNFL.

Both zones are significantly larger and occur more often in glaucomatous eyes than in normal eyes. A large β zone, also called "halo glaucomatous" when encircling the optic disc, is often associated with a marked degree of fundus tessellation, a shallow glaucomatous disc cupping, a relatively low frequency of disc haemorrhages and detectable localised defects of the RNFL, a mostly concentric loss of neuroretinal rim, and normal or almost normal intraocular pressure measurements. The location of parapapillary chorioretinal atrophy is spatially correlated with the neuroretinal rim loss in the intrapapillary region.[2] It is larger in that sector with the more marked loss of neuroretinal rim.

In contrast to glaucomatous optic neuropathy, non-glaucomatous optic nerve damage does not lead to an enlargement of parapapillary atrophy.[2]

Diameter of retinal arterioles

Diffuse narrowing of the retinal vessels is found in glaucomatous and nonglaucomatous optic neuropathies.[2] In glaucoma the vessel diameter reduces with decreasing area of the neuroretinal rim, diminishing visibility of the RNFL and increasing visual field defects. Since the reduction of the vessel calibre is also found in eyes with nonglaucomatous optic nerve damage, such as descending optic nerve atrophy and nonarteritic anterior ischaemic optic neuropathy, one inferred that a generalised reduction of the vessel diameter is typical for optic nerve damage, but not characteristic for glaucoma. From a pathogenetical point of view it suggested that vessel reduction was not

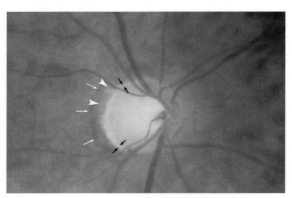

Figure 5.3 Glaucomatous optic disc with parapapillary atrophy.
White arrows α zone, white arrow heads β zone; black arrows, peripapillary scleral ring.

causative for glaucomatous optic nerve fibre loss, but, at least partially, secondary to a reduced demand in the superficial layers of the retina.

Besides diffuse narrowing, focal attenuation of the diameter of the retinal arterioles is found in eyes with glaucomatous and non-glaucomatous optic nerve atrophy.[2,14] Eyes with glaucoma and eyes with nonglaucomatous optic nerve damage do not vary significantly in the degree of focal narrowing. The degree of focal narrowing of the retinal arterioles increases with an increasing degree of optic nerve damage. In a fluorescein angiographic correlation, focal retinal arteriole narrowing in the parapapillary region of eyes with optic neuropathies represented a real stenosis of the vessel lumen and was not due to an ophthalmoscopic artifact.[2]

Visibility of the retinal nerve fibre layer

Visibility of the RNFL in normal eyes is regionally unevenly distributed.[2] The nerve fibre bundles are best visible in the inferotemporal sector, followed by the superotemporal area, the superonasal region and finally the inferonasal inferior sector. It corresponds with the normal configuration of the neuroretinal rim, the location of the foveola in relation to the centre of the optic disc, and the diameters of the retinal arterioles.

Visibility of the RNFL decreases with age. It correlates with an age-related reduction of the optic nerve fibre count with an annual loss of about 4,000–5,000 fibres/year, out of an original population of presumably 1.4 million optic nerve fibres.

The optic nerve fibre loss in diseases occurs in a diffuse way and/or in form of localised defects (Figure 5.4).[2,15–17] Localised defects of the RNFL are defined as wedge-shaped and not spindle-like defects, running towards or touching the optic disc border. If they are pronounced, they can have a broad basis at the temporal raphe of the fundus. Besides in glaucoma eyes, localised RNFL defects can be

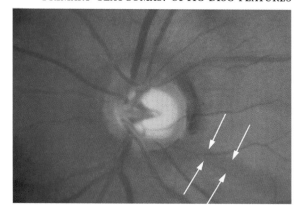

Figure 5.4 Glaucomatous optic disc with localised retinal nerve fibre layer defect (arrows), corresponding to a notch in the neuroretinal rim.

found in eyes with an atrophy of the optic nerve. This can be due to other reasons, e.g. optic disc drusen, toxoplasmotic retinochoroidal scars, ischaemic retinopathies with cotton-wool spots of the retina, after longstanding papilloedema or optic neuritis due to multiple sclerosis. Since the localised RNFL defects are not present in normal eyes, they almost always signify a pathological abnormality. This is important for subjects with ocular hypertension in which a localised RNFL defect points to optic nerve damage, even in the absence of perimetric abnormalities.[2,15–17]

The frequency of localised RNFL defects in glaucomatous eyes increases significantly from an "early" glaucoma stage to a stage with medium advanced glaucomatous damage and decreases again to a stage with very marked glaucomatous changes.[2] In eyes with very advanced optic nerve damage they are usually no longer detectable due to the pronounced loss of nerve fibres in all fundus sectors. In their vicinity at the optic disc border, one often finds notches of the neuroretinal rim, sometimes an optic disc haemorrhage, and a parapapillary chorioretinal atrophy which is more marked in that sector than in other sectors.

Besides localised RNFL defects, a diffuse loss of retinal nerve fibres occurs in eyes with damage of the optic nerve. It leads to a decreased visibility of the RNFL. Ophthalmoscopically the diffuse RNFL loss is more difficult to detect than a localised defect. It is helpful to use the variable "sequence of fundus sectors concerning the best RNFL visibility". If one detects in an eye without fundus irregularities that the RNFL is markedly better detectable in the temporal superior fundus region than in the temporal inferior sector, it points towards a loss of RNFL mainly in the temporal inferior fundus region. It is also helpful to evaluate if the retinal vessels are clearly and sharply detectable. The retinal vessels are normally embedded in the RNFL. In eyes with a diffuse RNFL loss, the retinal vessels are covered only by the inner limiting membrane resulting in a better visibility and a sharper image of the large retinal vessels.

Considering its great importance in the assessment of anomalies and diseases of the optic nerve and taking into account the feasibility of its ophthalmoscopical evaluation, the RNFL should be examined during every routine ophthalmoscopy. This holds true especially for patients with an early damage of the optic nerve. The importance of evaluating the RNFL is further examplified in studies in which glaucomatous damage of the optic nerve could be earlier detected by examination of the RNFL other than by conventional computerised perimetry.[2,15–17] It is of utmost importance for the detection of glaucoma in eyes with a pseudo-normal but glaucomatous minicup in minidiscs, and it is useful to classify an eye with a pseudoglaucomatous but normal large cup in a large disc as normal.[2] In eyes with advanced optic nerve atrophy, other examination techniques such as perimetry may be more helpful for the follow-up of the optic nerve damage.

Early or "preperimetric" diagnosis of glaucomatous optic nerve damage

For the early detection of glaucomatous optic nerve damage in ocular hypertensive eyes before the development of visual field loss, the most important variables are: shape of the

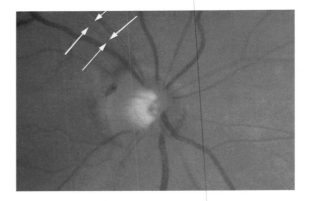

Figure 5.5 Optic disc with "early" glaucomatous optic nerve damage.
The neuroretinal rim is more or less even in width in all optic disc regions. Arrows: localised retinal nerve fibre layer defect.

neuroretinal rim, size of the optic cup in relation to the size of the optic disc, decreased visibility of the RNFL, and occurrence of localised RNFL defects and disc haemorrhages.[2,8–10] If the rim is not markedly broader in the inferior and superior disc regions compared to the temporal disc region (Figure 5.5), a glaucomatous loss of rim tissue may be suspected in the inferior and superior disc regions. In eyes with small discs, the neuroretinal rim cannot clearly be delineated from the optic cup, so that the shape of the rim cannot be well determined. The variable "cup size in relation to disc size" in these eyes is the most important intrapapillary factor to detect glaucomatous optic nerve damage.

Differentiation glaucomatous versus nonglaucomatous optic neuropathy

Glaucomatous and nonglaucomatous optic neuropathy have in common a decreased diameter of the retinal arterioles including the occurrence of focal arteriole narrowing, and a reduced visibility of the RNFL.[2] Localised RNFL defects can be found in glaucoma and in many types of nonglaucomatous optic nerve damage, e.g. in optic disc drusen and long-standing papilloedema. In glaucomatous optic neuropathy compared to nonglaucomatous optic nerve atrophy, the optic cup enlarges and deepens, and in a complementary manner the neuroretinal rim decreases. Besides in glaucoma, an enlargement of the optic cup and a loss of neuroretinal rim may be found in patients after arteritic anterior ischaemic optic neuropathy and in few patients with intrasellar or suprasellar tumours. With parapapillary atrophy usually not being markedly increased in eyes with nonglaucomatous optic nerve damage, it is helpful for the differentiation of glaucomatous versus nonglaucomatous optic neuropathy.

Morphologic classification of the glaucomas based on the morphologic variables of the optic nerve head

The chronic open angle glaucomas form a heterogeneous group of different types of glaucomas. These can be differentiated from each other by reason of elevation of intraocular pressure, level of intraocular pressure, age of the patients, refractive error, morphology of the anterior segment of the eye, and appearance of the optic nerve head and RNFL.[2,18–20]

The highly myopic type of primary open angle glaucoma (POAG) shows a secondary or acquired macrodisc of an abnormal shape, shallow and concentric disc cupping, and a large myopic crescent. Disc haemorrhages and localised RNFL defects are rarely detected, and intraocular pressure measurements are often in the normal range. In juvenile-onset POAG, optic disc cupping is steep and deep, and parapapillary atrophy is only slightly enlarged. Frequencies of disc haemorrhages, neuroretinal rim notches and broad localised RNFL defects are relatively low, and the minimal and maximal values of intraocular pressure measurements are high. Eyes with the sclerotic or "age-related atrophic" type POAG show a shallow and concentric disc cupping. Disc haemorrhages, rim notches and localised RNFL defects are seldom found, and intraocular pressure readings are in the lower range. In focal normal-pressure glaucoma, as originally described by Spaeth, Hitchings and Sivalingam,[18] intraocular pressure is normal and the optic disc shows focal emaciation of the neuroretinal rim typically in the inferotemporal and superiortemporal disc sector. Optic disc cupping can be steep and deep, and parapapillary atrophy is only slightly enlarged. Secondary open angle glaucomas such as pseudoexfoliative glaucoma and pigmentary glaucoma do not show clinically significant peculiarities in the morphology of the optic disc.

Optic nerve head imaging

Whereas clinical examination remains the mainstay in assessing the optic nerve head (ONH) for glaucomatous damage, a number of imaging devices are becoming available, capable of making quantitative measurements of nerve structure, and which may aid the clinician in making management decisions.

Confocal scanning laser ophthalmoscopy is one of these new imaging modalities. The technology permits a reconstruction of the surface shape of the ONH and surrounding retina. This enables measurement of a variety of new parameters, such as the shape of the ONH surface, the slope of the peripapillary retina, and the neuroretinal rim and optic cup volumes. This is in addition to conventional parameters such as the neuroretinal rim (NRR) and optic cup areas.

Several research groups have looked at the large number of measurement parameters generated by these devices to determine which are of most use to distinguish between normal and glaucomatous ONHs. Various approaches to data analysis have been taken: the generation a discriminant function from the normal and glaucomatous group data,[21–24] a comparison of the contour of the normal and glaucomatous peripapillary surface,[25] and the generation of confidence intervals for NRR area with respect to ONH size from a normal population.[26]

Reports suggest that high sensitivities and

specificities can be achieved in selected study populations, although it has yet to be shown that these results can be reproduced in clinical practice. If they can, the sensitivity and specificity values need to be interpreted in relation to individual patients.

When a measurement parameter that discriminates between two populations has been identified, a particular value for that parameter can be selected as a "cut-off". Typically, if the cut-off has a high specificity (fewer false positives), then the sensitivity will be lower (more false negatives). If the cut-off has a low specificity (more false positives), then the sensitivity will be higher (fewer false negatives) (Figure 5.6.). However, when applied to an individual, a single cut-off value merely gives the probability (given the disease prevalence) that an individual has a certain condition. For a test to be useful, the clinician needs to know with greater certainty whether or not the individual has the condition. To partially resolve this problem, two cut-off values can be used – one with high specificity and one with high sensitivity. If an individual's NRR area falls above the high sensitivity cut-off, then the clinician can be fairly sure that the ONH is normal. If the NRR area falls below the high specificity cut-off, then the clinician can be fairly sure that the

ONH is not normal. NRR areas lying between the cut-offs can be said to be "borderline". This approach has been applied to data derived from a scanning laser ophthalmoscope (Heidelberg Retina Tomograph – HRT), using the method of data analysis described by Wollstein et al.[26] Cut-off values were derived from the prediction intervals for NRR area, given the size of the ONH, in a group of normal subjects. A disc is considered borderline or abnormal if the NRR area falls outside a prediction interval (cut-off). Figure 5.7 illustrates the analysis for a glaucomatous ONH.

If this approach is applied to a population with a glaucoma prevalence of about 30% (typical for the population of "glaucoma suspects" referred to hospital eye services in the UK), then 85.5% of subjects will be categorised (63.8% as "normal" and 21.7% as "glaucomatous") and 14.5% will be "borderline". Of those categorised, the probability that the classification is correct is 97% (for both categories). Of those labelled "borderline", the probability that they are glaucomatous is 48%. This level of probability for correct classification should be clinically useful.

It should be noted that the process of categorising patients by means of imaging device measurements is not the same as diagnosis. Diagnosis requires the integration of all available information about a patient. This includes the clinical evaluation of the ONH and RNFL, visual field status, and risk factors such as intraocular pressure level, age, and family history.

The cost of scanning laser ophthalmoscopes has been high, and at present the clinical use, on cost grounds, is limited to larger glaucoma practices. As the benefits of the greater clinical information afforded by optic disc measurement become apparent, and as the cost of the instruments declines, the clinical use of scanning laser ophthalmoscopes is likely to expand.

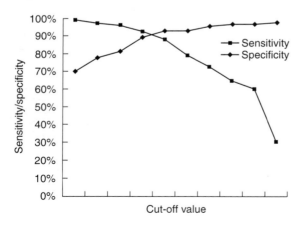

Fig 5.6 Plot of sensitivity and specificity for varying hypothetical cut-offs of a test.
As sensitivity increases, specificity decreases, and vice versa.

<u>C</u>ontourLine   <u>D</u>iagram   <u>C</u>oordinates   <u>R</u>eference   <u>M</u>easure   <u>L</u>oad   <u>B</u>ack

L4: 10°,   3.0mm,   04/07/95 BL   (17.44 227 228 229)

Rim Area		global	temporl	tmp/sup	tmp/inf	nasal	nsl/sup	nsl/inf
actual	[mm^2]	0.973	0.126	0.118	0.053	0.369	0.144	0.162
predicted	[mm^2]	1.632	0.292	0.196	0.215	0.451	0.223	0.232
actual/disc area	[%]	46.3	24.3	44.4	19.0	71.9	55.4	62.2
predicted	[%]	77.7	56.1	74.1	76.6	87.8	85.8	89.1
low 95% CI lim.	[%]	55.5	21.5	47.7	50.3	68.3	63.6	71.6
low 99% CI lim.	[%]	49.8	15.7	41.4	44.0	63.0	57.9	66.7
low 99.9% CI lim.	[%]	43.9	10.9	35.0	37.3	57.1	51.7	61.4

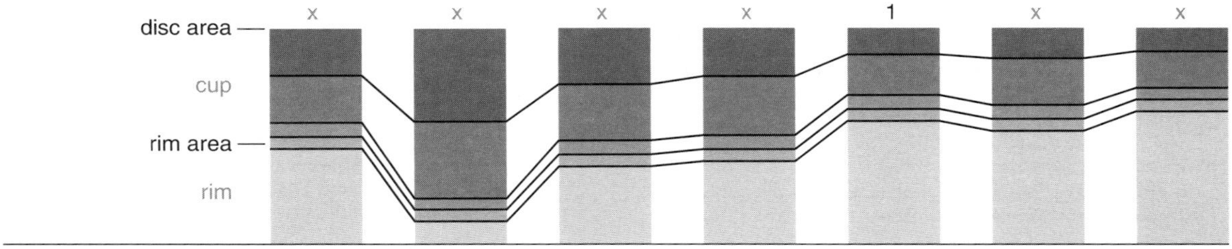

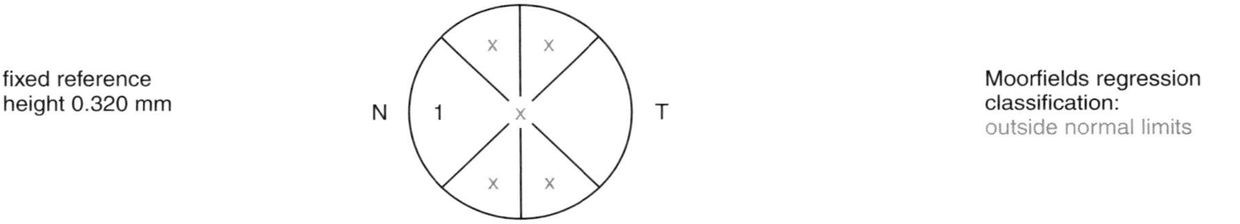

fixed reference
height 0.320 mm

Moorfields regression
classification:
outside normal limits

Figure 5.7 Analysis of HRT data according to the method described by Wollstein et al.[26] modified for two cut-offs.
The bars represent the ONH area for the whole ONH (first bar), and each segment predefined by the HRT software. The bar is divided into cup (red) and NRR (green). The top white line is the mean (predicted) NRR area for a normal ONH. The group of three lines at the lower end of the bars represents various cut-off levels. The upper of the three is the high sensitivity cut-off: a NRR area above this is considered normal. The lower of the three is the high specificity cut-off: a NRR area below this is considered abnormal. If the NRR area falls between these lines, the disc is considered borderline.

References

1 Varma R, Tielsch JM, Quigley HA, et al. Race-, age-, gender-, and refractive error-related differences in the normal optic disc. Arch Ophthalmol 1994; 112: 1068–76.

2 Jonas JB, Budde WM, Panda-Jonas S. Ophthalmoscopic evaluation of the optic nerve head. Surv Ophthalmol 1999; (In Press).

3 Chi T, Ritch R, Stickler D, Pitman B, Tsai C, Hsieh FY. Racial differences in optic nerve head parameters. Arch Ophthalmol 1989; 107: 836–9.

4 Spencer AF, Vernon SA. Optic disc measurement with the Zeiss four mirror contact lens. Br J Ophthalmol 1994; 78: 775–80.

5 Airaksinen PJ, Drance SM. Neuroretinal rim area and retinal nerve fiber layer in glaucoma. Arch Ophthalmol 1985; 103: 203–4.

6 Hitchings RA, Spaeth GL. The optic disc in glaucoma II: correlation of the appearance of the optic disc with the visual field. Br J Ophthalmol 1977; 61: 107–13.

7 Britton RJ, Drance SM, Schulzer MD, Douglas GR, Mawson DK. The area of the neuroretinal rim of the optic nerve in normal eyes. Am J Ophthalmol 1987; 103: 497–504.

8 Hitchings RA, Wheeler CA. The optic disc in glaucoma. IV: Optic disc evaluation in the ocular hypertensive patient. Br J Ophthalmol 1980; 64: 232–9.

9 Pederson JE, Anderson DR. The mode of progressive disc cupping in ocular hypertension and glaucoma. Arch Ophthalmol 1980; 98: 490–5.

10 Schwartz B. Optic disc changes in ocular hypertension. Surv Ophthalmol 1980; 25: 148–54.

11 Drance SM. Disc haemorrhages in the glaucomas. Surv Ophthalmol 1989; 33: 331–7.

12 Hitchings RA, Corbetz JJ, Winkleman J, Schwartz NJ. Haemorrhages with optic nerve drusen. A differentiation from early papilloedema. *Arch Neurol* 1976; **33**: 675–7.

13 Tezel G, Kolker AE, Kass MA, Wax MB, Gordon M, Siegmund KD. Parapapillary chorioretinal atrophy in patients with ocular hypertension. I. An evaluation as a predictive factor for the devlopment of glaucomatous damage. *Arch Ophthalmol* 1997; **115**: 1503–8.

14 Rader J, Feuer J, Anderson D. Peripapillary vasoconstriction in the glaucomas and the anterior ischemic optic neuropathy. *Am J Ophthalmol* 1994; **117**: 72–80.

15 Sommer A, Katz J, Quigely HA, *et al*. Clinically detectable nerve fiber atrophy precedes the onset of glaucomatous field loss. *Arch Ophthalmol* 1991; **109**: 77–83.

16 Tuulonen A, Airaksinen PJ. Initial glaucomatous optic disk and retinal nerve fiber layer abnormalities and the mode of their progression. *Am J Ophthalmol* 1991; **111**: 485–90.

17 Quigley HA, Katz J, Derick RJ, Gilbert D, Sommer A. An evaluation of optic disc and nerve fiber layer examinations in monitoring progression of early glaucoma damage. *Ophthalmology* 1992; **99**: 19–28.

18 Spaeth GL, Hitchings RA, Sivalingam E. The optic disc in glaucoma: Pathogenetic correlation of five patterns of cupping in chronic open-angle glaucoma. *Trans Am Acad Ophthalmol Otolaryngol* 1976; **81**: 217–23.

19 Geijssen HC, Greve EL. The spectrum of primary open-angle glaucoma I. Senile sclerotic glaucoma versus high tension glaucoma. *Ophthalmic Surg* 1987; **18**: 207–13.

20 Caprioli J. Correlation between disc appearance and type of glaucoma, in Varma R, Spaeth GL (eds). The optic nerve in glaucoma. Philadelphia: Lippincott, 1993; 91–8.

21 Mikelberg FS, Parfitt CM, Swindale NV, Graham SL, Drance SM, Gosine R. Ability of the Heidelberg Retina Tomograph to detect early glaucomatous visual field loss. *J Glaucoma* 1995; **4**: 242–247.

22 Iester M, Mikelberg FS, Drance SM. The effect of optic disc size on diagnostic precision with the Heidelberg retina tomograph. *Ophthalmology* 1997; **104** (3): 545–8.

23 Bathija R, Zangwill L, Berry CC, Sample PA, Weinreb RN. Detection of early glaucomatous structural damage with confocal scanning laser tomography. *J Glaucoma* 1998; **7** (2): 121–7.

24 Uchida H, Brigatti L, Caprioli J. Detection of structural damage from glaucoma with confocal laser image analysis. *Invest Ophthalmol Vis Sci* 1996; **37** (12): 2393–2401.

25 Caprioli J, Park HJ, Ugurlu S, Hoffman D. Slope of the peripapillary nerve fiber layer surface in glaucoma. *Invest Ophthalmol Vis Sci* 1998; **39** (12): 2321–8.

26 Wollstein G, Garway-Heath DF, Hitchings RA. Identification of early glaucoma cases with the scanning laser ophthalmoscope. *Ophthalmology* 1998; **105** (8): 1557–63.

6 Glaucoma perimetry

A HEIJL

Visual field testing has been an important part of the management of patients with glaucoma and suspect glaucoma for a very long time. The importance of perimetry has increased over the last decades, however, with the understanding of the importance of maintaining a very clear distinction between elevated intraocular pressure and glaucoma. It is now generally accepted that glaucoma may occur at any intraocular pressure (IOP) – also at levels that are lower than the mean IOP of a normal population – and that the majority of patients with "elevated" IOP will not develop glaucoma during their lifetime. Instead the diagnosis of glaucoma must rely on detection of glaucomatous damage.

Glaucomatous visual field defects are functional correlates of glaucomatous axonal loss. Visual field testing has the disadvantage of being subjective and often time-consuming, but also has several advantages: testing and test interpretation have become automated through computerisation and can be carried out by ancillary personnel, the instrumentation is readily available, and quite importantly, the normal visual field shows less inter-subject variability than normal optic nerve topography.

Glaucomatous visual field loss

The location of glaucomatous field defects

Glaucomatous visual field defects are the result of lesions at the level of the optic disc. The defects may occur anywhere in the visual field but are particularly common in the arcuate, so-called Bjerrum areas of the central 30° field and nasally. This is explained by the predilection for early glaucomatous optic disc lesions to occur around the poles of the optic disc. Early defects are somewhat more common in the superior than in the inferior hemifield. Only a very small percentage of glaucomatous eyes exhibit field defects in the peripheral field, while the central field is normal. This might be explained by the organisation of receptive fields in the retina. In the retinal periphery receptive fields are very large with signals from large numbers of photoreceptors converging on every retinal ganglion cell. As a result, only a small percentage of papillary axonal bundles stem from ganglion cells in the retinal periphery.

Typical glaucomatous field defects and their anatomical correlates

The typical glaucomatous visual field defects are paracentral scotomas, arcuate (Bjerrum) scotomas and nasal steps and wedges. Retinal and papillary neural anatomy and the nature of the glaucomatous optic disc lesions can explain these findings. Axons from the nasal, upper and temporal parts of the retina proceed almost directly to the disc, while those from the retina, temporal to the optic disc, curve around the macula and the papillomacular bundle. No axonal bundles cross the temporal raphe. Localised optic disc lesions around the optic disc poles will, therefore, result in loss of arcuate nerve fibre layer bundles. If the notch extends all the way or almost all the way to the disc margin, there will be a corresponding Bjerrum scotoma in the opposite hemifield (Figure 6.1).

Smaller lesions will result in paracentral scotomas. In the retinal nerve fibre layer shorter axons are more superficial, while longer axons are located deeper. A focal lesion at the optic disk involving, for example, only the middle part of the neuroretinal rim in a

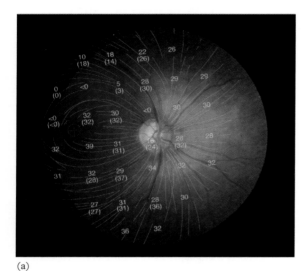

(a)

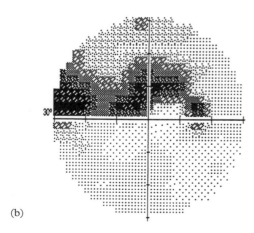

(b)

Figure 6.1 (a) Inverted fundus photograph including an optic disc with focal loss of the neuroretinal rim.

The normal retinal nerve fibre layer has been added including the approximate positions of corresponding test point locations in the Humphrey 30-2 test point pattern.

(b) The corresponding grey-scale representation of the threshold field.

certain direction may, therefore, only damage axons of intermediate length, while sparing longer and shorter axons; the latter are located closer to the scleral ring or to the optic cup, respectively.

Any widespread or relatively diffuse loss of axons that is not perfectly symmetrical across the horizontal meridian will lead to dissimilarities in axonal density above and below the temporal raphe. Such imbalances result in nasal steps, which are extremely common in glaucoma.

Localised and diffuse field loss

All field defects mentioned above are examples of localised field loss, i.e. reduction of differential light sensitivity that occur in or are more pronounced in one area of the visual field than in other areas. Such defects have shape and influence the shape of the hill of vision. Diffuse field loss, on the other hand, is a homogenous reduction of sensitivity depressing the whole hill of vision to the same extent. Cataract and pharmacologically induced miosis are very common reasons for such loss (Figure 6.2). It was often claimed that diffuse visual field loss is one, albeit not very common, type of glaucomatous visual field loss. While diffuse loss often accompanies localised loss in glaucoma, such pure loss is very rare or non-existent in glaucoma.[1] Diffuse visual field loss, therefore, is not a diagnostic sign of glaucoma, and the search for glaucomatous field loss should concentrate on localised defects.

Variability

Glaucomatous visual field defects are characterised by large fluctuations. This is already clear at the very earliest stages, and clear-cut defects are preceded by an increased sensitivity scatter in the areas where defects are developing (Figure 6.3).[2] This period with questionable perimetric results often lasts for two or three years.

Test-retest variability is larger in glaucomatous than in normal fields, and is not constant

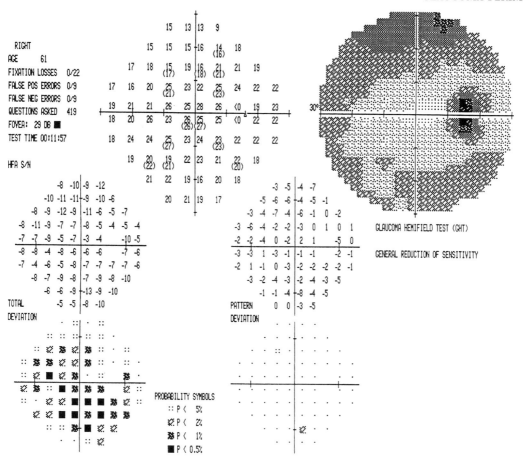

Figure 6.2 Test results from an eye with cataract and diffuse visual field loss.

Numerical pattern deviation and probability maps are both normal and the Glaucoma Hemifield Test classification is "General Reduction of Sensitivity" (see "Tools of computer-assisted visual field interpretation").

across the field. Test point status, normal or abnormal, is of importance; points with normal or almost normal differential light sensitivity vary less than locations with reduced sensitivity.[3,4] Furthermore variability increases with eccentricity just as in normal fields.

Visual field testing in Glaucoma

Computerised perimetry is definitely the method of choice in glaucoma management; manual perimetry will find defects later and is no longer a real alternative.[5] Threshold perimetry of the central 25–30° field has become the clinical norm and should be preferred. Threshold testing makes it possible to detect defects at the earliest stage, characterised by shallow relative defects that come and go. Peripheral testing can be omitted.

One standard threshold test, therefore, can be used for all tests, except in very advanced stages of the disease, when only a small number of test point locations of the standard test retain measurable sensitivities. In that situation one may choose a larger than standard stimulus size or concentrate the examination in the central 10°-field.

SITA and threshold tests

There are now many different threshold algorithms available. Choosing between them can

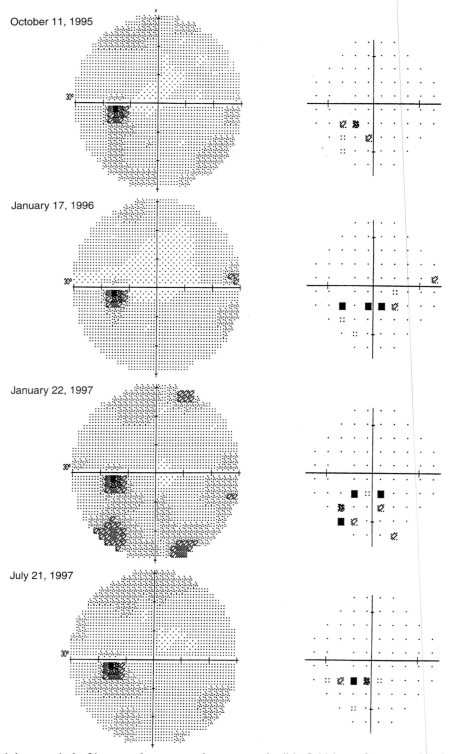

Figure 6.3 A long period of increased scatter and non-reproducible field loss often precedes the stage when clear glaucomatous defects can be found at every test.

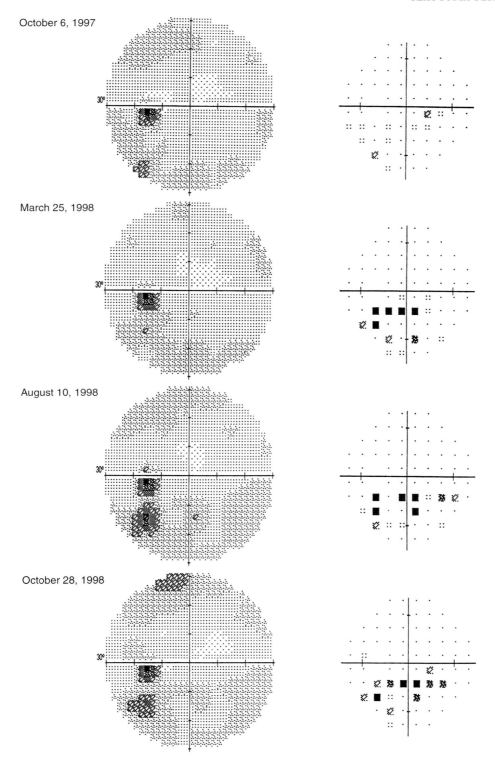

October 6, 1997

March 25, 1998

August 10, 1998

October 28, 1998

be difficult for anybody without a special interest in perimetry, particularly since names and marketing often seem to indicate that they are all equally dependable and differ only in terms of test time.

The traditional threshold tests in the Humphrey perimeter have been Full Threshold and Fastpac. Full Threshold is slightly more time-consuming and accurate, but both algorithms provide true threshold-measuring tests. The new SITA Standard and SITA Fast algorithms[6,7] have been designed to replace the Full Threshold and Fastpac respectively. By continuously estimating threshold values and threshold error using maximum posterior probability calculations in visual field models, they provide tests with the same accuracy as their predecessors while saving about 50% of the test time.[7,8] Many of the approaches used in SITA are entirely new; earlier efforts to reduce test time, for example, by using larger stimulus steps and/or fewer staircase reversals, lead to decreased accuracy.[9]

The Octopus perimeter also has several different threshold tests. The traditional threshold strategy, used, for example, in the G1 and G1X programs[10] are similar to Humphrey's Full Threshold. The Dynamic Strategy[11] is a faster threshold test. Test time is reduced by approximately 40–50% compared to the Humphrey Full Threshold strategy, by using larger stimulus steps in areas with decreased sensitivity.[12] The new Tendency Oriented Perimetry (TOP) test presents just one stimulus at every tested point regardless of response. Sensitivity values are then estimated by interpolating answers from a group of locations. This strategy has little similarity to true threshold tests.

Because of visual fatigue,[13] shorter tests on average indicate somewhat smaller and/or shallower glaucomatous field defects than more time-consuming tests. The reduced test time and smaller fatigue may also provide smaller inter-subject variability among normal subjects and thus narrower normal limits. This increases the statistical significance of measured field defects. In SITA, for example, the narrower limits ensure that the shorter tests yield at least as much significant glaucomatous field loss as the older more time-consuming tests.

Non-standard techniques

Short-wavelength automated perimetry (SWAP)

The very great majority of clinical perimetry is performed with white stimuli of Goldmann size III. Several other perimetric techniques have been used or advocated during the last years, in the hope of increasing the sensitivity of the perimetric test to facilitate earlier detection of the disease. The most successful of these techniques is blue-yellow perimetry or SWAP. SWAP is performed with size V blue stimuli on a high luminosity (314 asb) yellow background. With this technique glaucomatous perimetric loss can often be detected several years before field defects appear on standard white-on-white perimetry.[14] Unfortunately SWAP is associated with some new problems. Normal inter-subject variability and age-induced reduction of sensitivity are both much larger with SWAP than with standard white stimuli (Figure 6.4).[15] Lens opacities are also considerably more disturbing for blue-yellow perimetry than for standard techniques. SWAP is currently more time-consuming than the older standard and many patients find the bright background unpleasant. These factors may explain why SWAP has not yet gained large clinical acceptance. It is unlikely that blue-yellow perimetry in its current form will play an important role in clinical glaucoma management. The test needs to be made more time-effective, dynamic range must be increased and better means must be developed to compensate for media opacities.

Frequency-doubling contrast test

Frequency-doubling contrast test (FDT) is an even more novel technology developed to detect glaucomatous field loss.[16] It uses the so-called frequency-doubling illusion which

Test time 16:41

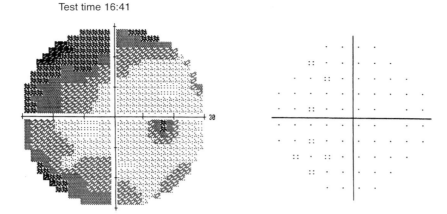

Figure 6.4. Glaucomatous visual field defect plotted with SWAP.
Despite the fact that defects appear very large in the grey-scale representation, with many test point locations where not even the strongest stimuli have been seen, many points in such absolute field defects fail to reach high statistical significance.

has been attributed to a small subset of magnocellular ganglion cells. Functional deficits in magnocellular pathways are believed to occur in early stages of the disease. FDT is available commercially in two forms, as a supraliminal screening test and as a threshold test. Seventeen to nineteen large areas in the central 20–30° field are tested. A clinical study comparing the screening test with conventional Humphrey threshold testing indicated that FDT is a promising method for glaucoma screening.[17] Further studies will show its role in the future.

Motion detection perimetry

Motion detection is another visual function relying on magnocellular pathways. It was demonstrated 10 years ago that peripheral motion detection thresholds are influenced by glaucoma.[18] Motion detection perimetry is not widely available, and large clinical experience is therefore lacking, but automated motion perimetry has been demonstrated to identify early glaucomatous field loss.[19] As with FDT and SWAP we still cannot know whether motion detection perimetry will be part of regular glaucoma management in the future.

Recognising glaucomatous visual field loss and field progression

The recognition of glaucomatous visual field loss is usually straightforward. At the stage when defects were detected by manual methods, they were usually already very clear-cut in the grey-scale representations of computerised perimeters. It is important to remember, however, that non-glaucomatous field defects are quite common in the population. Therefore, one should look for reasons other than glaucoma if field defects appear non-specific, particularly if they respect the vertical meridian or if the optic disc looks normal. Some common false positive patterns caused by test artefacts are also characteristic and worth recognising (see below).

Tools of computer-assisted visual field interpretation

Modern computerised perimeters provide computer-assisted analyses.[20,21] Measured threshold values are compared to age-corrected normal mean values and the differences displayed as deviation maps (Figure 6.5, C, D).

45

Probability maps and the Glaucoma Hemifield Test

The statistical significance of each measured threshold value is shown in probability maps[22] (Figure 6.5, E, F). These are quite helpful, since those distributions of deviations from the age-corrected normal mean values that form the basis for significance limits are non-Gaussian and vary with test point location.[23] Significances of deviation values are thus not intuitively clear. Probability maps are of great help for identification of early visual field loss, particularly if such loss occurs within the central 15–20° of the visual field, where significance limits are quite narrow (Figure 6.3). They also help de-emphasise common false positive patterns in the periphery of the tested field (Figure 6.8).

In the Humphrey perimeter such statistical significances form the basis for a small system of artificial intelligence, the Glaucoma Hemifield Test (Figure 6.5, G), that allows sensitive and specific recognition of glaucomatous field loss.[21,24]

Pattern deviation and diffuse field loss

The total deviation from the mean age-corrected normal values are shown in the total deviation numerical (Figure 6.5, C) and probability (Figure 6.5, E) maps. Eliminating homogenous, diffuse visual field loss will also eliminate most of the influence of any media opacities. Any general difference in height between the measured field and the age-corrected normal reference hill of vision is removed. The remaining pattern deviation maps indicate the shape and extent of localised field defects, numerically (Figure 6.5, D) and statistically (Figure 6.5, F). Differences in total and pattern maps are small (Figure 6.5), showing the test result from a patient with clear media. The corresponding differences are large (Figure 6.2), from a patient with a cataract and significant diffuse field loss.

Visual field indices

Visual field indices summarise the field test results into a single number (Figure 6.5, H).

Indices can be used for coarse classification of fields into stages of disease. They are more suited for following glaucoma than for diagnosing the disease.

Reliability parameters

Patient reliability is estimated by a number of so-called reliability parameters: fixation losses, false positive (FP) and false negative (FN) responses. These parameters are of limited value, however. Thus frequencies of FN answers have traditionally been estimated by catch trials – extra questions added to the test. The numbers of catch trials have been kept low because of time constraints. These small samples make the resulting errors in estimated frequencies very large. Frequencies of FN errors also depend on visual field status being considerably higher in pathological than in normal fields – thus further limiting the clinical value of the FN estimate. False positive errors are not associated with field status and high frequencies of FP answers can make the test result completely valueless. Fields from "trigger-happy" patients can often be identified by almost white areas in grey-scale printouts, and in the Humphrey perimeter, by the Glaucoma Hemifield Test statement "abnormally high sensitivity" (Figure 6.6). The SITA algorithms calculate frequencies of false answers in new ways. Frequencies of FP answers are estimated with no cost in test time and higher accuracy using periods during the test when no true answers to stimuli are expected.[25]

Most perimeters use the blind spot technique for fixation monitoring. If fixating correctly the patient should not perceive the fixation stimuli projected in the blind spot of the tested eye. The technique is quite sensitive but not entirely dependable. When fixation check stimuli are located outside the blind spot of the tested eye, the method may indicate faulty fixation even in a perfect observer. An additional way of judging fixation is to see whether the blind spot has been found in the test. With most test

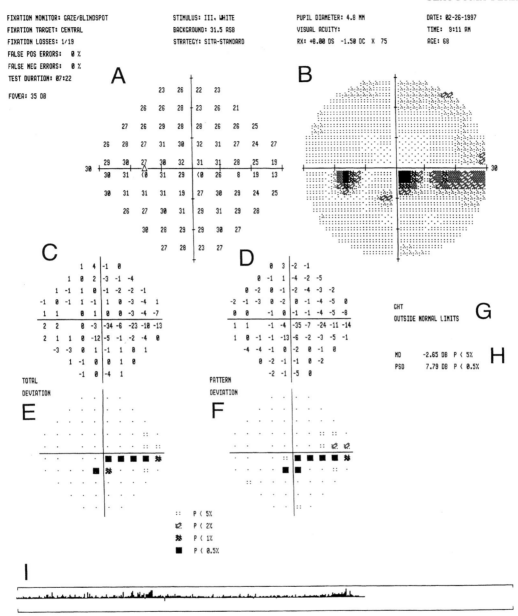

Figure 6.5 Single field Statpac printout from a 30-2 SITA Standard field.
[20]Explanation under "Tools of computer-assisted visual field interpretation".

programmes an absolute defect in the blind spot indicates that the patient has maintained fixation in an acceptable way. Some new Humphrey HFA-II perimeters monitor fixation for each test stimulus presentation using a gaze monitor performing real-time image analysis of an image of the patient's eye.[26] The gaze tracker record is displayed at the bottom of the field chart (Figure 6.5).

The intra-test threshold variability, short-term fluctuation, is of little interest and relevance as a reliability parameter. Short-term fluctuation increases in pathological visual fields, yet not in a way that makes it diagnostically interesting.

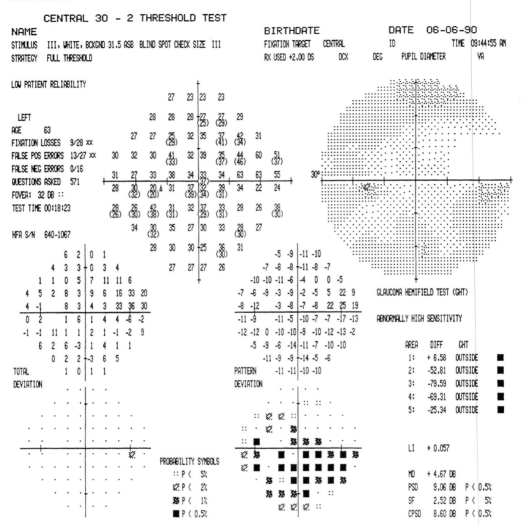

Figure 6.6. Visual field printout from a patient with a high percentage false positive answers.
The FP and fixation losses frequencies are both high. Several areas are abnormally pale in the grey-scale printout where measured sensitivity values are higher than normal. The GHT classification is "abnormally high sensitivity".

Common false positive patterns

Some FP patterns are quite common and characteristic. Recognising them will spare patients and doctors from faulty diagnoses and unnecessary anxiety (Figure 6.6).

Perimetric learning

Earlier experience with computerised perimetry is of importance for test results. A sizeable minority of normal subjects do not produce a normal test result at the first test.[27] The FP pattern of such inexperienced fields is characteristic. Sensitivity values are below normal in the periphery of the test point pattern, i.e. usually in the mid periphery of the field, while the paracentral area is entirely normal (Figure 6.7). In most cases the results of a subsequent test on another day will be normal. Most perimetric learning takes place between the first and the second test session, and few normal subjects need more than two tests to

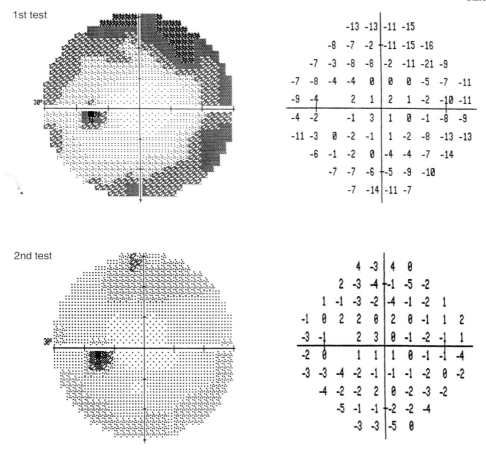

Figure 6.7   Typical untrained pattern of the first field eye from a patient needing more perimetric experience. Sensitivities are depressed in the midperiphery while the paracentral area is entirely normal. The second test of the same eye is normal.

produce a normal result. Very seldom is the untrained concentric pattern seen as a result of glaucoma damage. Thus, if such concentric contraction is encountered in a first test of a patient with suspect glaucoma, one can almost always regard the result as an indication of a normal field, which can most likely be confirmed at the next visit.

Experience with one type of perimetry may not be sufficient for normal results with a different technique. The patient's experience during a supraliminal screening test is very different from that of a threshold test. Despite previous experience with conventional white-on-white threshold perimetry, further learning can be necessary before representative results are obtained with blue-yellow perimetry.[28]

Ptosis and droopy lids

Slight depressions in the superior field are very common and usually caused by slight ptosis (Figure 6.8). Encouraging the patient to keep his eye well open between blinks, or taping of the lid, may alleviate at least part of the problem and may be motivated if the area of depressed sensitivity is large, causing diagnostic problems.

Correcting lens defects

Artefacts caused by the correcting lens holder or rim are also situated in the mid periphery,

49

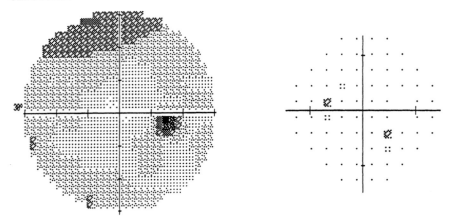

Figure 6.8   Slight depression of sensitivity in the upper field due to a droopy lid.

This false positive pattern is so common that it may be regarded as falling within normal variability. This is obvious from the corresponding probability map; in no test points do encountered depressions of sensitivity reach high significance.

often with a row of seriously depressed test point locations (Figure 6.9). The problem is more common with high plus corrections, but can occur with any correction if the patient becomes decentred or if the corrective lens is placed too far from the eye.

Thus the false positive defects of the untrained field and those caused by lids or correction lenses, all occur in the periphery. They all illustrate the lower quality of field data obtained further from the point of fixation. They also to some extent contribute to the larger normal inter-subject variability and normal limits of the midperipheral as compared to the central and paracentral field (see above). The larger midperipheral variability is not caused by these artefacts, but is also present in perfect observers tested without correction lenses. There is a clinically valuable and clear message here; visual field defects appearing in the paracentral field are statistically more significant and clinically more credible, than peripheral or midperipheral defects.

"Trigger-happy" fields

Fields produced by patients with high frequencies of FP answers (Figure 6.7) are quite characteristic and easy to recognise (see above).

Finding the earliest field loss

To find the earliest field loss in glaucoma, one must find the defects at the early stage, characterised by increased scatter – shallow defects that come and go. This requires true threshold testing and also access to results from several field tests. If early field disturbances can be identified in the same area, but not at exactly the same test point locations, at several tests, the test results judged as a whole can often prove convincingly abnormal even if none of the fields when judged alone can prove glaucomatous damage (Figure 6.3).

When such early glaucomatous field disturbances occur in the paracentral field they are often first evident in probability maps. This is particularly clear in SITA tests,[6,7] where the narrow normal limits can make early, but significant field defects almost, or sometimes entirely, non-visible in greyscale printouts.

It is almost always preferable to concentrate on pattern deviation probability maps.[20] Media opacities are common in those age groups where glaucoma is common, and removing cataract-induced general depression of sensitivity will help ensure sufficient specificity.

November 16, 1987

January 15, 1988

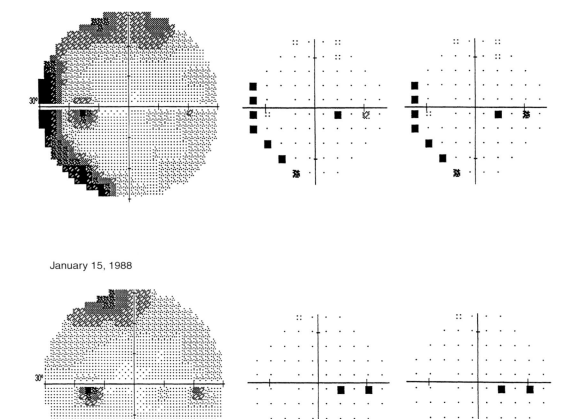

Figure 6.9 Typical correction lens artefact. A series of severely depressed points in the midperiphery. In the following test of the same eye the artefact is gone.

Following glaucomatous field loss

Once field loss has been established, continued visual field testing is the best method to follow the development of the disease. Regular white-on-white static perimetry has a large dynamic range and is preferable to the newer tests for follow-up. It can be used until very late stages of glaucoma, when it may become necessary to shift to manual kinetic perimetry. Statokinetic dissociation is the reason that a field may often be plotted with the latter technique even

when the field appears entirely black on computerised static perimetry.

In follow-up it is important to always use the same type of visual field test. Tests of different lengths are influenced by visual fatigue[13] to a different magnitude, and will therefore produce slightly different results.

Glaucomatous visual fields will show considerable test-retest variability, however, even when the same test is used for all examinations. This variability is complex, depends on initial test point status and eccentricity and on general field status, and makes intuitive analyses of visual field progression difficult.[23] Computer-assisted visual field interpretation can offer help. With few available tests one may use glaucoma change probability maps,[21,29] with six or more fields. Visual field development may also be judged with the help of linear regression analysis, of index values such as Mean Deviation or based on threshold values from individual test point locations.[20,30]

Glaucoma eyes are subject to even more perimetric learning than normal ones and occur in most eyes.[31] Usually learning is complete or almost complete at the second test, but some glaucoma eyes show slow improvements due to learning over as many as four or five tests. The regular occurrence of perimetric learning makes it necessary to discard the results of the first or the first two tests, when establishing an optimal baseline to identify disease progression.

Concomitant glaucoma and cataract complicate interpretation of follow-up fields. The pattern deviation concept is of great value in this situation, i.e. field interpretation is often facilitated when the homogenous field loss component[29] is removed.

A few simple rules of thumb can be very helpful, also when computer-assisted analysis is lacking. The large test-retest variability of glaucoma fields makes it necessary to almost always base judgements of progression on a series of fields instead of on only one or two suspicious test results. Regression analysis for visual field analysis requires rather frequent field testing.[32] Defective test points vary more than normal ones, and initially normal points showing decreased sensitivity over time, therefore, are much stronger indicators of field progression than encountered sensitivity decrements occurring at already initially disturbed test point locations. Variability in glaucomatous as well as normal fields is smaller paracentrally than further peripherally and encountered changes have larger significance if occurring in the central 20°-field.

The role of perimetry in Glaucoma management

Many diagnostic techniques are available today both for diagnosing and for following glaucoma, and it might be relevant to reflect on the position of perimetry in glaucoma management. Modern computerised threshold perimetry is certainly a much more sensitive diagnostic tool than earlier manual techniques.[5] The new standard perimetry regularly detects field defects several years before the stage at which they were identified with the older techniques. Yet considerable axonal loss has taken place before the newer standard techniques will reliably detect functional losses, less if the damage is focal and more if it is widespread. Some non-standard techniques will detect glaucoma damage considerably earlier than the current standard static white-on-white perimetry. However, problems with the new techniques still prevent them from widespread clinical usage.

Short-wavelength automated perimetry (SWAP)

SWAP is probably already useful as a better detection tool in young patients, but the majority of glaucoma suspects are older. It is in this group the interpretation of test results are so difficult that the technique as it currently stands cannot be recommended for routine clinical usage, except maybe in younger glaucoma suspects. If better means to compensate for media opacities are developed, if the dynamic range of the instruments is increased, and if the test time could be reduced drastically, the situation could change. Thus, SWAP might develop into a standard or even preferred tool for detection of glaucoma damage in most patients. Any new technique will have the drawback of lacking the long clinical usage and extensive research of standard white-on-white computerised static perimetry, which form the basis for our current quite thorough understanding of the results obtained with it.

Normal limits, specificity and clinical value

New diagnostic techniques are often released without, or with too narrow, normal limits, established on an elite material of normal subjects. They will then seem to be more sensitive than existing standard techniques thus permitting earlier detection of damage. When such limits are applied in clinical routine usage, one will detect that the methods are non-specific. The limits used in the standard Statpac programmes[20,21] for static perimetry, on the other hand, have been developed taking into account the considerable inter-individual and inter-centre variability of obtained perimetric results, and are specific also in regular clinical settings. The clinical value of new techniques can only be ascertained by thorough clinical studies where both specificity and sensitivity figures are compared to those obtained by established standard techniques in well-defined materials of patients and normal subjects.

Perimetry versus ophthalmoscopy and fundus imaging

Glaucoma damage is often visible by ophthalmoscopy before clear field loss is present with standard techniques. A glaucoma specialist will often detect glaucoma damage in this way, but a general ophthalmologist will miss more often. Normal optic nerve head topography is highly variable, however, and depends on optic disc size. Eyes with large discs are often falsely labelled as glaucomatous. In eyes with small discs, field defects are often present while optic disc topography is still being judged as normal.[33]

Computerised image analysis of optic disc topography can identify glaucomatous eyes with visual field with relatively high sensitivity and specificity. However, these imaging techniques do not yet permit earlier diagnosis than standard perimetry. Optic disc imaging also requires expensive equipment and suffers from lack of general availability and standardisation,

and it is therefore still not an alternative to perimetry. There is no doubt that the advantages of imaging may become more apparent with further research and further technical development.

It could be ideal to base glaucoma diagnoses on identification of retinal nerve fibre layer defects, particularly since available data indicate that such defects precede glaucomatous visual field defects, at least when visual field testing is performed with standard white-on-white perimetry. Unfortunately, it is presently almost impossible to rely on the results of nerve fibre layer examinations. Thus, nerve fibre layer photography is difficult, is performed at only a few glaucoma centres in the world and yields a relatively large number of FP defects, even in expert hands.[34] Visualising the nerve fibre layer during ophthalmoscopy is also often impossible in elderly Caucasian patients. Modern methods for quantitative nerve fibre layer assessment, laser polarimetry and optic coherence tomography, are still not developed for routine clinical usage.

The clinical bottom line

An interested clinician using standard white-on-white threshold perimetry and computer-assisted analysis can identify glaucomatous damage with high sensitivity and specificity. The same method can be used to follow the patient through all stages of the disease except the most advanced. Diagnosing glaucoma with ophthalmoscopy is associated with moderate sensitivity and less than ideal specificity. Computerised imaging techniques are not yet ready for routine clinical usage, but hold a lot of promise for the future.

In clinical practice it may be best to avoid the concept of preperimetric glaucoma and instead establish the diagnosis at the stage of manifest glaucoma with field defects. Such security of diagnosis is preferable particularly in elderly patients. Glaucoma progresses very slowly and standard perimetry will detect glaucomatous damage many years before the patient will experience any deterioration of vision caused by the disease. Specificity of diagnosis will save patients unnecessary inconvenience, cost, side-effects of treatment, and most importantly, anxiety – all factors that could negatively affect the patient's quality of life.

References

1 Åsman P, Heijl A. Diffuse visual field loss and glaucoma. *Acta Ophthalmol* 1994; **72**: 303–8.

2 Werner EB, Drance SM. Early visual field disturbances in glaucoma. *Arch Ophthalmol* 1977; **95**: 1173–5.

3 Heijl A, Lindgren A, Lindgren G. Test-retest variability in glaucomatous visual fields. *Am J Ophthalmol* 1989; **108**: 130–5.

4 Flammer J, Drance SM, Schulzer M. Covariates of the long-term fluctuation of the differential light threshold. *Arch Ophthalmol* 1984; **102**: 880.

5 Katz J, Tielsch JM, Quigley HA, Sommer A. Automated perimetry detects field loss before manual Goldmann perimetry. *Ophthalmology* 1995; **102**: 21–6.

6 Bengtsson B, Olsson J, Heijl A, Rootzén H. A new generation of algorithms for computerised threshold perimetry, SITA. *Acta Ophthalmol Scand* 1997; **75**: 368–74.

7 Bengtsson B, Heijl A. SITA Fast, a new rapid perimetric threshold test. Description of methods and evaluation in patients with manifest and suspect glaucoma. *Acta Ophthalmol* 1998; **76**: 431–7.

8 Bengtsson B, Heijl A. Evaluation of a new perimetric threshold strategy, SITA, in patients with manifest and suspect glaucoma. *Acta Ophthalmol* 1998; **76**: 268–72.

9 Johnson CA, Chauhan BC, Shapiro LR. Properties of staircase procedures for estimating thresholds in automated perimetry. *Invest Ophthalmol Vis Sci* 1992; **33**: 2966–74.

10 Messmer C, Flammer J. Octopus program G1X. *Ophthalmologica* 1991; **203**: 184–8.

11 Weber J. Eine neue Strategie für die automatisierte statische Perimetri. *Fortsschr Ophthalmol* 1990; **87**: 37–40.

12 Weber J, Klimaschka T. Test time and efficiency of the dynamic strategy in glaucoma perimetry. *German J Ophthalmol* 1995; **4**: 25–31.

13 Heijl A, Drance SM. Changes in differential threshold in patients with glaucoma during prolonged perimetry. *Br J Ophthalmol* 1983; **67**: 512–6.

14 Johnson CA, Adams AJ, Casson EJ, Brandt JD. Blue-on-yellow perimetry can predict the development of glaucomatous visual field loss. *Arch Ophthalmol* 1991; **111**: 645–50.

15 Wild JM, Cubbidge RP, Pacey EY, Robinson R. Statistical aspects of the normal visual field in short-wavelength automated perimetry. *Invest Ophthalmol Vis Sci* 1998; **39**: 54–63.

16 Johnson CA, Samuels SJ. Screening for glaucomatous visual field loss with frequency-doubling perimetry. *Invest Ophthalmol Vis Sci* 1997; **38**: 413–25.

17 Quigley HA. Identification of glaucoma-related visual field abnormality with the screening protocol of frequency doubling perimetry. *Am J Ophthalmol* 1998; **125**: 819–29.

18 Fitzke F, Poinoosawmy D, Nagasubramanian S, Hitchings RA. Peripheral displacement thresholds in glaucoma and ocular hypertension. In: Heijl A, ed. Perimetry Update 1988/89; 399–405, Kugler & Ghedini, Amsterdam, 1989.

19 Bosworth CF, Sample PA, Gupta N, Bathija R, Weinreb RN. Motion automated perimetry identifies early glaucomatous field defects. *Arch Ophthalmol* 1998; **116**: 1153–8.

20 Heijl A, Lindgren G, Olsson J. A package for the statistical analysis of computerized visual fields. *Doc Ophthalmol* proc series 1987; **49**: 153–68.

21 Heijl A, Lindgren G, Lindgren A, *et al*. Extended empirical statistical package for evaluation of single and multiple fields in glaucoma: Statpac 2. *Perimetry Update* 1990/91, 303–15. Proceedings of the IXth International Perimetric Society Meeting. Kugler, Amsterdam, 1991.

22 Heijl A, Lindgren G, Olsson J, Åsman P. Visual field interpretation with empirical probability maps. *Arch Ophthalmol* 1989; **107**: 204–8.

23 Heijl A, Lindgren G, Olsson J. Normal variability of static perimetric threshold values across the central visual field. *Arch Ophthalmol* 1987; **105**: 1544–9.

24 Åsman P, Heijl A. Glaucoma hemifield test; automated visual field evaluation. *Arch Ophthalmol* 1992; **110**: 812–9.

25 Olsson J, Bengtsson B, Heijl A, Rootzén H. An improved method to estimate frequency of false positive answers in computerized perimetry. *Acta Ophthalmol Scand* 1997; **75**: 181–3.

26 Anderson DR, Patella VM. Automated Static Perimetry, 2nd edition, p. 90. Mosby, 1999.

27 Heijl A, Lindgren G, Olsson J. The effect of perimetric experience in normal subjects. *Arch Ophthalmol* 1989; **107**: 81–6.

28 Wild JM, Moss ID. Baseline alterations in blue-on-yellow normal perimetric sensitivity. *Graefes Arch Clin Exp Ophthalmol* 1996; **234**: 141–9.

29 Bengtsson B, Lindgren A, Heijl A, Lindgren G, Åsman P, Patella M. Perimetric probability maps to separate change caused by glaucoma from that caused by cataract. *Acta Ophthalmol Scand* 1997; **75**: 184–8.

30 Noureddin B, Poinoosawmy D, Fitzke FW, Hitchings RA. Regression analysis of visual field progression in low tension glaucoma. *Br J Ophthalmol* 1991; **75**: 493–5.

31 Heijl A, Bengtsson B. The effect of perimetric experience in patients with glaucoma. *Arch Ophthalmol* 1996; **114**: 19–22.

32 Viswanathan AC, Hitchings RA, Fitzke FW. How often do patients need visual field tests? *Graefes Arch Clin Exp Ophthalmol* 1997; **2354**: 563–8.

33 Heijl A, Mölder H. Optic disc diameter influences the ability to detect glaucomatous disc damage. *Acta Ophthalmol* 1993; **71**: 122–9.

34 Airaksinen PJ, Drance SM, Douglas GR, Mawson DK, Nieminen H. Diffuse and localized nerve fiber loss in glaucoma. *Am J Ophthalmol* 1984; **98**: 566–71.

7 Intraocular pressure

J C TSAI

Since the study of glaucoma deals primarily with the effects of elevated intraocular pressure (IOP), an understanding of the physiological factors that control IOP is essential. The Goldmann equation (P0 = (F/C) + Pv) summarises the relationship between these factors and the measured IOP in the undisturbed eye. In this equation, P0 is the IOP value in millimetres of mercury (mm Hg), F is the rate of aqueous production in microlitres per minute (ul/min), C is the facility of outflow in microlitres per minute per millimetre of mercury (ul/min/mm Hg), and Pv is the episcleral venous pressure in millimetres of mercury. Thus, IOP is a function of the rate of aqueous inflow into the eye balanced against the rate of aqueous outflow drainage from the eye.

Fluorophotometry is the most commonly used method to measure aqueous humour formation. Aqueous production is calculated by measuring the rate by which the concentration of fluorescein dye, administered systemically or topically, decreases in the anterior chamber. In normal eyes, aqueous inflow is approximately 2–3 ul/min, thereby signifying a 1% turnover in aqueous volume per minute. Aqueous production exhibits diurnal variation with decreased inflow observed during sleep. Aqueous inflow also declines with age, ocular inflammation, carotid occlusive disease, and with certain medications such as β-antagonists, carbonic anhydrase inhibitors, and systemic hypotensive agents.

Whereas inflow is solely dependent on the rate of aqueous humour production by the ciliary processes, the outflow component is dependent on both the resistance to aqueous outflow (outflow facility) and the episcleral venous pressure. Episcleral venous pressure is between 8–12 mm Hg in most individuals. Variations from this range are rare and occur when alterations in body position and/or diseases of the orbit, head and neck obstruct venous flow to the heart or shunt blood from the arterial directly to the venous system. In acute conditions, for every 1 mm Hg increase in episcleral venous pressure, the IOP rises by approximately 1 mm Hg. In chronic conditions increases in episcleral venous pressure may result in IOP changes that are of greater, lesser, or the same magnitude.

Compared to aqueous inflow and episcleral venous pressure, outflow facility (C in the Goldmann equation) varies widely among individuals and ranges from 0.22–0.28 ul/min/mm Hg. Outflow facility is affected by various factors including age, surgery, medications, trauma, and endocrine factors. In most cases, patients with elevated IOP and/or glaucoma have decreased outflow facility rather than increased aqueous inflow or elevated episcleral venous pressure.

Outflow facility is composed of both trabecular and uveoscleral outflow components. Most of the aqueous humour outflow (from 80–90%) exits via the trabecular meshwork and Schlemm's canal system. The primary resistance to outflow in this system occurs at the juxtacanalicular tissue. Once aqueous passes through this interface, it moves into Schlemm's canal and then the episcleral venous plexus by way of scleral collector channels. The remaining 10–20% of aqueous humour leaves the eye by nontrabecular means via the uveoscleral system. In this system aqueous passes initially from the anterior chamber into the ciliary muscle and then into the suprachoroidal spaces, eventually exiting the eye through intact sclera. The amount of uveoscleral outflow is increased by cycloplegic agents, epinephrine, and α-agonists and is decreased by miotic agents.

Intraocular pressure distribution in the population

Large epidemiological studies have indicated that mean IOP for the general population is approximately 15.5 mm Hg.[1] The frequency distribution of IOP is not precisely Gaussian in character, but has a right skew toward higher pressures for patients over 40 years of age (Figure 7.1). This apparent skew appears to be associated with a reduced facility of aqueous

outflow after age 40, despite a decline in aqueous humour production.[2] It is interesting that a recent study found that IOP in the Japanese population decreases with age in both sexes, but to a greater extent in men.[3]

Aside from age, numerous other internal and external factors are felt to influence the level of IOP (to variable degrees in each individual). These factors include genetic factors, diurnal factors, season of the year, postural variation, exercise, lid and eye movement, anaesthesia, fluid intake, stress, and topical and systemic medications. For instance, higher eye pressures are more common in relatives of patients with primary open angle glaucoma (POAG). Alcohol consumption decreases IOP, while caffeine causes a slight transient rise in IOP.

Two standard deviations to either side of the mean IOP value produce a "normal" IOP range of about 10–21 mm Hg. Since IOP distribution in the general population is skewed to higher pressures, this statistical principle provides only a rough approximation of normal limits. In fact, many eyes do not appear to develop glaucomatous optic atrophy or visual field loss despite IOPs well above 21 mm Hg, while others will develop progressive field and optic disc damage at pressures well below 21 mm Hg.

In normal individuals diurnal variation of IOP varies from 3–6 mm Hg.[4] This cyclical fluctuation results from aqueous humour production changes over a 24 hour period. Many individuals have their peak IOPs in the morning hours, though a significant few reach their peak pressures in the afternoon or evening hours or have short-term fluctuations throughout the day. A diurnal variation > 10 mm Hg is suggestive of glaucoma. Moreover, glaucomatous eyes have been reported to exhibit diurnal IOP fluctuations > 30 mm Hg.[5]

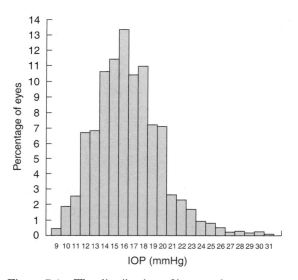

Figure 7.1   The distribution of intraocular pressures in the general population.
Reproduced with permission from Colton T, Ederer F. The distribution of intraocular pressures in the general population. *Surv Ophthalmol* 1980; **25**: 123–9.

Ocular hypertension: definition and relationship to glaucoma

Ocular hypertension is defined as any ocular condition presenting with an IOP > 21 mm Hg (without apparent cause), but with normal appearing optic discs and visual fields. Some investigators have labelled this condition "early open angle glaucoma without damage" to emphasise that a certain percentage of these patients will eventually develop glaucomatous damage. Still others have preferred the term "glaucoma suspect", though this term may also describe eyes that possess other risk factors for glaucoma such as suspicious appearing optic nerve heads.

In the majority of patients, an elevated IOP is the most important single prognostic risk factor in the development of POAG. One study of 307 patients revealed that the higher the presenting IOP, the greater the percentage of patients noted to have optic nerve head damage.[6] Another study reported that the probability of glaucoma is near zero at IOPs < 18 mm Hg, is about 0.5 at 27–28 mm Hg, and approaches almost 1 at approximately 35 mm Hg.[7] In general, the higher the presenting IOP level, the greater the likelihood of optic nerve damage. In addition, the prevalence of glaucoma increases in relation to screening IOP (Figure 7.2).

However, this correlation of presenting IOP and the probability of glaucoma has substantial limitations. Due to diurnal fluctuations of IOP, elevations of IOP may occur only intermittently in some patients with glaucomatous damage. Thus, single IOP measurements, taken alone for the purpose of screening, may be misleading and inaccurate. In one population-based survey, more than half of all glaucomatous eyes had screening pressures < 22 mm Hg.[8] Moreover, some patients are able to tolerate significant IOP elevations without detectable optic nerve or visual field damage, while others sustain substantial disc defects and/or visual field loss with IOPs in the normal range. Therefore,

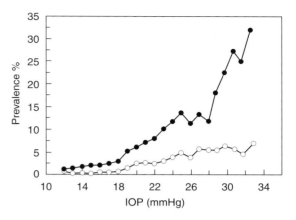

Figure 7.2 Prevalence of primary open angle glaucoma in relation to screening IOP.
Reproduced from Sommer A, Tielsch JM, Katz J, et al. Relationship between intraocular pressure and primary open angle glaucoma among white and black Americans. The Baltimore Eye Survey. *Arch Ophthalmol* 1991; **109**: 1090–5 with permission from Elsevier Science.

careful evaluation of the optic nerve head and visual field should be performed along with IOP measurement in all patients evaluated for glaucoma.

Several large population-based surveys have attempted to determine the prevalence of POAG and ocular hypertension in a given population.[9–11] Though the methodologies of these studies vary, the prevalence of POAG in most of these studies is reported to be between 1–2%, while the prevalence of ocular hypertension is considerably higher. Overall, nearly 4% per year of all individuals with elevated IOP will develop glaucomatous damage.[12–13]

Though a relationship between increased IOP and glaucomatous neuropathy exists, there is marked individual variation in the susceptibility of the optic nerve to IOP-induced damage. One recent population-based study found that only 10% or less of patients with elevated IOP have glaucomatous field loss.[8] Other studies have attempted to determine the rate of occurrence of primary open angle glaucoma in untreated groups of ocular hypertension patients. Data from longitudinal studies, spanning observation periods of 5–20 years, report an incidence of approximately 1% per year for the development of glaucomatous field loss in these patients. One study suggested that only one-tenth of ocular hypertension patients will develop visual field loss within a ten year period.[14]

Investigators have reported an increased central corneal thickness in eyes of patients with ocular hypertension. In one study the mean central corneal thickness of eyes with ocular hypertension was significantly greater (0.606 mm) than that of glaucomatous eyes (0.554 mm) and of normal controls (0.561 mm).[15] As a result, increased central corneal thickness may cause an artificially high IOP measurement by applanation tonometry. In developing a treatment approach for patients with ocular hypertension, the likelihood of this artefact must be considered.

In summary, a strong relationship exists between increased IOP and a greater risk of developing glaucomatous neuropathy. However, great individual variation in the apparent susceptibility of ocular hypertension patients to IOP-related damage is observed. Since elevated IOP is a major risk factor in the pathogenesis of glaucoma damage and amenable to treatment, consideration should be given to lowering IOP to halt or retard such damage (see below).

Parameters for intraocular pressure treatment

There has been considerable controversy regarding the management of individuals with the diagnosis of ocular hypertension. Three predominant schools of thought have arisen:

1 Treat all of these patients in the hope of preventing the occurrence of POAG. However, some of these patients may be needlessly exposed to the side effects, risks, and economic expense of therapy.
2 Treat none of these patients, thus risking the development of potentially preventable glaucomatous optic atrophy and visual loss.
3 Selectively treat patients who appear at greatest risk for developing glaucoma since elevated IOP is one of the few risk factors amenable to intervention. Treatment is initiated in the hope of halting or retarding glaucomatous damage. This is currently the most favoured approach.[16]

Before a treatment decision is made, a comprehensive baseline examination should be undertaken. A thorough review of family, ocular, and systemic history should be performed. The physical examination should entail pupil examination, IOP, slit lamp examination, gonioscopy, evaluation of optic disc rim and nerve fibre layer, evaluation of cup:disc ratio, fundus evaluation, and visual field assessment. The IOP should be measured preferably with a Goldmann-type applanation tonometry prior to dilation or gonioscopic examination. Due to diurnal IOP variation, the time of the day should be recorded. Diurnal IOP measurements may be indicated when patients have optic disc damage not expected with the initial IOP recording.

The ophthalmologist must look carefully for signs of early damage to the optic nerve head or visual field. Early signs of optic disc damage include progressive enlargement of the cup:disc ratio, focal notching and/or thinning of the optic rim tissue, asymmetry of disc cupping, splinter disc haemorrhage, and dropout of the nerve fibre layer. Early signs of visual field damage (on standard automated and/or kinetic perimetry) include overall field depression, paracentral defect, arcuate defect, nasal step and/or depression, and subtle field constriction. If any of these ocular signs are present, the patient should no longer be considered as having ocular hypertension, but rather an early case of POAG and treated accordingly.

The most reliable findings of glaucoma are documented changes in the optic disc rim or nerve fibre layer or reproducible visual field abnormalities consistent with glaucomatous damage. However, visual field abnormalities may occur only after significant optic nerve damage has occurred. One study found that some glaucoma suspects lose up to 50% of their optic nerve axons while maintaining normal kinetic visual fields.[17]

If no signs of early disc or field damage are present, the ophthalmologist should determine whether the patient has significant risk factors for developing POAG in the foreseeable future. Strong risk factors include elevated IOP, advanced age (especially over 50 years of age), family history of glaucoma, and Afro-American or Afro-Caribbean descent. Other possible risk factors include myopia, migraine headaches, peripheral vasospasm, and systemic medical conditions such as hypertension, diabetes mellitus, and cardiovascular disease.

An individual's overall risk of developing glaucoma increases with the number and strength of risk factors. Patients with significant risk factors should be treated in the hope of preventing or delaying the development of POAG. However, the treatment decision should be individualised, taking into account the potential efficacy and side effects of treatment, the probability of glaucoma damage, the likelihood of visual impairment, and the patient's tolerance for treatment. Since the likelihood of developing glaucomatous optic nerve damage is in part related to the overall duration of risk factors, patients with a longer life expectancy require more vigorous treatment. The patient's willingness to participate in the prescribed medical regimen should also be assessed. Treatment should be postponed for patients with minimal risk factors. However, these low-risk patients should continue to undergo periodic ocular examinations to evaluate their disease status. High-risk glaucoma suspect patients would require more frequent and comprehensive follow-up examinations.

The Ocular Hypertension Treatment Study[18] is currently under way in the United States. This controlled clinical study, sponsored by the National Eye Institute (NIH), seeks to understand whether treatment of patients with ocular hypertension and IOP levels between 22–34 mm Hg will reduce the incidence of POAG. Approximately 1,500 patients with ocular hypertension will be randomised to medicine or no treatment and followed for 5 or more years. Results from this study, as well as other controlled clinical studies, will help elucidate the parameters for IOP treatment in ocular hypertension.

A practical approach to intraocular pressure reduction

As outlined above, the level of IOP is an important predictor of the presence or the development of glaucomatous optic atrophy and corresponding visual field loss. The higher the IOP, particularly in those patients presenting with IOP > 30 mm Hg, the greater the risk of future glaucomatous damage. In the presence of other significant risk factors, elevated IOP should be lowered since it is one of the few risk factors amenable to intervention.

Ocular hypertension can be classified into four different categories based on risk factors associated with the level of IOP elevation:

Minimal risk factors with elevated intraocular pressure consistently < 30 mm Hg

These patients should not be treated, but followed every 6–18 months, depending on the level and duration of elevated IOP and appearance of the optic disc. Baseline optic disc photographs and/or accurate disc drawings should be obtained for future comparison.

Moderate risk factors with elevated IOP consistently < 30 mm Hg

These patients should have closer follow-up of every 3–12 months. Treatment should be considered if the patients cannot be closely followed. If placed on treatment, these patients require frequent follow-up examinations to monitor their response to therapy.

Significant risk factors with elevated intraocular pressure consistently < 30 mm Hg

These patients should be strongly considered for treatment (see below).

Elevated intraocular pressure consistently > 30 mm Hg

These patients should be treated since there is a strong relationship between elevated IOP and optic nerve damage (Figure 7.2).

Once treatment is deemed necessary, the following steps should be instituted for patients with ocular hypertension:

Estimate a target intraocular pressure level below which optic nerve damage is unlikely to occur

Though target IOP levels may vary among individual practitioners, a reasonable level would be at least 20–30% below the pretreatment IOP level. Additional factors that may influence the target IOP sought include the severity of the existing optic disc damage, the height of the IOP, the duration in which the optic disc and/or visual field damage occurred (if known), and risk factors such as family history, race, and myopia. In general, the more advanced the glaucomatous damage observed, the lower the initial target pressure should be set.

Attempt to maintain intraocular pressure at or below the target intraocular pressure level with the appropriate therapeutic interventions

The potential risks and benefits of these interventions should be considered. The patient should be educated and counselled regarding the disease. The current IOP should be compared to the target level at each visit.

Since the target intraocular pressure level is an estimate, it should be periodically refined and based on the visual fields and the appearance of the optic discs

If the target IOP is not easily attained, the ophthalmologist should reassess the validity of the target pressure given the visual field and optic disc status compared to baseline measurements.

If deterioration is noted in either the visual field or optic nerve head

In this case the diagnosis of POAG should be made, and the target IOP should be lowered to treat this diagnosis.

References

1 Colton T, Ederer F. The distribution of intraocular pressures in the general population. *Surv Ophthalmol* 1980; **25**: 123–9.
2 Becker B. The decline in aqueous secretion and outflow facility with age. *Am J Ophthalmol* 1958; **46**: 731.
3 Shiose Y. The aging effect on intraocular pressure in an apparently normal population. *Arch Ophthalmol* 1984; **102**: 883–7.
4 Kitazawa Y, Horie T. Diurnal variation of intraocular pressure in primary open angle glaucoma. *Am J Ophthalmol* 1975; **79**: 557–66.
5 Newell FW, Krill AE. Diurnal tonography in normal and glaucomatous eyes. *Trans Am Ophthalmol Soc* 1964; **62**: 349.
6 Pohjanpelto PE, Palva J. Ocular hypertension and glaucomatous optic nerve damage. *Acta Ophthalmol* 1974; **52**: 194–200.
7 Davanger M, Ringvold A, Bilka S. The probability of having glaucoma at different IOP levels. *Acta Ophthalmol* 1991; **69**: 565–8.
8 Sommer A, Tielsch JM, Katz J, *et al.* Relationship between intraocular pressure and primary open angle glaucoma among white and black Americans. The Baltimore Eye Survey. *Arch Ophthalmol* 1991; **109**: 1090–5.
9 Kahn HA, Leibowitz HM, Ganley JP, *et al.* The Framingham Eye Study. I. Outline and major prevalence findings. *Am J Epidemiol* 1977; **106**: 17–32.
10 Klein BEK, Klein R, Sponsel WE, *et al.* Prevalence of glaucoma. The Beaver Dam Eye Study. *Ophthalmology* 1992; **99**: 1499–504.
11 Dielemans I, Vingerling JR, Wolfs RCW, *et al.* The prevalence of primary open angle glaucoma in a population-based study in the Netherlands. The Rotterdam Study. *Ophthalmology* 1994; **101**: 1851–5.
12 Perkins ES. The Bedford glaucoma study. I. Long-term follow-up of borderline cases. *Br J Ophthalmol* 1973; **57**: 179–85.
13 Armaly MF, Krueger DE, Maunder LR, *et al.* Biostatistical analysis of the collaborative glaucoma study. I. Summary report of the risk factors for glaucomatous visual-field defects. *Arch Ophthalmol* 1980; **98**: 2163–71.

14 Quigley HA, Enger C, Katz J, *et al.* Risk factors for the development of glaucomatous visual field loss in ocular hypertension. *Arch Ophthalmol* 1994; **112**: 644–9.

15 Herndon LW, Choudhri SA, Cox T, Damji KF, Shields MB, Allingham RR. Central corneal thickness in normal, glaucomatous, and ocular hypertensive eyes. *Arch Ophthalmol* 1997; **115**: 1137–41.

16 American Academy of Ophthalmology. Primary Open-Angle Glaucoma Suspect, Preferred Practice Pattern, San Francisco. Am Acad Ophthalmol 1995.

17 Quigley HA, Addicks EM, Green WR, *et al.* Optic nerve damage in human glaucoma. II. The rate of injury and susceptibility to damage. *Arch Ophthalmol* 1981; **99**: 635–49.

18 American Academy of Ophthalmology. Primary Open-Angle Glaucoma, Preferred Practice Pattern, San Francisco. Am Acad Ophthalmol 1996.

8 Principles of treatment of glaucoma

G L SPAETH

This chapter will deal with principles of treatment of glaucoma. Although it addresses the problems posed by primary open angle glaucoma (POAG), the principles are applicable to all varieties. It will discuss the timing as well as the consequences of treatment before addressing the major clinical trails of therapy completed or currently underway.

What is glaucoma?

Glaucoma is a condition in which damage occurs to the optic nerve, the damage being at least partially related to intraocular pressure (IOP).[1] It should be remembered that other ocular tissues may be damaged by raised IOP and it is appropriate that treatment be directed at preventing or minimising such other types of damage.[2] For example, the corneal endothelium is severely damaged when IOP goes from normal levels to elevated levels Hg. Indeed, corneal damage occurs in patients with glaucoma even in the absence of such markedly elevated IOP.[3] The treating physician should be aware of the possibility of corneal endothelial changes, recognising that such patients need to have special approaches to cataract extraction, and that therapeutic agents with the potential to cause corneal endothelial damage should be used with especial caution.

Despite the fact that glaucoma can cause damage to many different tissues in the eye, the major concern rests with damage that occurs to the ganglion cells and the optic nerve, and for simplicity and clarity we will here define open angle glaucoma as damage to the optic nerve associated with a characteristic deformation known as glaucomatous cupping at least partially related to IOP.

The significance of glaucoma

The significance of glaucoma is that it can in some instances make people sick.[4] Glaucoma does not always make people sick. In fact, in the common types of glaucoma it is not until the optic nerve has become severely damaged that any actual symptomatic illness develops. In many patients with glaucoma such marked damage never occurs, even in the absence of treatment. One of the most important principles, then, that must be clearly defined by both the patient and the physician, deals with the appropriate goal of treatment. This issue of defining what glaucoma is and of being clear with regard to therapeutic goals is so critically important that the principles must be firmly established and agreed upon before proceeding further with discussions of treatment of glaucoma.

One must keep the objective of treatment in mind when deciding on the needs of the individual patient.

The proper intent: preservation of health

For most people the ultimate objective of treatment is to maintain or enhance the person's health. The means by which a person's health is maintained, with regard to glaucoma, is far more complex than frequently considered. Clearly preservation of "vision" is an essential part of the way a person with glaucoma remains healthy (Tables 8.1, 8.2). But also important is avoidance of damage to the person's health, psychologically and physically. If one considers the situation regarding the treatment of glaucoma around 50 years ago at the mid-point of the 20th century, the amount of damage to American patients caused by treatment was probably greater than that caused by the glaucoma itself. This was because treatment was based on a definition of glaucoma that did not require damage and considered that glaucoma was present if the IOP was elevated.[5–7] Most Americans who were found to have IOPs, then, were treated. However, had they not been treated, around 90% of those individuals never would have developed damage, so whatever problems, the treatment caused were unnecessary problems. Health also involves emotional and spiritual factors. To maintain or enhance the health of a person with glaucoma requires restoring or at least preventing visual loss, relieving pain, and enhancing the person's emotional and spiritual health without causing damage by the therapies utilised. This is a tall task.

If preservation of health is the ultimate objective, and maintenance of vision without induction of problems is the primary means to achieve the objective, the method of preserving vision is to prevent damage to the optic nerve. To date, the only proven method to prevent damage to the optic nerve is reducing IOP. Although neuroprotective agents may be available in the future, for the present, however, the only proven therapy is to lower IOP.

Risks of treatment: the treatment is not needed

How does one reduce IOP without causing unwanted problems? This question raises the issue of the so-called risk-benefit ratio. One assesses as well as possible the estimated risk of the treatment and weighs that against the estimated benefit of the treatment. To get an idea of the estimated benefit, one must know what will happen to the person if no treatment is given.[2,4] Benefit cannot be estimated unless this information is known. For many years, for example, it was assumed that treating patients with elevated IOP was beneficial, because it was believed that those with elevated IOP developed visual field loss and became blind. It was not until the natural history of ocular hypertension had been defined,[8–10] and it was recognised that only 5–10% of patients with ocular hypertension actually develop visual field loss, that the possible benefit of therapy could be meaningfully assessed.

Table 8.1 Objectives of the care of a patient with glaucoma

Step	Objective	Purpose of achieving objective
1	Reduce intraocular pressure	Achieving step 2 ↓
2	Prevent optic nerve damage	Immediate objective of step 2 and method of achieving step 3 ↓
3	Preserve vision	Immediate objective of step 3 and method of achieving step 4 ↓
4	Be healthy	Ultimate objective (purpose)

Table 8.2 Outcomes of treatment of a patient with glaucoma

Step	Objectives	
1	Perform surgery ↓	
2	Develop non-healing fistula ↓	
3	Develop bleb < >	
	< >	
	< >	
4	Reduce intraocular pressure ↓	Cause hypotony, endophthalmitis, etc ↓
5	Preserve health	Make person sick

How to determine if treatment is needed

How does one determine the course of glaucoma in a particular patient? There are three separate parts to the answer to this question. The first has to do with what has already occurred, the second with what is occurring, and the third with what will occur in the future.

What has happened in the past is indicated by the amount of damage already present. What is happening at the present time is suggested by establishing what has happened in the past and then determining if the same set of circumstances continues to exist. What is going to happen in the future can be extrapolated by knowing what was happening in the past, what is happening at present, and the duration that the process will continue.

A few specific examples may bring life to these abstract principles. Consider the patient who, when first seen, has no visual symptoms, an IOP of 30 mm Hg in the right eye and 25 mm Hg in the left, and optic nerve with a round cup occupying approximately 70% of the optic nerve head, and a rim without notches or pallor in the right eye, and a similar-appearing optic nerve in the left eye, with a smaller cup occupying approximately 50% of the optic nerve head. There is no visual field loss in either eye. The patient is a healthy 55 year old woman who does not smoke or drink and whose parents lived into their 90s. It is reasonably likely that the difference in the optic nerves is a reflection of the difference in the IOP between the two eyes. It is impossible to determine whether the presumed change in the right eye took place over a period of a month, a year, or ten years. It is, then, reasonable to presume with relative certainty that the right eye has developed damage, but the rate at which the damage is occurring cannot be determined. It is impossible to establish what is presently happening, and as far as the future is concerned, one cannot make meaningful predictions, since one does not know the rate of change of the condition.

Now consider the same patient with exactly the same findings. However, there is an additional piece of information. The patient was examined two years previously, at which time the findings were exactly the same, except for the fact that the patient was two years younger and that the optic nerves of the two eyes seemed identical to each other. Given this information, one can now state that it is highly likely that the patient has developed damage within a period of two years, that the damage occurred because the IOP was around 30 mm Hg in the right eye, that the damage is continuing to occur since the pressure is at the same level, and that the damage will continue to occur in the future at roughly the same rate unless something changes. Because this patient has a life expectancy of around 40 years it is likely that the patient will lose significant vision in the right eye unless something is done to alter the course.

Establishing the course of glaucoma

The course of the glaucoma, then, is defined by establishing the nature of the patient for at least two different points in time. The accuracy with which the course can be determined relates to the accuracy of the findings and the number of times those findings have been repeated in order to establish certainty and to allow developing an accurate estimate of the rate of change.

The findings utilised to determine the clinical course are the nature of the optic disc in the early stage of the glaucoma, the visual field in the middle stages, and the history in the late stages of the disease. Once the optic nerve has become severely cupped it is usually too difficult to see changes in the optic disc to use the disc as a means of establishing continuing change. Once the visual field has become severely damaged, it is frequently too difficult to use the visual field as a means of establishing further change. At every stage the history is important, but in the final stages of the glaucoma, the history is by far the most important determination of the course (Table 8.3).

Table 8.3 Appropriate methods to monitor the course of glaucoma

Stage	Method required to monitor the change
At risk or pre-glaucoma	History and serial studies of optic disc, nerve fibre layer, and angle.
Asymptomatic damage	
Early glaucoma	Serial studies of optic disc, nerve fibre layer, and angle
Moderate glaucoma	Serial studies of optic disc and visual field
Symptomatic damage	
Advanced glaucoma	History and serial studies of visual fields and optic discs
Far advanced glaucoma	History and serial studies of visual field

The glaucoma graph

Figure 8.1 illustrates a graph that is helpful in establishing the course of the glaucoma, and the likelihood that the patient will have an interference with his or her health in response to the effects of the glaucoma. This graph on the y-axis indicates the stage of the glaucoma, and on the x-axis the duration that the glaucoma will affect the patient, specifically, the patient's longevity. The initial stage of glaucoma is one that is best characterised as "suspect." The findings are suggestive of glaucoma but not definitive. Table 8.4 lists findings that indicate that a patient is suspect for having glaucoma. The second stage is the stage of definite damage. Initially the damage is asymptomatic, but eventually the patient starts to lose function, and if the progress of the damage continues, the patient may become incapacitated. This symptomatic stage of glaucoma in which the symptoms are caused by glaucoma damage, is the third stage of the condition.

In order to determine the significance of the glaucoma for the patient's health, the patient's longevity must be estimated (Tables 8.5, 8.6). The factors that must be taken into account are the stage of the glaucoma at present, the rate with which the glaucoma is changing, the pattern of change, and the patient's longevity.

Unfortunately the current labels used to describe glaucoma provide little information regarding the clinical course. A patient with the exfoliation syndrome may have no glaucoma at all, may have a slowly progressing glaucoma that never causes significant damage, or may have a glaucoma in which there is precipitous loss of function. Thus, saying that a patient has glaucoma associated with the exfoliation syndrome provides useful information as to the cause for the glaucoma, but gives little information of value with regard to understanding the course of the glaucoma in that particular individual. This lack of correlation between diagnostic labels and clinical course applies to the other glaucomas as well, including POAG, pigmentary glaucoma, chronic POAG, and even some of the secondary glaucomas, such as neovascular glaucoma following retinal vein occlusion.

The risk-benefit ratio, then, requires establishing the likelihood that the patient will become damaged if no treatment is given.

Can glaucoma treatment be helpful?

Is there evidence that many patients with glaucoma can benefit from treatment? The answer here is an overwhelming "yes."[11–16] Glaucoma, then, is a condition in which an apparently undamaged nerve becomes damaged by IOP higher than the nerve can tolerate. In response to lowering the IOP the damage can disappear in some cases, in some cases further damage can be prevented, and in most cases the rate of damage can be slowed. While it has been assumed that treatment benefited patients with glaucoma, until relatively recently there has been no proof of this assumption.

Why do some people with glaucoma get worse despite treatment?

There still are many cases in which glaucoma progresses despite treatment. How can this be? Table 8.7 lists the reasons why a patient diagnosed with glaucoma may have progressive optic nerve damage, or more broadly, may get worse despite of or even because of treatment:

Table 8.4 Findings that indicate a patient is at risk for developing damage or has damage from glaucoma

At risk for developing damage
Lower Likelihood
1. Positive family history of glaucoma damage
2. Intraocular pressure 21–24 mm Hg
3. Exfoliation syndrome with intraocular pressure < 20 mm Hg
4. Pigment dispersion syndrome with intraocular pressure < 20 mm Hg
5. Myopia with intraocular pressure < mm Hg
6. Disc asymmetry of 0.1 c/d

Higher Likelihood
1. Gene associated with development of glaucoma
2. Intraocular pressure 25–30 mm Hg
3. Exfoliation syndrome, pigment dispersion syndrome, or myopia with intraocular pressure 5 mm Hg higher than previously measured, or intraocular pressure > 20 mm Hg
4. Disc asymmetry of 0.2 cd
5. Cup/disc ratio > 0.6
6. Visual field loss of:
   a. nasal hemifield loss, one spot 5–10 dB
   b. paracentral hemifield loss, one spot 5–10 dB
   c. generalised loss 1–5 dB

Asymptomatic damage
Questionable Damage
1. Intraocular pressure 31–40 mm Hg
2. Disc appearance
   a. asymmetry 0.2–0.3 C/D
   b. rim width 0.1–0.2 C/D
   c. questionable notch
   d. questionable saucer
   e. temporal/inferior rim ratio < 1/2
   f. temporal/superior rim ratio < 2/3
3. Visual field loss
   a. nasal hemifield loss, 2 contiguous spots, 5–10 dB
   b. nasal hemifield loss, 1 spot, 10–15 dB
   c. paracentral hemifield loss, 2 contiguous spots, 5–10 dB
   d. paracentral hemifield loss, 1 spot, 10–15 dB
   e. generalised loss, mean defect 5 dB
4. Optically closed angle with questionable peripheral anterior synechiae

Definite Damage
1. Intraocular pressure > 40 mm Hg

2. Disc appearance
   a. asymmetry 0.3 or greater
   b. rim lost in no more than one quadrant
   c. definite notch
   d. definite acquired pit of optic nerve
   e. disc haemorrhage crossing rim edge
3. Visual field loss
   a. nasal hemifield loss, 3 contiguous spots, 5–15 dB
   b. nasal hemifield loss, 2 contiguous spots, 10–20 dB
   c. arcuate loss, 3 contiguous spots, 10–20 dB
   d. arcuate loss, 4 contiguous spots, 10–15 dB
   e. generalised loss, mean defect 5–10 dB
4. Peripheral anterior synechiae < 50% of angle

Symptomatic damage
Early
1. Intraocular pressure > 51 mm Hg
2. Disc appearance
   a. rim lost in more than one quadrant
   b. superior and inferior notch
3. Visual field loss
   a. nasal hemifield loss, 4 contiguous spots, 5–15 dB
   b. nasal hemifield loss, 3 contiguous spots, 15–20 dB
   c. arcuate loss, 4 contiguous spots, 10–20 dB
   d. arcuate loss, 3 contiguous spots, 20–30 dB
4. Questionable symptoms
   a. no limitation of function, but sense that vision is not "right"
   b. intermittent minimal discomfort
5. Early functional loss
   a. unable to do activities requiring good vision: loses place on page, sees poorly in dark, etc
   b. Mild, definite pain or discomfort

Moderate and Advanced
1. Moderate functional loss
   a. major change in lifestyle required because of loss of vision: can no longer drive, difficulty reading, etc
   b. pain severe enough to interfere with daily activities
   c. incapacitated by visual loss and/or pain
2. Severe functional loss
   a. incapacitated by visual loss and/or pain

Because the patient does not have glaucoma

One reason why a patient believed to have glaucoma may continue to get worse is that the optic neuropathy is not pressure-related. That is, the patient does not actually have glaucoma. The optic nerve may be similar in appearance to the change that occurs in glaucoma, but has some other cause. Recognised causes for optic neuropathy include those entities listed in Table 8.8. Of these, masses in the region of the pituitary gland, and anterior ischaemic optic neuropathy deserve especial mention. These entities are not rare and can mimic the disc and field changes in patients with glaucoma. Their possible existence needs to be remembered, especially patients in whom glaucoma appears to be progressive despite what is considered to be adequate lowering of IOP.

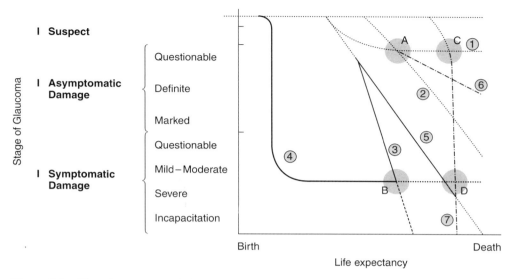

Figure 8.1   The glaucoma graph is a way of determining and understanding the clinical course of glaucoma in an individual patient.

On the y axis of the graph is the stage of the glaucoma, and on the x axis is the life expectancy. The slope and the curve of each of the individual lines are determined and graphed in different ways: dotted lines indicate that the slope and the curve have been determined by plotting the results of serial studies, such as repeated disc photographs taken yearly or repeated visual field examinations; solid lines depict the clinical course as described in the patient's history; dashed lines are extrapolations that are presumed to represent what will happen in the future. These hypothetical, extrapolated future courses are based on the nature of the previous courses and on knowledge of what has happened since a known point in time.

This illustration shows the courses of seven different patients with different manifestations of glaucoma: point A – this patient has minimal glaucoma, and about one third of his/her life still to live; point B – this patient has advanced glaucoma and has about one third of his/her life still to live; point C – this patient has very early glaucoma and only a few years to live; point D – this patient has advanced glaucoma and only a few years to live.

- Patient 1, considered at point A, has one third of his/her life to live and is in an early stage of glaucoma. About one third of his/her life earlier, this patient was noted to have elevated pressure and followed without treatment. The patient continued to be followed without treatment and no damage to the optic nerve or visual field was ever noted. It is reasonable to assume that, if the patient continues to have intraocular pressures around the same level as those noted initially, he/she will probably follow the course described by line 1, and will die without any evidence of glaucoma damage.
- Patient 2, also considered at point A, i.e. having minimal damage with one third of his/her life left to live. In this case, however, the patient's intraocular pressure rose continuously, and the patient was noted to develop early disc and field damage, which then continued at the rate depicted by the dashed line 2. This patient, if untreated, would develop definite asymptomatic damage. However, the patient would have no functional loss at the time of his/her death.
- Patients 3 and 4, at point B both have advanced glaucoma and one third of their lives left to live. However, patient 3 is deteriorating rapidly and will be blind long before he/she dies, whereas patient 4, who had a blow to the eye as a child and lost vision to a steroid-induced glaucoma at that time, has had stable vision for most of his/her life, and it is reasonable to expect that it will continue to be stable.
- Both patients at points C and D have only a few years to live, but those at point C (like patients 1 and 2 at point A) have minimal damage, and those at point D (like patient 4 at point B) have marked damage.
- Patient 5 started with a clinical course similar to that of patient 3 (advanced glaucoma and deteriorating rapidly), but around the midpoint of his/life, the glaucoma became less severe. Nevertheless, this patient will be blind at the time of his/her death unless there is effective intervention. Compare patient 4, who at point D has the same life expectancy and the same amount of damage as patient 5 (only a few years to live and advanced glaucoma). Patient 4, however, has a stable clinical course and does not appear to need a change in therapy. In contrast, patient 5 needs lowering intraocular pressure urgently.
- Patient 6, at around point C also has only a few years of life remaining, but has a glaucoma that is getting worse a little more slowly than that affecting patients 2 and 5. However, since patient 6 has so little damage to

Fig 8.1 continued

start with, no treatment is necessary, even though he/she is getting worse. Even without treatment, he/she will not have enough damage or visual loss due to glaucoma at the time of death that he/she will have any awareness of being sick, and will have no limitation in function.

- Patient 7 at point C has only a few years left to live, but has a type of glaucoma that is deteriorating so rapidly that even though he/she has only a short period of time to live, he/she will be blind well before the time of death.

Using the glaucoma graph to define and characterise the nature of the clinical course helps the physician and patient to understand that:

- Patients 1, 4, and 6 do not need any treatment at all; patient 1 will never develop damage, patient 4 has marked damage but it is not getting worse, and patient 6 is getting worse so slowly that it will not interfere with his/her life.
- Patients 3, 5, and 7 can be seen to need treatment urgently in order to prevent them from becoming totally blind prior to the time of their deaths.
- Patient 2: The need for treatment is controversial. Since this patient would never develop glaucoma, perhaps he/she should not be treated at all. But since he/she would develop *some* damage, those who want to prevent any damage at all would advise therapy.

Table 8.5 Estimate of life expectancy

Genetic factors
    longevity of parents
    age of siblings
    health of siblings

Health of person
    known illnesses that affect life expectancy
        heart disease
        cirrhosis
        other
    level of energy
    blood pressure
    pulse
    weight (relative to height)
    mental outlook
    emotional illness, especially depression
    lifestyle of person
        ability of manage his/her life
        history of cigarette or cigar smoking
        excessive alcohol intake
        drug usage
        amount of exercise
        nature of diet
        state of marriage
        mental outlook
        level of activity
    person's own estimate of longevity

Table 8.6 Most Important factors regarding life expectancy

Long-lived family?
Healthy person?
Good self-management skills?
Healthy lifestyle?
Happy person?

Table 8.7 Reasons why patients with glaucoma get worse

Patient does not have glaucoma.

Patient has glaucoma and another entity as well.

The intraocular pressure is higher than the neurons can tolerate.

The damage is so marked that the neurons continue to be damaged regardless of the level of intraocular pressure.

The normal occurrence of cell death due to ageing.

Effects of treatment
  A. Toxic effects
    Examples:
      1. Cell death due to mitomycin
      2. Decreased function of carbonic anhydrase
  B. Side effects
    Examples:
      1. Dellen due to high bleb
      2. Fatigue due to beta-blocker
  C. Excessive effects
    Examples:
      1. Hypotony with macular oedema
      2. Hypotony with more rapid loss of visual field
      3. Intraocular pressure lower than actually needed with consequent unnecessary side effects from use of treatment
  D. Psychological effects
    Examples:
      1. Anxiety caused by knowing that one has glaucoma
      2. Psychological effects of becoming visually handicapped

Table 8.8 Conditions that mimic glaucoma

1. Chorioretinal lesions
   juxtapapillary chorioretinitis
   melanocytoma
   previous photocoagulation
   retinal vein occlusion
   retinal artery occlusion
2. Optic nerve disease
   anterior ischaemic optic neuropathy
   disc drusen
   disc anomalies
     myopia
     congenital pits
     morning glory syndrome
   chronic papilloedema
   "toxic" amblyopia (alcohol, etc)
   optic nerve compression
   multiple sclerosis
3. Intracranial lesions
   chiasmal disease
     pituitary adenoma
     meningioma
     etc.
   optic tract and radiation abnormalities
     occipital lobe ischaemia, etc

The patient has glaucoma as well as a different condition

A second reason why a patient with glaucoma can continue to get worse is that the patient has two conditions, specifically, glaucoma and an additional condition such as a pituitary adenoma. Glaucoma can coincide with other diseases and should not be considered as inevitably occurring alone.

The intraocular pressure is too high for the patient (not an absolute number)

A third reason why a patient with glaucoma continues to get worse is that the IOP is higher than the nerve can tolerate. It appears that lowering IOP around 30–40% is effective in most patients in arresting progressive optic nerve damage.[17] However, this is merely a supposition and merely an estimate that applies to populations. How much the IOP needs to be lowered in an individual patient in order to prevent further optic nerve damage or to allow recovery of previous damage is unknown. It is likely that the larger the cup, the thinner the rim, and the greater the amount of damage, the more sensitive the optic nerve is to continu-

ing damage. This can be supported theoretically[18] as well as by clinical impression.[19] Patients who have developed marked damage may have been predisposed to developing such damage all along, and the fact that such patients tend to get worse more rapidly than patients who have not developed marked damage, is not a proof that the marked damage itself sensitises the patient to further damage. Nevertheless, it seems prudent to acknowledge the studies that have shown that patients who have become worse tend to continue to get worse, and the more markedly they have become worse,[4, 20] the greater is the likelihood that they will continue to deteriorate. Thus, IOP lowering presumably needs to be greater for patients with marked damage than in those with less damage.

Is there an IOP below which damage is not likely to continue to occur? The answer to this is "yes" and "no." By and large, lowering IOP below 15 mm Hg appears to be adequate to prevent the majority of patients from developing further optic nerve damage.[20] But it is not adequate to prevent all patients from developing further optic nerve damage. Some patients will get worse at pressures of 15 mm Hg but not get worse at pressures of 13 mm Hg. Some will get worse at pressures of 15 mm Hg and not 10 mm Hg. There are, at present, no definitive ways of establishing exactly what pressure will be adequate to prevent further damage in a specific patient. It has been suggested that an improvement in the optic disc or the visual field is an indication that the pressure has been lowered adequately.[21,22] This is an attractive thesis and has some support. However, establishing an actual improvement in the optic disc or visual field is not an easy matter. There is much variability in subjective tests such as visual field tests and even in so-called objective tests, such as disc photographs or images.

Advanced optic nerve damage: the neurons are mortally wounded

A fourth reason why patients with glaucoma have progressive damage is a theoretical one, but almost certainly valid. Specifically, when the optic nerve has become severely deformed it is likely that the neurons continue to be compressed and deprived of neuronal and vascular nourishment. Additionally, an insult to the nerve, such as could be caused by an IOP of 80 mm Hg for one hour, may be severe enough to damage the neuron irreversibly. Thus, it is reasonable to assume that there is a point at which optic nerve damage becomes so severe that neurons will continue to die regardless of the level of IOP.

The intraocular pressure is too low

Can the IOP be lowered too much? The answer here is also a decided "yes." Lowering IOP can be associated with swelling of the optic nerve head, an increased incidence of retinal vein occlusion,[23] and perhaps an increased rate of visual field deterioration.[24] There is a theoretical basis for this in that the optic disc oedema can be associated with IOPs below around 10 mm Hg. Such oedema can theoretically cause increasing compression of the optic neurons and compression of the central retinal vein, predisposing to the problems just mentioned. Optic disc oedema following lowering of IOP is more likely to occur in patients with early or moderate disc damage. For patients with far-advanced glaucomatous nerve damage there is so little glial tissue left that papilloedema is rarely seen in association with low IOPs. Thus, the patients who are at the greatest risk for this type of problem are those with early or moderate optic nerve damage. It is probably imprudent to lower IOP below 10 mm Hg in such cases. As far as patients with far-advanced damaged are concerned, it may conceivably be better to have an IOP of 6 mm Hg than 10 mm Hg, but this has not been established with certainty.

How does one determine what intraocular pressure is low enough?

The traditional way of determining that a specific level of IOP is satisfactory for a certain patient is to assess progression of the disease or lack of it. This is ascertained by repeat diagnostic studies such as visual field examinations and optic disc photographs. The aim of treatment is to lower the IOP until the visual fields and optic disc become stable. However, since damage occurs slowly and there is a limited sensitivity of disc and field examinations, further damage may occur undetected. It is only when a rather marked amount of damage is apparent that the conclusion is then made that the IOP is not low enough, and a lower IOP is selected as a new goal. If that pressure is also not low enough, the patient continues to be damaged while it is being established that that new goal is also not low enough. On the other hand, if an IOP is selected that is actually lower than necessary, the patient is treated with methods that are more vigorous than required to prevent further deterioration. Since every method used to lower IOP carries a cost to the patient in terms of inconvenience and side effects, one wishes to use as little treatment as possible. Thus, selecting an IOP that is lower than necessary may also not be a prudent decision either. It may be comfortable from the ophthalmologist's point of view because the patient's glaucoma may stop getting worse, but it is not likely to be comfortable from the patient's point of view, because of the problems associated with the vigorous treatment. If it is indeed possible to select an IOP that is satisfactory for a certain patient by some other method than simply guessing and then watching to see whether one's guess is correct, a great advance will have been made in making glaucoma treatment both rational and successful. One way of achieving this aim is to use "improvement" in the appearance of the disc or visual field as a means of determining "what pressure is low enough". Therefore, the matter of disc and field improvement will be discussed further.

The initial observation that the optic disc could improve in patients with glaucoma was made by von Jaeger in 1869.[25] Isolated reports followed sporadically. Almost 100 years later it became clear that improvement in the appearance of the optic disc was a quite routine finding following lowering of IOP in patients with congenital glaucoma. That the phenomenon was not rare, however, was not established until a review was done of a large number of patients who had been followed for 10 years.[27] It was noted that where the IOP was lowered by 30% or more, around one third of the patients showed a definite improvement in the appearance of the optic disc. It is likely that this represented a marked underestimation of the patients who actually showed disc changes, as the methodology was routine monoscopic disc photography. Since then, using more refined techniques, an even higher incidence of improvement in the appearance of the optic disc has been documented,[28–30] and the mechanism accounting for this has been thoroughly reviewed.[31]

Following IOP reduction there can be considerable change (improvement) in the appearance of the optic disc (Figures 8.2, 8.3).

Improvement in the visual field has also been documented.[32,33] However, changes here are more difficult to evaluate because of the more subjective nature of the visual field. For example, it was recently suggested that a major proportion of the visual fields obtained for patients in the Ocular Hypertension Treatment Study showed an improvement, even in the absence of treatment.[34] The reasons for this apparent change were due to improvement in the patients' performance on the perimeter, rather than better retinal function.

More refined methods of recognising changes in the nature of the optic nerve and nerve fibre layer, would allow a change in the appearance of the nerve or the nerve fibre layer to be a way to identify adequate reduction of IOP. One study has suggested that patients in whom the optic disc has shown an improvement, have a better prognosis than those in whom an improvement has not been noted, unrelated to the amount of pressure reduction.[35]

Because it is clear that different individuals need different levels of IOP in order to have

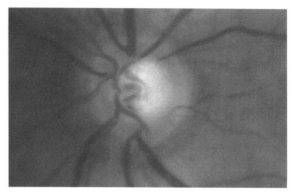

(a)

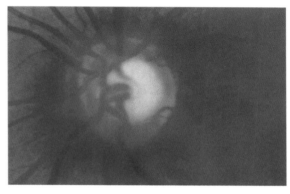

(b)

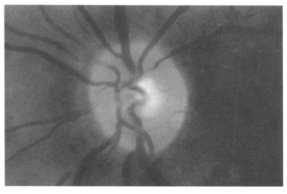

(c)

Figure 8.2 The optic disc of a middle-aged woman with early onset primary open angle glaucoma and intraocular pressures in the upper 30s (mm Hg).

Despite treatment the amount of cupping progressed from that shown in (a) to that illustrated in (b). Glaucoma surgery lowered intraocular pressure to the upper teens (mm Hg), at which time the disc showed a marked improvement (c).

71

their glaucomatous damage arrested, the idea of setting of a "target pressure" for each individual case has been developed. This method has been adopted in several studies.[40] A method of determining target pressure is to determine that pressure at which the glaucoma is deteriorating, and to use that as a percentage of desired reduction of IOP[41]. Thus, if a person has an IOP of 40 mm Hg, the IOP should be reduced 40% or 16 mm Hg, and the target pressure would be 24 mm Hg. On the other hand, if the person was getting worse at a pressure of 20 mm Hg, then lowering the pressure 20% (or 4 mm Hg) would result in a target pressure of around 16%. "Fudge factors" can be added to this, so that where there is advanced damage, additional IOP lowering is considered.

There are disadvantages to target pressures. The attribution of a specific number suggests validity, when in fact it is only a guess. To meet or fail to meet a target pressure does not have an inevitable result. The target pressure is just an estimate and must be considered as such. Thus, should it be concluded that the target pressure for a particular patient is 16 mm Hg and the pressure is easily lowered to 14 mm Hg, it seems unwise to cut back on the therapy, just because one is below target. Similarly, if the target pressure is 16 mm Hg and vigorous therapy lowers the pressure to only 18 mm Hg, it is wise to consider the risks of further IOP reduction if there is considerable extra ocular morbidity involved.

Clinical trials of treatments for glaucoma

Several studies are presently under way which will provide information that will allow more rational decision-making regarding when and how to treat patients believed to have glaucoma. These studies will not give all the answers that are needed. In fact, they will provide only a small portion of the information that is needed to provide truly rational treatment for patients with glaucoma. But they will improve the

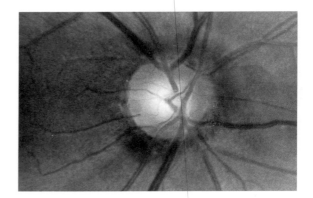

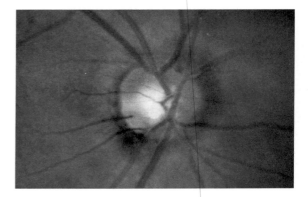

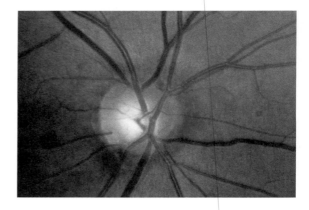

Figure 8.3 (a) The optic disc of a middle-aged woman with moderate glaucoma and no detectable visual field loss. (b) The same optic nerve two years later, with progressive cupping inferiorly and the development of superior visual field loss. Note the disappearance of the inferotemporal artery. (c) Postoperative appearance with lower intraocular pressure. Note the very slight change in the position of the inferotemporal artery, which is again visible. Note also the straightening of the tiny blood vessel in the base of the cup at the 7 o'clock position, especially compared with this vessel.

clinician's ability to make decisions. Consequently, a brief review of these studies is appropriate. Table 8.9 summarises some of the more important studies.

The Scottish Glaucoma Treatment Trial[12] found that trabeculectomy lowered IOP more than did medicinal therapy. Additionally, the group treated with drops lost more visual function than did those treated with trabeculectomy.

The Moorfields Primary Treatment Trial[14] compared drops versus laser trabeculoplasty versus a guarded filtration procedure. The guarded filtration procedure lowered IOP more than did drops or argon laser trabeculoplasty and the patients treated with guarded filtration procedure lost less visual field than did those receiving drops or argon laser trabeculoplasty.

The Glaucoma Laser Trial and the Glaucoma Laser Trial follow-up Study[15,36–38] demonstrated that initial treatment with an argon laser trabeculoplasty was at least as effective as initial treatment with topical timolol in lowering IOP and preserving visual field. The results of this trial have been criticized[39] because the method of medical treatment was not entirely typical of that used by many practising ophthalmologists. However, despite that drawback, they suggest that argon laser trabeculoplasty should be strongly considered as the initial treatment in patients with early or moderate glaucoma who have moderate pigmentation of the posterior trabecular meshwork.

Initial results from the Advanced Glaucoma Intervention Study have been reported.[40] There is a suggestion that for black patients there was better visual preservation when argon laser trabeculoplasty was performed before a guarded filtration procedure, whereas in white patients there appeared to be better visual preservation when the trabeculectomy was performed first, followed by argon laser trabeculoplasty where needed. For both black and white patients, the general reduction of IOP tended to be greater with trabeculectomy than with argon laser trabeculoplasty. However these are initial results and the final analyses from this trial are still awaited.

The Normal-Tension Glaucoma Study demonstrated that reduction of IOP, even in those with IOPs in the "normal" range slowed the rate of glaucomatous deterioration.[16] This study demonstrated that reduction of IOP slowed glaucomatous damage in many patients, even when the IOP started in the "normal" range.

The Ocular Hypertension Treatment study

Table 8.9* Controlled clinical trials, types of glaucoma being studied, enrolment goals, and projected follow up

Name	Acronym	Type of Glaucoma	Enrolment	Follow-up
Scottish glaucoma trial	–	Newly diagnosed POAG	99 patients	3–5 years
Moorfields Primary Treatment Trial	–	Newly diagnosed POAG	168 patients	5+ years
Glaucoma Laser Trial	GLT	Newly diagnosed POAG	271 patients (542 eyes)	2.5–5.5 years
Glaucoma Laser Treatment Follow-up Study	GLTFS	Participants in the GLT	203 patients (406 eyes)	6–9 years
Advanced Glaucoma Intervention Study	AGIS	OAG after medical treatment failure, no previous surgery	591 patients (789 eyes)	4–9 years
Normal Tension Glaucoma Study	NTGS	POAG in eyes with normal IOP	202 patients	5+ years
Ocular Hypertension Treatment Study	OHTS		1637 patients	5+ years
Early Manifest Glaucoma Trial	EMGT	Newly diagnosed POAG	300 patients	4+ years

*Adapted from Wilson RM, Gaasterland D. Translating research into practice: controlled clinical trials and their influence on glaucoma management. J Glaucoma 1996; 5: 139–146 (p. 140).

has recruited 1637 patients.[42] The study is still ongoing, but when completed should give some guidance regarding the transformation from ocular hypertension to glaucoma and the degree to which treatment is effective. Additionally, the study will provide information regarding the effect of medications on corneal endothelial cell density, whether short-wave automated perimetry detects visual field defects earlier than does standard white-on-white perimetry, and whether scanning laser ophthalmoscopy detects glaucomatous damage to the optic disc earlier than sequential stereo photographs.

The Early Manifest Glaucoma Treatment Trial[43] also has not yet concluded and the results are not yet known. The design of this study is different than that in the Ocular Hypertension Treatment study as is the treatment employed. The study outcome is deterioration, based on Humphrey visual field analysis and masked evaluations of disc photographs.

Finally, the Collaborative Initial Glaucoma Treatment Study should provide meaningful information on the effect of glaucoma and various treatments for glaucoma on the quality of life of the patients, as well the relative effectiveness of the different treatments.[44]

Overall principles of management

The major principle that must guide the treatment of glaucoma is awareness that the goal of therapy is maintenance or improvement of the patient's health. Because all treatments, even argon laser trabeculoplasty, have side effects, no treatment can be justified unless it is clear that the side effects are justified.

It is essential to establish with at least relative certainty the course of the glaucoma prior to considering initiation of treatment. In the early stages of the disease there is usually ample time to make a decision without irreversible damage to the patient. Even should irreversible damage occur, this will be asymptomatic, and will not result in reduced visual function. Consequently, there is little risk in carefully establishing the

clinical course, and there is great risk in failing to do so.

For patients with moderate glaucoma damage, small amounts of further damage are frequently tolerated without difficulty. It is useful, where possible, to establish the clinical course before initiating therapy. However, here the room to manoeuvre is less and it becomes increasingly important to notice and meticulously document small changes that indicate that the patient is deteriorating.

There can be a number of milestones in visual deterioration. These will vary according to the patient and to his or her needs. For example the patient who loses sufficient vision in both eyes so that his binocular field is insufficient to meet standards set down for driving, will suffer considerably from any small amount of additional visual loss that could bring this about.

When the patient has reached the symptomatic stages of glaucoma, i.e. the advanced stages of the disease, any further deterioration will increase the amount of symptoms. There is a need to prevent any further damage if possible. There is no justification for allowing the disease to progress at this stage. The clinical course of the entity needs to be established on the basis of past historical information, not on continuing deterioration. Thus, the critical questions that need to be asked are something like the following: "Are you getting worse?" "How are you now in comparison to one week ago?" "How are you now in comparison to a month ago, or a year ago, or 10 years ago?" "Is the vision in your right eye getting worse?" "Is the vision in your left eye getting worse?" How well are you functioning now in comparison to a week ago, a month ago, a year ago, 10 years ago?"

The clinical course of the disease can usually be established accurately by taking a careful history. When a patient says, "I'm getting worse," the patient is in fact getting worse and it is the physician's job to establish the cause for that deterioration. The cause may be glaucoma, or may be some other condition, mental or physical. Whatever the cause or causes, they need addressing appropriately and caringly, with the objective of enhancing or at least maintaining the patient's health.

Keeping in mind that the objective of care is the maintenance of enhancement of the patient's health, question the patient appropriately, listening carefully, and using present-day methods of examination and treatment, it should be possible for ophthalmologists to successfully treat most patients with glaucoma.

References

1 Shields MB, Ritch R, Krupin T. Classification of the glaucomas. In: Ritch R, Shields MB, Krupin T (eds). *The Glaucomas* St Louis: Mosby 1996; 717–29.

2 Spaeth GL. Glaucoma. In: Spaeth GL, Katz LJ, Wilson RP, Moster M, Terebuh AK. Glaucoma. In: Atlas of Ophthalmology. Tasman W, Jaeger E (eds). Philadelphia: Lippincott-Raven 1995.

3 Gagnon MM, Boisjoly HM, Brunette I, Charest M, Amyot M. Corneal endothelial cell density in glaucoma. *Cornea* 1997; **16**: 314—8.

4 Spaeth GL, Hwang S, Gomes M. Disc damage as a prognostic and therapeutic consideration in the management of patients with glaucoma. In: Gramer E, Grehn F (eds). *Pathegenesis and Risk Factors of Glaucoma.* Berlin: Springer-Verlag 1999.

5 *Random House Webster's College Dictionary.* NY: Random House 1991: 567.

6 *The Wellness Encyclopedia.* Boston: Houghton Mifflin Co; 1991: 314.

7 Sugar HS. *The Glaucomas* 2nd edn. NY: Hoeber-Harper 1951; 151.

8 Linnér E, Strömberg U. Ocular hypertension: A five year study of the total population in a Swedish town, and subsequent discussions. In W. Leydhecker (ed), Glaucoma: Tutzing Symposium. Basel: Karger; 1967: 187.

9 Perkins ES. Recent advances in the treatment of glaucoma. *Trans Ophthalmol Soc UK* 1966; **86**: 199.

10 Wilensky JT, Podos SM, Becker B. Prognostic parameters in primary open angle glaucoma. *Arch Ophthalmol* 1974; **91**: 200.

11 Shiose Y, *et al.* (1978): Glaucoma and the optic disc. I. Studies on cup and pallor in the optic disc. *Jpn J Ophthalmol* 1978; **32**: 51.

12 Jay L, Allan D. The benefit of early trabeculectomy vs conventional management in primary open-angle glaucoma relative to the severity of the disease. *Eye* 1989; **3**: 528–35.

13 Araujo SV, Spaeth GL, Roth SM, Starita RJ. A Ten-year Follow-up on a Prospective, Randomized Trial of Postoperative Corticosteroids after Trabeculectomy. *Ophthalmology* 1995; **102**: 1753–9.

14 Migdal C, Gregory W, Hitchings RA. Long-term functional outcome after early surgery compared with laser and medicine in open-angle glaucoma. *Ophthalmology* 1994; **101**: 1651–6.

15 Glaucoma Laser Trial Research Group. The Glaucoma Laser Trial (GLT). 2. Results of argon laser trabeculoplasty vs topical medications. *Ophthalmology* 1990; **97**: 1403–13.

16 Normal-Tension Glaucoma Study Group. Results of the Normal-Tension Glaucoma Study. *Am J Ophthalmol* (in press).

17 American Academy of Ophthalmology. 1) Primary Open-Angle Glaucoma (1996). 2) Primary Open-Angle Glaucoma Suspect (1995). Preferred Practice Patterns. San Francisco: Am Acad Ophthalmol.

18 Burgoyne CF, Quigley HA, Thompson HW, Vitale S, Varma R. (1995) a): Early changes in optic disc compliance and surface position in experimental glaucoma. *Ophthalmology* 1995; **102**: 1800–09.

19 Chandler P, Grant WM. Lectures on Glaucoma. Philadelphia: Lea 14.

20 Grant WM, Burke JF Jr. Why do some people go blind from glaucoma? *Ophthalmology* 1982: **89**: 991–8.

21 Spaeth GL. Reversible changes in the optic disc and visual field in glaucoma. *Curr Opinion Ophthalmol* 1994; **5**: 36–56.

22 Spaeth GL, Fellman RL, Starita RL, *et al.* A new management system for glaucoma based on improvement of the appearance of the optic disc or visual field. *Trans Am Acad Ophthalmol* 1985; **83**: 269–84.

23 Baker KS, Condon GP, Lehrer RL. Occurrence of branch retinal vein and central retinal vein occlusion following trabeculectomy surgery. *Invest Ophthalmol Vis Sci* 1996; **37**: S250.

24 Lin SA, David S, Ta C, Singh K. Progressive visual field loss following mitomycin trabeculectomy in normotensive patients. *Invest Ophthalmol Vis Sci* 1996; **37**: S28.

25 von Jaeger E. (1869): *Ophthalmoskopischer Handatlas* Plate 52. Druck und Verlag der K. K. Hof und Staatsdruckerei, Wien.

26 Hetherington J Jr, Shaffer RN, Hoskins HD Jr. (1975): The disc in congenital glaucoma. In: XXII Congress International of Ophthalmology. Paterson ER (ed), pp. 127–51, Generale de Librairie.

27 Katz LJ, Spaeth GL, Cantor LB. Reversible optic disc cupping and visual field improvement in adults with glaucoma. *Am J Ophthalmol* 1989; **107** (5): 485–92.

28 Raitta C, Tomita G, Vesti E, Harju M, Nakao H. Optic Disc Topography Before and After Trabeculectomy in Advanced Glaucoma. *Ophthalmic Surg* 1996; **27**: 349–54.

29 Shin DH, Bielik M, Hong YJ, Briggs KS, Shi DX. (1989): Reversal of glaucomatous optic disc cupping in adult patients. *Arch Ophthalmol* 1989; **107**: 1599–603.

30 Lesk MR, Spaeth GL, Azuara-Blanco A, *et al.* Reversal of optic disc cupping after glaucoma surgery, analysed with a scanning laser tomograph. *Ophthalmology* (In press).

31 Azuara-Blanco A, Spaeth GL. Methods to objectify reversibility of glaucomatous cupping. *Curr Opinion Ophthalmol* 1997, **8**: 50–4.

32 Paterson G. Effect of intravenous acetazolamide on relative arcuate scotomas and visual field in glaucoma simplex. *Proc Roy Soc Med* 1970; **63**: 865–69.

33 Spaeth GL. The effect of change in intraocular pressure on the natural history of glaucoma: Lowering intraocular pressure in glaucoma can result in improvement of visual fields. *Trans Ophthalmol Soc UK* 1985; **104**: 256–64.

34 Kass MA. Primary therapy is medical. Glaucoma 1998: Controversies and Update in Conjunction with the American Glaucoma Society Subspecialty Day, November 7, 1998. Am Acad Ophthalmol, San Francisco.

35 Spaeth GL. The course of glaucoma in patients whose disc has improved is better than in those in whom the disc has not improved. Presented at the Joint Meeting of the American and European Glaucoma Societies, Reykjavik, Iceland, 1993.

36 Glaucoma Laser Trial Research Group. The Glaucoma Laser Trial (GLT) 3. Design and methods. Control Clin Trials 1991; **12**: 504–24.

37 Glaucoma Laser Trial Research Group. The Glaucoma Laser Trial (GLT) 6. Treatment group differences in visual field changes. *Am J Ophthalmol* 1995; **120**: 10–22.

38 Glaucoma Laser Trial Research Group. The Glaucoma Laser Trial (GLT) and Glaucoma Laser Trial Follow-up Study: 7. Results. *Am J Ophthalmol* 1995; **120**: 718–31.

39 Lichter P. Practice implications of the Glaucoma Laser Trial. *Ophthalmology* 1990; **97**: 1401–2.

40 The Advanced Glaucoma Intervention Study Group. The Advanced Glaucoma Intervention Study (AGIS): 4. Comparison of treatment outcomes within race. Seven-year results. *Ophthalmology* 1998; **105**: 1146–64.

41 Zeyen, T. Target pressures in glaucoma. *Ball Soc Belge Opthalmol* 1999; **274**: 61–5.

42 Kass MA. The Ocular Hypertension Treatment Study. *J Glaucoma* 1994; **3**: 97–100.

43 Heijl A. The Early Manifest Glaucoma Trial. National Eye Institute Home Page. The Internet 1998.

44 Wilson MR, Gaasterland D. Translating research into practice: controlled clinical trials and their influence on glaucoma management. *J Glaucoma* 1996; **5**: 139–46.

9 Medical treatment of glaucoma

G K KRIEGLSTEIN

This chapter looks at the rationale for medical treatment of primary open angle glaucoma (POAG). It discusses the various classes of hypotensive medications currently available before passing on to the potential role for neuroprotective agents.

The decision to treat

Once a decision has been taken that treatment is needed to lower intraocular pressure (IOP), the initial therapy will be one or more hypotensive drops[1]. It is quite unusual to start with primary laser, and less common still to operate. The continuous introduction of powerful, easy to use and relatively side effect-free drops has ensured that this approach remains the choice of ophthalmologists worldwide. Only availability, affordability and uncommon but specific indications, dictate otherwise. The decision to treat (see Chapter 8) will depend upon the clinician's appreciation of risk. The type of medical treatment will be influenced by the state of the eye and the expected response of the patient, both locally and systemically.

A simple rule of thumb for instituting treatment would be: if IOP levels are > 27 mm Hg, irrespective of other potential risk factors; IOP levels are > 23 mm Hg if there are other risk factors apart from elevated IOP; and any IOP level if glaucomatous damage to the optic nerve is present.

A "non-aggressive approach" to therapy is warranted: in the very old, and visual loss is unlikely to affect the patient's quality of life in their expected lifetime; there is little progression over time and, if there is only moderately elevated IOP, and no other risk factors.

General aspects of medical treatment

Medical treatment of glaucoma continues to be an art as much as a science. It is necessary to tailor the treatment to the needs of the patient.[2] When so doing the following rules need to be remembered:

- The target tissues of topically applied ocular hypotensives are within the eye so that ocular conditions which limit bioavailability may exist. These can include tear film deficiency, corneal scarring, chronic non-specific blepharoconjunctivitis, and intraocular inflammation.
- The compliance of the patient with instructions for instilling their eye drops are improved by: patient education about the nature of their disease; telling the patient about the need for lifelong treatment; making sure that the patient (or a carer) has the ability to instil eye drops correctly and according to a dosage schedule; making the patient aware of possible side effects; avoiding eye drops with specific side effects on the individual patient; and using drops which have little affect on the patient's daily routine, either visually or from frequency of instillation.

- Can the treatment regime maintain a target IOP for 24 hours a day?
- Can the patient be followed frequently enough to ascertain the success of treatment?

Whereas separate preparations offer selective dosing and selective discontinuation if necessary.

The simpler the treatment regime, the greater the likelihood of good compliance. Similarly the fewer the side effects the better. Doubts about compliance will arise if the patient complains about either side effects or antisocial times of instillation. A "get up and go to bed" regime is simplest for the patient to follow, for the timing of drop instillation follows the patient's own fixed daily routines. Drops which do not need to be instilled at fixed intervals (such as 12 hourly) are better still, as none of us has such set routines. Multiple drops are less likely to be correctly instilled than single preparations. This means that combinations of drops are more likely to be correctly instilled than drops from several different bottles. In addition, fixed drug combinations offer the additional advantages of less toxicity by preservatives and lower costs, than separate preparations. However, combination therapy drops with identical mechanisms of action should be avoided. If, despite good compliance, the IOP remains uncontrolled, then it will be necessary to increase the number, strength and frequency of instillation, with the attendant worries about compliance.

Although there are numerous medications available having different modes of action, about two thirds of patients require combination treatment. Using monotherapy approximately a 25% reduction can be expected in the relative IOP. From combination therapy 35%, and from maximum medical therapy a 40% IOP reduction from baseline, can be expected.[3] "Maximum medical therapy" is a term used for a combination of drugs which act in all possible ways to lower IOP. Any complex combination of drugs can have a negative effect on compliance and quality of life. Multi-

ple preparations can produce toxic reactions in the conjunctiva, increase the risk of allergic reactions and reduce the success rate of subsequent glaucoma surgery (see Chapter 11). Additionally, the costs to the patient and the healthcare providers may be prohibitive.

Classes of hypotensive agents

Cholinergic agents

Cholinergic agents (parasympathomimetics and miotics) have been used in glaucoma therapy for more than a century. Despite new drug developments they still have a place in modern glaucoma practice. The pharmacological action is to improve trabecular outflow via ciliary muscle contraction, which in turn stretches

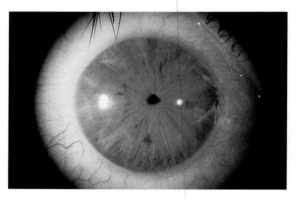

Figure 9.1 Extreme miosis in a glaucoma patient with carbachol 3% eye drops.

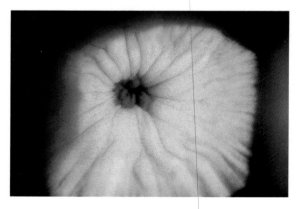

Figure 9.2 Pupillary cysts in patient treated with ecothiophate eye drops. The cysts of the iris pigment epithelium nearly close up the pupillary area.

the trabecular meshwork and opens the Schlemm's canal. Additionally, there is a decrease in uveoscleral outflow and some decrease of aqueous inflow in eyes with chronic treatment.

The visual consequence of ciliary muscle contraction is accommodative myopia, which in conjunction with pupillary constriction produces the major visual side effects of miotics.

Pilocarpine is the most commonly used drug in this class of compounds. Dual action miotics such as carbachol or Aceclidine, can replace pilocarpine. Indirect cholinergic agents (so-called because of their mechanism of action) which inhibit the enzyme that breaks down the physiological cholinergic transmitter (acetylcholine), are rarely used today due to their toxicity, i.e. physostigmine or echothiophate in aphakic or pseudophakic glaucomas.[4,5,6]

The duration of action of topical pilocarpine requires four applications a day in a concentration range of 1–4% aqueous solution. Pilocarpine 2% four times a day is considered to be adequate for most open angle glaucomas. In heavily pigmented eyes higher concentrations may be indicated. The miotic effect of pilocarpine is used to pull the iris root away from the chamber angle in prevention of acute pupillary block glaucoma; the 1% concentration is preferable for this indication. Different pharmaceutical preparations have been developed to prolong bioavailability of the drug at the target tissue, such as soluble polymers, gels, ointments, oily solutions or membrane-controlled delivery systems (Figure 9.3). The magnitude of pilocarpine medicated IOP reduction is about 20% from baseline.

Side effects of Pilocarpine are: ciliary muscle spasm with brow-ache and accommodative myopia; miosis with constriction of visual field; increased risk of retinal detachment; blood-aqueous-barrier instability; keratopathy; and hypersensitivity.

There are much more severe side effects encountered with the indirect acting cholinergic agents which make their clinical use in most glaucoma patients obsolete. These include: systemic toxicity; cataractogenity; intraocular inflammation; iris cysts (Figure 9.3); and ocular pseudopemphigoid.

Adrenergic agents

Dipivalyl-Epinephrine

Epinephrine compounds (bitartrate, borate or hydrochloride formulations) in a clinically relevant concentration range of 0.5–2%[7] are inferior to the pro-drug Dipivalyl-epinephrine 0.1% with respect to their extraocular and systemic side effects. Dipivalyl-epinephrine, which is biotransformed within the cornea, has a 17-fold better corneal permeability than the traditional epinephrine preparations, thus a much smaller external concentration is required to produce an equivalent intraocular response. However, a topical allergic response with conjunctival follicle remains annoyingly common.

The mechanism of epinephrine related IOP reduction[7] is threefold initially by decreased aqueous inflow due to vasoconstrictive properties of the drug; an early increase in trabecular and uveoscleral outflow; and a late increase in outflow facility. Despite a reduction in the extraocular and systemic side effects with use of the pro-drug, epinephrine treatment of open angle glaucoma lost a lot of its popularity since the introduction of newer medications which are not only safer in clinical use but also more

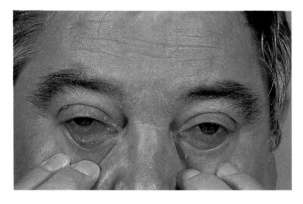

Figure 9.3 Reactive conjunctival hyperaemia in a patient on chronic topical epinephrine therapy.

potent. The epinephrine response in the 15–20% range is additive together with miotics or carbonic anhydrase inhibitors. It seems that there is much less of an additive effect with topical β blockers.

Untoward side effects associated with epinephrine therapy may be: systemic – elevated blood pressure, tachycardia, arrhythmia, headache, anxiety; extraocular – burning, stinging, reactive hyperaemia, adrenochrome deposits (Figure 9.4), epidermalisation of lacrimal punctum, madarosis, pseudopemphigoid; intraocular – mydriasis (be aware of occludable angles), maculopathy, endotheliopathy, vasoconstriction related ocular hypoxia.

Agonists

This group of antiglaucomatous agents can be pharmacologically differentiated by α_2-receptor specifity, CNS permeability, development of subsensitivity, incidence of ocular allergy.

Adequate clinical experience is available with clonidine, apraclonidine and brimonidine. Clonidine eye drops lower IOP in a 1/16–1/2% concentration range. The compound has considerable α1-agonistic side effects (vasoconstriction) and crosses the blood-brain-barrier due to its lipophilicity. Its mode of action is complex since peripheral and central nervous effects on IOP overlap.[9]

The response of clonidine eye drops absorbed systemically on the vasomotor centre of the brainstem is a fall in blood pressure resulting in a reduction of ocular perfusion pressure. Dry mouth, sedation and fatigue are other side effects encountered with clonidine eye drops which limit its clinical value.

Apraclonidine is much more hydrophylic than clonidine, thus entering the brain very little and not sharing the cardiovascular drawbacks of clonidine. As with other α2-agonists it lowers IOP by reduction of aqueous humour production.[10] The occurrence of dry mouth, mydriasis, eyelid retraction and conjunctival blanching indicates relevant α 1-agonistic side effects. The main limitation for long-term use in open angle glaucoma is, however, the high incidence of follicular conjunctivitis and periocular dermatitis as well as development of subsensitivity. Therefore the main indication of apraclonidine 1% eye drops is prevention of short term IOP elevation, i.e. following laser treatment.

Brimonidine is a highly specific α2-agonist. It has some systemic effects (contralateral IOP effect on untreated eye, systolic blood pressure reduction) and lowers IOP via aqueous humour suppression with an IOP decrease of around 25% with four times a day application. It is additive with other IOP lowering agents. In experimental models brimonidine has shown to have neuroprotective properties. Side effects reported with brimonidine are dry mouth, conjunctival blanching (α1-effects), follicular conjunctivitis (10% in long-term use), fatigue, drowsiness and blood pressure reduction (CNS responses). There is no subsensitivity observed from bromonidine.

Beta-blockers

Beta-blockers have been the dominating glaucoma medications for more than 20 years with timolol being the leading compound and reference drug.[12] They can be differentiated pharmacologically by their β-blocking potency, receptor sensitivity, membrane stabilising activity, intrinsic sympathomimetic activity, lipophilicity and plasma half-life. β-blockers

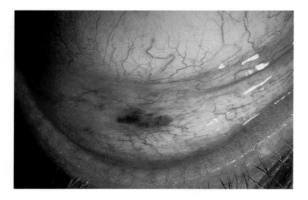

Figure 9.4 Adrenochrome deposits in the conjunctiva of a patient on chronic epinephrine therapy.

lower IOP around 20–25% via inhibition of aqueous humour secretion, except at night-time when flow rate drops physiologically by 40–50%.[11] The duration of IOP reduction after single dose application is 12–24 hours. β-blockers are usually applied twice daily, however, some patients do as well with once daily treatment. The IOP responses of β-blockers are usually not stable during chronic treatment. Different mechanisms of receptor adaptation can result in loss of response within a few days of treatment ("short-term escape") or within months ("long-term drift") with a broad inter-individual variety of the phenomenon. β-blockers are additive with miotics, α 2-agonists, carbonic anhydrase inhibitors and prostaglandins. Additivity with epinephrine compounds or oral β-blockers is doubtful. The spectrum of side effects of ophthalmic β-blockers differs with their pharmacological profile, however, the following are possible with all of them:

- Ocular: corneal hypaesthesia, superficial punctate keratopathy, dry eye syndrome, burning upon instillation, pseudopemphigoid
- Systemic in patients at risk: severe brady-cardia, arrhythmia, systemic hypotension, heart failure, syncope, dyspnoea, asthmatic attacks
- CNS: depression, anxiety, dysarthria, hallucinations, disorientation. Decrease in HDL cholesterol levels, gastrointestinal stress, dermatological disorders, loss of libido and masking of hypoglycaemic episodes in diabetics.

Careful general history taking in the glaucoma patient can avoid most of the severe ocular and systemic side effects of ophthalmic β-blockers.

Besides timolol the β-blockers betaxolol, levobunolol, carteolol and metipranolol are in worldwide use for glaucoma treatment.[14] Betaxolol, a cardioselective β-blocker is less potent than timolol in reducing IOP, but offers more safety with respect to respiratory side effects. The non-selective β-blockers leve-obunolol, carteolol and metipranolol are comparable to timolol in IOP lowering potency. While levobunolol shares the same side effect profile with timolol, carteolol offers some advantage due to its intrinsic sympathomimetic activity affecting LDL cholesterol levels less than timolol. Metipranolol has membrane sta-bilising activity which increases ocular irritation in predisposed patients.

Oral carbonic anhydrase inhibitors (CAIs)

This group of sulphonamide derivatives lowers IOP by inhibition of isoenzyme II of carbonic anhydrase in the ciliary processes. Clinically, relevant IOP reduction requires more than 90% enzyme inhibition which can be achieved by tablets, sustained-release cap-sules or intravenous solution, in appropriate doses.[13] Most of our clinical experience relates to acetazolamide Methazolamide, Dichlorphe-namide and ethoxyzolamide differ in the risk profile but not in therapeutic efficacy. Carbonic anhydrase inhibitors are used in the treatment of various clinical forms of glaucoma, if man-agement with topical medications has been unsuccessful and surgery would be too risky. They can also be used for a limited period in those forms of glaucoma for which surgery is inevitable, i.e. infantile, neovascular, angle clo-sure glaucoma.

The following daily doses produce maximum IOP reductions:[14]

- Acetazolamide: 4 × 250 mg (2 × 500 mg sustained-release capsules)
- Methazolamide: 2 × 50 mg
- Dichlorphenamide: 3 × 100 mg
- Ethoxyzolamide: 4 × 125 mg.

Methazolamide is supposed to have less renal side effects, dichorphenamide should cause less metabolic acidosis, ethoxyzolamide is reported to be equivalent to acetazolamide in efficacy and safety. Side effects of carbonic anhydrase inhibitors are frequent, partially severe and very seldom life threatening.

Elderly glaucoma patients are less tolerant of these drugs if they are on concomitant diuretics, or aspirin therapy.[16] The young patient seems more liable to develop feelings of exhaustion and depression coming on soon after starting the drug, but happily this reverses after discontinuing it.

The following side effects describe the risk profile of CAIs:

- Ocular: transient myopia (shallowing of the anterior chamber)
- Systemic: paraesthesia of the extremities, urinary frequency, metabolic acidosis (causing malaise, fatigue, weight loss, anorexia, depression, loss of libido), loss of serum potassium, abdominal discomfort, metallic taste, nausea, diarrhoea, renal calculi, blood dyscrasias (thrombocytopaenia, agranulocytosis, aplastic anaemia, neutropaenia), exfoliation dermatitis, hypersensitive nephropathy.

Carbonic anhydrase inhibitors should not be given to pregnant women or breast-feeding mothers because of potential teratogenicity. Severe potassium loss may occur if the patient is on additional diuretics. Carbonic anhydrase inhibitors are additive with most topical anti-glaucomatous medications.

Topical carbonic anhydrase inhibitors

The severity and frequency of side effects of the oral CAIs prompted intensive research efforts to find an effective topical CAI. The goal was well defined: acceptable ocular tolerance, sufficient corneal permeability and enzyme inhibition > 90%. Numerous sulphonamide derivatives, formulations and pharmaceutical preparations were tested before dorzolamide was introduced to clinical practice.[15]

Dorzolamide 2% ophthalmic solution three times daily has shown to produce a maintained IOP reduction of 18%, additivity with miotics, β-blockers, α_2-agonists and epinephrine. The magnitude of the IOP reduction is less than that seen with oral CAIs. This may be due to

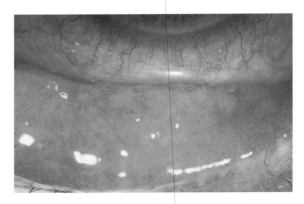

Figure 9.5 Follicular conjunctivitis in patient on topical carboanhydrase therapy.

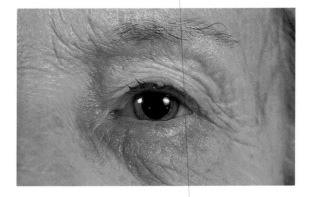

Figure 9.6 Periocular allergic dermatitis in the same patient as in Figure 9.5.

the metabolic acidosis seen with the oral preparations which have an IOP lowering effect independent of carbonic anhydrase inhibition.

Although most of the systemic side effects encountered with oral CAIs were not found with dorzolamide, some can, theoretically, still occur. These include sulphonamide hypersensitivity, Stevens–Johnson syndrome, toxic epidermal necrosis and aplastic anaemia.

Dorzolamide has the same indications, contraindications and precautions as oral CAIs. Preliminary clinical studies have suggested that dorzolamide has a beneficial effect on circulatory parameters of the eye. It has been suggested that this has been caused by local tissue acidosis producing vasodilation.

In approximately 5% of patients chronically treated with dorzolamide, treatment has to be discontinued because of side effects which include: transient burning, stinging and discomfort upon instillation (33%); bitter taste (26%); ocular allergy, superficial punctate keratitis (10%); and blurred vision, dryness, tearing, photophobia (1–5%).

It should be remembered that as a topically applied CAI, dorzolamide could be expected to have an effect on the metabolism of the corneal endothelium. Although this is not a problem for the normal cornea, the eye with an unhealthy endothelium can develop corneal thickening with loss of clarity from topical CAIs. Care needs to be taken in its use for treating some secondary glaucomas (see chapter 21).

Prostaglandin analogues (PGs)

Prostaglandins are ubiquitous local hormones involved in many body functions. The ocular responses of higher doses of prostaglandins comprise hyperaemia, breakdown of blood-aqueous-barrier, hypertension and miosis. Using very small doses, tailoring the molecule to appropriate receptor specificity and esterifying it for adequate corneal permeability, renders an IOP lowering agent that has a low incidence and minimal intensity of conjunctival hyperaemia, foreign body sensation and photophobia.[17,18] These prerequisites were ideally fulfilled by the prostaglandin F2α-isopropylester (latanoprost) as a 0.005% ophthalmic solution.

The esterified prostaglandin is hydrolised within the cornea and the free active acid released into the anterior chamber. Latanoprost 0.005% eye drops given once daily in the evening lowers IOP about 30% without signs of drift of the response, thus being more potent than all the other topically applied drugs. The other PG in clinical use for glaucoma treatment is isopropyl-unoprostone, a modified prostaglandin F2α-metabolite, used twice daily, it is well tolerated and less potent via a lower level receptor specificity. Latanoprost has no effect on blood-aqueous-barrier verified by fluo-photometry, laser-flare meter or fluorescein angiography. However, caution is indicated in aphakic or pseudophakic patients since cystoid macular oedema can develop leading to blurring of vision. Latanoprost has a half-life time in the plasma after systemic absorption of 17 minutes making systemic side effects quite unlikely. Prostaglandins lower IOP by increasing uveoscleral outflow, the effect by day or night. Thus (in contrast to the β-blocker drugs) an IOP lowering effect will be maintained during sleep. The mechanism of action is unique within the antiglaucomatous medications giving several options for additivity. This has even been shown to occur with miotics even though these drugs, by contracting ciliary muscle, should partially close uveoscleral outflow routes.

The improvement in uveoscleral outflow may be explained by ciliary muscle relaxation or by changes in the extracellular matrix of the ciliary body.

There are some ocular side effects of glaucoma with latanoprost which include: mild conjunctival hyperaemia; mild punctate keratopathy; foreign body sensation; ocular irritation; and increased iris pigmentation.

Increased iris pigmentation is expected in about 20% of patients with mixed colour irides (green-brown, blue/gray-brown). As the cell cycle of melanocytes is not affected, neuro-humoural or hormonal mechanisms regulating melanin content of melanocytes will be the cause of the phenomenon. Recent observations have been made on changes in eyelashes (growing longer and curlier, with new eyelashes medial of the lacrimal punctum). This phenomenon is not yet understood.

Future developments

Pharmacotherapy of the glaucomas has up until now focused exclusively on IOP reduction. Much of our current research has been focused around new agents to lower IOP. New areas of research have included classes of "non IOP lower drugs" such as those involved in neuro-protection.[19] Other research has looked at drugs which could biochemically modify the outflow structures to improve or restore outflow facility (the so-called "medical trabeculotomy").[20]

Several different classes of drugs are being studied to try and develop new IOP lowering medications. These include cannabinoids, vasoactive peptides, dopaminergic agents, glucocorticoid receptor antagonists, organic nitrates and antihistaminic drugs. Many have shown promise as IOP lowering agents, but so far none has yet been developed sufficiently for clinical use.

Neuroprotective therapy is designed to interfere with different pathways of neuronal death in glaucoma. Excitatory amino acids like glutamate and aspartate have well understood roles causing cell death. There are specific inhibitors that show promise and which should undergo clinical trials in the near future. Calcium-channel blockers have already shown to be beneficial in some forms of normal tension glaucoma. Oxygen radical scavengers are another class of drug that could find a clinical role.

Many classes of drugs have been investigated to see whether they can restore aqueous outflow in glaucoma. These have included enzymes that are supposed to clear the meshwork from extracellular debris such as α-chymotrypsin. Additionally, calcium chelators, cytochalasins, colchicine, ethacrynic acid and sulphydril-reactive agents have also been tried. Most of these agents produce severe toxic effects on the cornea or other structures not involved in glaucoma, and have not entered clinical trials.

References

1 Krieglstein GK. When to start ocular hypotensive therapy? In: Bucci MG. ed. Glaucoma–Decision Making in therapy. Springer/Milano 1997; 97–99.

2 Krieglstein GK. Medical Therapy of Glaucoma Patients. In: Haefliger IO, Flammer J. (eds.) Nitric Oxide and Endothelin in the Pathogenesis of Glaucoma. Lippincott-Raven/Philadelphia-New York 1998; 230–3.

3 Krieglstein GK. Current Concepts of Medical II Combination Therapy. Glaucoma World 1998; 13: 7–9.

4 Nardin GF, Zimmerman TJ, Zaita AH, Felts K. Ocular cholinergic agents. In: Ritch R, Shields MB, Krupin TH, (eds.) The Glaucomas St Louis: CV Mosby 1989; 515–21.

5 Leopold IH. The uses and side effects of cholinergic agents in the management of intraocular pressure. In: Drance SM, Neufeld AH, (eds.) Glaucoma: Applied Pharmacology in Medical Treatment. Orlando: Grune and Stratton 1984; 357–93.

6 Kaufman PL, Wiedman, T, Robinson TR. Cholinergics. In: Sears ML, (ed.) Handbook of Experimental Pharmacology. Berlin: Springer 1984; 149–91.

7 Becker B, Pettit TH, Gay AJ. Topical Epinephrine Therapy of Glaucoma. Arch Ophthalmol 1961; 66: 219.

8 Bigger JF. Dipivefrin and Glaucoma. Perspect Ophthalmol 1980; 4: 85.

9 Krieglstein GK, Langham, ME, Leydhecker W. The peripheral and central neural actions of clonidine in normal and glaucomatous eyes. Invest Ophthalmol Vis Sci 1978; 17: 149–58.

10 Kaufman PL, Gabelt B. Alpha-adrenergic agonist effects on aqueous humor dynamics. J Glaucoma 1995; 4(suppl): 8–14.

11 Neufeld AH, Bartels SP, Liu JH. Laboratory and clinical studies on the mechanism of action of Timolol. Ophthalmology 1983; 28: 286–90.

12 Zimmerman TJ. Topical ophthalmic beta-blockers: a comparative review. J Ocul Pharmacol Ther 1993; 9: 373–84.

13 Maren TH. Carbonic anhydrase: chemistry, physiology, and inhibition. Physiol Rev 1967; 47: 595–781.

14 Lichter PR, Musch DC, Medzihradsky F, Standardi CL. Intraocular pressure effects of carbonic anhydrase inhibitors in primary open angle glaucoma. Am J Ophthalmol 1989; 107: 11–17.

15 Lippa EA. Dose response and duration of action of dorzolamide, a topical carbonic anhydrase inhibitor. Arch Ophthalmol 1992; 110: 495–9.

16 Anderson CJ, Kaufman PL, Sturm RJ. Toxicity of combined therapy with carbonic anhydrase inhibitors and aspirin. Am J Ophthalmol 1978; 86: 516.

17 Bito LZ. Prostaglandins: old concepts and new perspectives. Arch Ophthalmol 1987; 105: 1036–9.

18 Camras CB, Alm A. Initial clinical studies with prostaglandins and their analogues. Surv Ophthalmol (suppl) 1997; 41: 61–8.

19 Iversen LL. Pharmacological approaches to the treatment of ischemic neuronal damage. Eye 1991; 5: 193–7.

20 Kaufman PL, Svedbergh B, Lütjen-Drecoll E. Medical trabeculocanalotomy in monkeys with cytochalasin B or EDTA. Ann Ophthalmol 1979; 11: 795–6.

10 Laser treatment of primary open angle glaucoma

C MIGDAL

The use of light energy to treat glaucoma has been one of the most innovative additions to the therapeutic management of this disease in recent times. Initial enthusiasm and promise has been followed by evidence-based trial results, suggesting a specific place for laser therapy in individually selected patients.

Lasers emitting different wavelengths of light are used in glaucoma patients with angle closure to perform iridotomies, and iridoplasties. They have been used in open angle glaucoma to create sclerostomies, but without lasting success. This chapter will deal with two common uses of lasers to treat open angle glaucoma; laser trabeculoplasty and laser cyclophotocoagulation.

Argon laser trabeculoplasty

Argon laser trabeculoplasty (ALT) was introduced in the late 1970s as a treatment option for glaucoma.[1] Although this method of treatment is simple and cost-effective, the effect ALT has on intraocular pressure (IOP) decreases over time in many patients.[2] This fact needs to be considered when assessing an individual for treatment.

Mechanism

Argon laser trabeculoplasty would appear to lower the IOP by improving aqueous humour outflow,[3] although the precise effect of treatment on the trabecular meshwork (TM) is unclear. Two hypotheses have been put forward. The mechanical theory suggests that scar tissue contraction at the coagulation site lowers IOP by pulling open adjacent intertrabecular spaces. The second hypothesis moots that an increased rate of trabecular cell replication precipitated by the laser increases the number of cells involved in maintaining the appropriate TM outflow facility.

Method

The angle structures are viewed through a goniolens (Figure 10.1) after the instillation of a topical anaesthetic. The laser burns should be placed between the anterior pigmented TM and the non-pigmented TM. Burns sited too posteriorly will result in peripheral anterior synechiae (PAS) formation. For this reason, narrow drainage angles are not suitable for this form of treatment, as they tend to develop PAS.

The amount of laser energy delivered to the TM is a function of power, duration and spot size. Suggested settings are: spot size (50 μm), duration (0.1 s), and power (500–1200 mW).

The power is adjusted to cause minimal blanching or minute gas bubble formation. The reaction seen will depend on the amount of pigmentation on the TM. Excessive power should not be used as this causes unnecessary scarring and subsequent increase in IOP. Most studies of ALT have used the argon laser (blue-green spectrum), although recent studies have shown that the diode laser may be equally effective.[4] In most instances approximately 50 burns are applied to each half of the circumference of the TM.

Most clinicians treat 360° of the circumference in two separate sessions separated by approximately two weeks, with 180° being treated in each session. Others treat the second half of the angle only if the initial treatment does not adequately lower IOP, or if the pressure increases again at a later date.

To prevent a post-treatment spike in IOP the patient can be treated with pilocarpine 2% or apraclonidine 1% instilled immediately before/after the laser. The IOP should be checked approximately $\frac{1}{2}$ –1 hour post-laser.

Indications

Argon laser trabeculoplasty may be considered for patients with primary open angle glaucoma (POAG), pigmentary glaucoma or pseudoexfoliation syndrome glaucoma when the IOP is not adequately controlled with medical therapy (usually up to two topical medications). In selected patients, such as the elderly with poor compliance or the inability to use β-blockers, ALT may be used as the initial form of treatment. The Primary Treatment Study[5] which compared medical therapy, ALT or trabeculectomy as the initial treatment in patients with open angle glaucoma, showed that ALT performed less adequately than surgery or medicine in terms of maintenance of IOP control over time (Figure 10.2). Laser had a similar

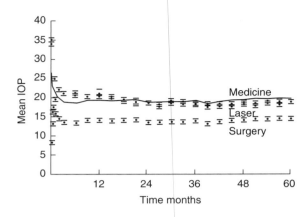

Figure 10.2 Moorfields Primary Therapy Trial – mean intraocular pressure for laser, medicine and surgery groups over five years.

effect to medically treated patients in terms of mean IOP and visual field. After a follow-up of five years, only 60% of laser patients had their IOP controlled at less than 21mm Hg. Initial reports from the Glaucoma Laser Trial showed that initial treatment of newly diagnosed open angle glaucoma with ALT was at least as effective as initial treatment with eye drops.[6]

Laser trabeculoplasty is contraindicated for patients with uveitic, rubeotic, angle-recession, and infantile and juvenile onset glaucomas. Repeat laser trabeculoplasty is not recommended in most cases. The reduction in IOP is usually smaller and short-lived and considerable increases in IOP may occur after retreatment.

Complications

The most common complication is a transient IOP rise within the first six hours after treatment. This spike may be minimised by treating only half the angle at one sitting and by using apraclonidine hydrochloride 1% or pilocarpine 2% prophylactically.[7] The acute rise in IOP may pose a risk for loss of central vision for those eyes with severely damaged optic nerves.

Mild iritis is also common after ALT. Gutt Predsol 0.5% q.i.d. is prescribed routinely for five days after laser to suppress this.

A sudden sustained rise in IOP may occur

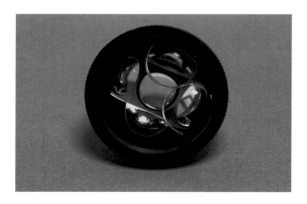

Figure 10.1 Ritch laser trabeculoplasty gonioscopy lens – containing 2 basic mirrors and 2 additional mirrors (the latter effectively reduce spot size and increase laser energy by a factor of two).

some time after ALT in some patients, probably due to scarring of the TM. It is thus essential to keep patients under routine regular long-term follow-up.

Efficacy

Argon laser trabeculoplasty reduces IOP in approximately 85% of treated eyes, with the hypotensive effect usually evident within four weeks of treatment. Studies have shown an initial reduction in the IOP of approximately 20–30% (6–9 mm Hg).[1,8] Patients in the Glaucoma Laser Trial had a mean reduction in IOP of 9 mm Hg.[9] Large reductions in IOP may be seen in patients with pseudoexfoliation or pigmentary glaucomas, although the loss of IOP control may also occur sooner in these groups. Aphakic eyes tend to respond less well than phakic ones.[10]

Other than reduction of IOP, a treatment's clinical effectiveness must also be judged on the ability to preserve the disc and field. In one study of 118 eyes treated with 360° ALT, 52% of eyes had an IOP ≤ 19 mm Hg (mean pretreatment IOP 26.1 mm Hg), a stable disc and field and no need for further surgery after four years follow-up. If subsequent drainage surgery is required, a previous ALT may increase the chance of failure.

It may be possible to reduce or stop adjunctive glaucoma medication after ALT, thus improving the quality of life of the patient. However, several studies have shown a diminished IOP effect over time, so that by 10 years, more than half of the treated eyes required further surgery. In the Primary Therapy Study only 60% of laser patients were still controlled, despite adjunctive pilocarpine 2% when necessary.[5] The two year follow-up of the Glaucoma Laser Trial showed that initial laser alone controlled IOP in 44% of eyes, while laser trabeculoplasty combined with a β-blocker controlled the IOP in 70% of eyes, and this was increased to 89% when up to two adjunctive medications were used. Comparing medical therapy without laser, a single drug controlled IOP in 66%.[9]

The initial report of the Advanced Glaucoma Intervention Study, in which patients with uncontrolled glaucoma despite maximal medical therapy were randomised to receive either ALT or trabeculectomy as their next treatment, shows some interesting findings, namely that black patients did better with ALT, compared with trabeculectomy performing better in white patients.[13]

Although ALT is simple to perform and cost-effective, the question of long-term control of IOP by this procedure remains and patients do need to be monitored continuously as IOP control can be lost suddenly. Ophthalmologists carrying out ALT must have a good knowledge of the anatomy of the drainage angle and be competent at gonioscopy.

Laser cyclophotocoagulation

Ciliary body ablation with laser has been used effectively to treat eyes with severe refractory glaucoma for many years. Although the exact mechanism of action is unknown, IOP is lowered by reducing aqueous production, probably by destruction of the ciliary epithelium of the ciliary body. Currently the most commonly used laser sources are the transscleral application of the Nd:YAG laser and the semiconductor diode laser. The Nd:YAG lasers deliver infrared (1,064 mm) light energy either by fibre-optic contact or through air in a free-running coagulative mode. The reports of long-term success are variable.[14,15] These lasers are large and expensive.

More recently semiconductor diode laser systems, which are more compact, lightweight and therefore portable, have been employed. The near infrared wavelengths (approximately 800 nm) appear to be effective in coagulating ciliary tissue.

Indications

Cyclodestruction in its various forms has traditionally been restricted to eyes with end-stage glaucoma and otherwise poor visual prognosis. Previous medical therapy or filtering surgery has usually failed in these cases and further such intervention contraindicated or impractical. Often these patients have virtually no functional vision. The relief of IOP-induced pain is also an important consideration.

The types of glaucoma which may be considered for cyclophotocoagulation include neovascular glaucoma, patients with scarred conjunctiva due to multiple previous surgical procedures, aphakic or uveitic glaucoma, patients with conjunctival cicatricial disease, or patients who are surgical risks because of systemic disease, i.e. patients who are unsuitable candidates for a surgical trabeculectomy.

Anaesthesia

Treatment is carried out under peribulbar or retrobulbar anaesthesia using a mixture of xylocaine and bupivacaine. Topical amethocaine is applied.

Method

Nd:YAG laser

The laser energy can be applied by either the contact or non-contact method. The contact laser is applied via a fibre-optic hand-held probe directly to the surface of the globe. The non-contact laser delivers energy via a slit lamp delivery system using the thermal or free-running mode. Thirty to forty evenly spaced burns (but avoiding the 3 and 9 o'clock positions because of the underlying long ciliary nerves and vessels) are applied over 360° with a power setting of 4–9 joules (Figure 10.3). Each burn causes a blanching of the conjunctiva. It is useful to transilluminate the area to assess the exact situation of the ciliary body, which can vary anatomically particularly in buphthalmic eyes, or eyes that have undergone considerable previous surgery. This is done using a hand-held transilluminator (Figure 10.4). When using the non-contact method, the Nd:YAG is used in the free-running

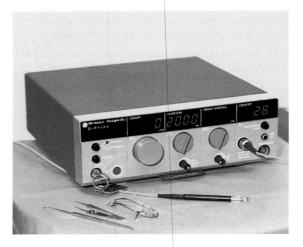

Figure 10.3   Diode laser control box and probe.

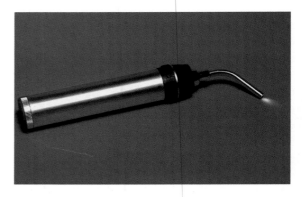

Figure 10.4 Hand-held transilluminator used for assessing the position of the ciliary body.

mode and maximally defocused for optimal effect.

The audible "pop" sometimes heard during transscleral laser cyclophotocoagulation represents a small zone of intraocular tissue disruption. If extensive, this could cause inflammation, hypotony or phthisis. The laser power should thus be decreased slightly.

Semiconductor diode laser

In the non-contact mode, a power of 1200–1500 mW, a duration of 1 second and a spot size of 100–400 μm are used. Thirty to forty applications are placed 1 mm posterior to the limbus over 360°. The contact diode laser places approximately 20 burns over 270° of the circumference, using a power of 1.5–2.0 W, a duration of 1.5 seconds, approximately 1.5 mm posterior to the limbus (again, transillumination should be performed first to assess the position of the ciliary body). A special G-probe (Figure 10.5) facilitates orientation in the correct axis. The power can be adjusted until a popping is heard and then reduced to just below the popping sound level.

Postoperative treatment

After treatment a subconjunctival steroid injection helps reduce postoperative pain and inflammation. Gutt Pred Forte is prescribed for 2–4 weeks.

Efficacy

The success rate depends on the type of glaucoma, preoperative IOP, race and other factors. About one third of patients will require one or more subsequent treatments. Reported success rates in lowering IOP vary between 44–66%.[15,16]

Although the short-term success rate for laser cyclodestruction is relatively good, the majority of patients have to continue taking medications. In addition, the long-term IOP levels after laser are not as low as those achieved by filtering surgery with antimetabolites.

Complications

This varies from mild to severe anterior segment inflammation, mild pain, to less frequent but more severe problems (including loss of vision, hyphaema, hypopyon, corneal decompensation, scleral thinning, retinal or choroidal detachment, phthisis bulbi, and sympathetic ophthalmia).

Transscleral laser cyclophotocoagulation is a relatively safe and effective method of lowering IOP pressure in eyes with complicated and uncontrolled glaucoma. This method should be used with caution in those patients who stand to lose useful vision.

Endoscopic laser cyclophotocoagulation

One possible reason for the failure of transscleral cyclophotocoagulation, particularly in congenital glaucoma, may be displacement of the ciliary processes. Indirect treatment may thus miss the appropriate area. Endoscopic laser cyclophotocoagulation allows direct visualisation, with treatment being accurately applied to the ciliary processes, using a diode laser. The procedure has been combined with cataract extraction, and has mostly been used in refractory cases of glaucoma where other treatments have failed.[17]

Complications reported include inflammation, hypotony, retinal detachment, loss of acuity, and vitreous haemorrhage. Safety and efficacy need to be assessed with proper trials and longer follow-up.

References

1 Wise JB, Witter SL. Argon laser trabeculoplasty for open-angle glaucoma: a pilot study. *Arch Ophthalmol* 1979; **97**: 3199–22.

2 Schwartz AL, Love DC, Schwartz MA. Long-term follow-up of argon laser trabeculoplasty for uncontrolled open-angle glaucoma. *Arch Ophthalmol* 1985; **103**: 1482–4.

3 Van Buskirk EM. Pathophysiology of laser trabeculoplasty. *Surv Ophthalmol* 1989; **33**: 264–72.

4 Brancato R, Trabucchi G. Diode laser compared with argon laser trabeculoplasty. *Am J Ophthalmol* 1991; **112**: 50–5.

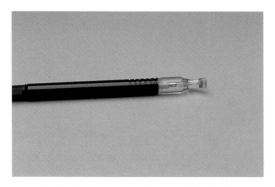

Figure 10.5 Diode laser with hand-held G-probe.

5 Migdal C, Gregory W, Hitchings R. Long-term functional outcome after early surgery compared with laser and medicine in open-angle glaucoma. *Ophthalmology* 1994; **101**: 1651–7.

6 Glaucoma Laser Trial Research Group. The Glaucoma Laser Trial (GLT) and Glaucoma Laser Trial Follow-up Study: 7. Results. *Am J Ophthalmol* 1995; **120**: 718–31.

7 Robin AL. The role of apraclonidine hydrochloride in laser therapy for glaucoma. *Trans Am Ophthalmol Soc* 1989; **87**: 729–61.

8 Shingleton BJ, Richter CV, Bellows AR, *et al.* Long-term efficacy of argon laser trabeculoplasty. *Ophthalmology* 1987; **94**: 1513–8.

9 Glaucoma Laser Trial Research Group. The Glaucoma Laser Trial (GLT): 2. Results of argon laser trabeculoplasty versus topical medicines. *Ophthalmology* 1990; **97**: 1403–13.

10 Weinreb RN, Ruderman J, Justen R, *et al.* Immediate intraocular pressure response to argon laser trabeculoplasty. *Am J Ophthalmol* 1983; **95**: 279–86.

11 Shingleton BJ, Richter CV, Dharma SK, *et al.* Long-term efficacy of argon laser trabeculoplasty: a ten year follow-up study. *Ophthalmology* 1993; **100**: 1324–9.

12 Richter CV, Shingleton BJ, Bellows AR, *et al.* The development of encapsulated filtering blebs. *Ophthalmology* 1998; **95**: 1163–8.

13 The AGIS Investigations. The advanced Glaucoma Study (AIGS): 4. Comparison of Treatment Outcomes Within Race. *Ophthalmology* 1998; **105**: 1146–64.

14 Dickens CJ, Nguyen N, Mora JS, *et al.* Long-term results of non-contact transscleral neodymium:YAG cyclophotocoagulation. *Ophthalmology* 1995; **102**: 1777–81.

15 Kosoko O, Gaasterland DE, Pollack IP, Enger CL. Long-term outcome of initial ciliary ablation with contact diode laser transscleral cyclophotocoagulation for severe glaucoma. *Ophthalmology* 1996; **103**: 1294–302.

16 Bloom PA, Tsai JC, Sharma K, Miller MH, *et al.* "Cyclodiode". Transscleral diode laser cyclophotocoagulation in the treatment of advanced refractory glaucoma. *Ophthalmology* 1997; **104**: 1508–20.

17 Chan J, Cohn RA, Lin SC, Cortes AE, Alvarado JA. Endoscopic photocoagulation of the ciliary body for treatment of refractory glaucoma. *Am J Ophthalmol* 1997; **124**: 787–96.

11 Glaucoma surgery

A BÉCHETOILLE, R A HITCHINGS

This chapter looks at the practice of glaucoma surgery and the principles behind it. The chapter describes the techniques behind the guarded sclerostomy, as well as results and complications. It then looks at "non-penetrating" or deep sclerectomy contrasting techniques and compares these with results from the guarded sclerostomy. Finally it looks at glaucoma tubes, placing these in perspective in the hierarchy of surgical procedures for glaucoma.

Fistulising surgery is an effective way to decrease intraocular pressure (IOP) in glaucoma patients. Trabeculectomy, which is the standard of practice for surgery in adults, is more efficient than medical and/or laser treatment both in lowering IOP and in preserving visual function in the long term.[1,2] The advantage of glaucoma surgery is that when successful in reducing IOP, it is not necessary to rely on patient compliance with treatment. The major disadvantages are the complications as well as failure of the procedure to maintain control of IOP and thus to prevent disease progression.

We will consider techniques of modern glaucoma surgery and recent modifications, including non-penetrating sclerectomy, and combined cataract with glaucoma surgery. Then we will look at current methods of preventing scar tissue formation, and at glaucoma tube surgery, before discussing results and complications of these procedures.

With the exception of operations on children and perhaps complex tube surgery, all the procedures described here can be performed as day case surgery using topical anaesthesia.

Basic trabeculectomy

In 1856 von Graefe described iridectomy as the first surgical treatment for glaucoma. It is still used today in the treatment of angle closure glaucoma when laser iridectomy is not available. At the turn of the century up until the 1960s, full thickness fistulising surgery was the standard approach, first as the trephine procedure,[3,4] and then the thermal sclerostomy.[5] These operations could successfully lower IOP and keep it within the normal range for many years. However the initial bulk outflow of aqueous caused major problems in a significant proportion of patients. The "guarded sclerostomy" described by Cairns, reduced bulk outflow in the immediate postoperative period and allowed good long term IOP control.[6] In this operation aqueous leaves the anterior chamber around the superficial scleral flap (which provides initial outflow resistance), to enter the subconjunctival space from which it is absorbed. This process leads to the formation of what is described clinically as the "filtration bleb". By the 1980s this approach had largely replaced the full thickness procedure and is still the primary glaucoma operation of choice today (Figure 11.1).

The basic trabeculectomy procedure starts with the opening of a conjunctival flap, followed by a 5–6 mm limbus-based scleral flap that

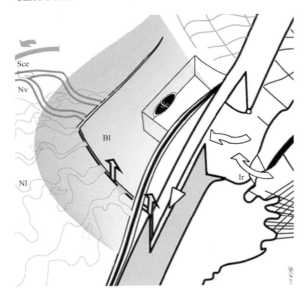

Figure 11.1 Illustration of the exit route of aqueous from the anterior chamber after trabeculectomy surgery. **Ir**, iridectomy; **Sc**, Schlemm's canal; **Sce**, drainage channels from Schlemm's canal; **Nv**, aqueous veins; **Nl**, neolymphatics; **Bl**, filtration bleb

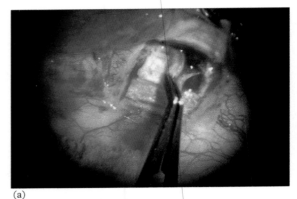

(a)

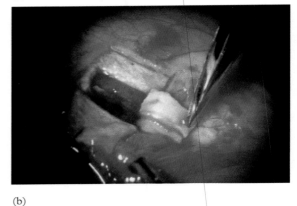

(b)

Figure 11.2 (a) Dissection of deep scleral tissue at the time of trabeculectomy. The attachment of ciliary body to scleral spur is shown (b), and the appearance of trabecular tissue after disinsertion of ciliary body.

allows an access to the periphery of the anterior chamber. Then the anterior chamber is entered and a deep block of sclera, cornea, and some trabecular tissue is removed. The deep block lies anterior to scleral spur, thus avoiding the creation of a cyclodialysis with the risk of later hypotony. The anatomical difference between the two approaches is shown in Figure 11.2. A peripheral iridectomy is then performed before suturing the scleral and the conjunctival flaps back into place.

The forms of the conjunctival and scleral flap openings are varied (Figures 11.3 and 11.4), as are the techniques of trabecular block removal. However, these variations have little if any effect on the postoperative results and are largely performed at the convenience of the surgeon. But the way the conjunctival and the scleral flaps are closed, including tight sutures (with further laser suture lysis[7]) or adjustable sutures,[8,9] has a direct influence on the results, and especially on the complication rate (Figure 11.5).

Non-penetrating sclerostomy

Non-penetrating surgery, so-called because the primary intention is not to create a direct entry at the time of surgery into the anterior chamber, allows filtration of aqueous through the inner trabecular meshwork (TM) into a space left after removal of the overlying sclera. The basic procedure, as originally described in Russia, was called a sinusotomy. Today's operations carry a number of names, depending on modifications of this basic procedure. These include the so-called "deep sclerectomy", and "viscocanalostomy".[10–12]

The potential advantages for the "non-penetrating" approach are twofold. Firstly, because the bleb (if any) is low lying and diffuse,

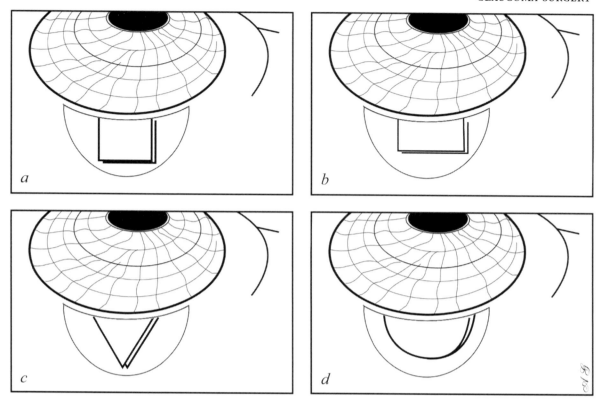

Figure 11.3   Forms of scleral flap used for trabeculectomy surgery.

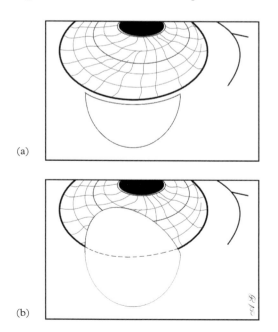

Figure 11.4   Different types of conjunctival flap (a) fornix based, (b) limbal based.

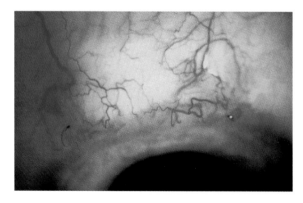

Figure 11.5 A "successful" drainage bleb, with reduced vascularity.

there should be fewer long-term "bleb-related" problems, such as discomfort, over-drainage and infection (Figure 11.5). Secondly, because the anterior chamber is not disturbed, there should be a lower incidence of lens opacification than seen after "penetrating" surgery.

The common approach for all these operations is to expose and then "deroof" Schlemm's canal by reflecting the scleral tissue above it. Then the internal wall of Schlemm's canal and the external part of the trabeculum are either mechanically aspirated[13] or removed by peeling away with forceps. Finally, the deep scleral flap is excised creating a cavity in the sclera, the roof of which is the superficial scleral flap (Figure 11.6).

The deep sclerectomy creates a trabeculectomy-like conjunctival flap and then a superficial limbus-based scleral flap. The viscocanalostomy involves injection of a viscoelastic into the perceived cut ends of Schlemm's canal, exposed after "deroofing" Schlemm's canal. Finally the procedure can be further modified by inserting a collagen "wick" into the empty space left by tissue removal, for some consider it to help filtration of aqueous to the subconjunctival space.[14]

It is probable that in all these procedures the aqueous percolates out to the subconjunctival space in the same way as for a trabeculectomy. However viscocanalostomy is supposed to work without the development of a filtration bleb[12] (Figure 11.7).

Combined glaucoma and cataract surgery

Because the maximum incidence of both cataracts and glaucoma occurs within the same age range, the two conditions not infrequently coexist. Additionally, it is well recognised that fistulising surgery is often followed by a "speeding-up" in the development of pre-existing cataract, leading to a second operation one to two years later. These effects have been recently documented in two controlled trials involving antiproliferatives (see below). Finally the glaucoma operation seems not to work so well after subsequent cataract surgery.[15] As a result, surgical procedures have been devised combining cataract and glaucoma surgery (the "combined operation").[16,17] Cumulative experience with combined procedures has led to specific techniques combining phacoemulsification and fistulising surgery (the "phacotrabeculectomy"). This can be either at one, or separate sites.[17,18] In "one site", the operation is started by a funnel-type scleral incision, after which a phacoemulsification is performed, followed by insertion of a foldable intraocular lens into the capsular bag. The process is completed by the trabeculectomy, frequently performed with a scleral punch. With the "two site" operation a standard trabeculectomy flap is first prepared, usually the twelve o'clock meridian; then phacoemulsification is performed at the second (usually) temporal site. Finally, the trabeculectomy is completed at the original site. The IOP control is probably enhanced when peroperative antimetabolites are used.[19] In similar fashion "same-site" surgery has been proposed for the cataract surgery and non-penetrating sclerectomy.[20]

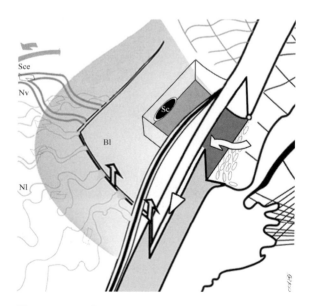

Figure 11.6 Suggested aqueous exit route after non penetrating surgery. **Sce**, drainage channels from Schlemm's canal; **Nv**, aqueous veins; **NL**, neolymphatics; **Bl**, filtration bleb.

Antimetabolites

Fistulising surgery involves the creation of a low resistance aqueous exit route from the anterior chamber to the subconjunctival space (Figure 11.7). Resistance to aqueous egress develops as a result of fibroblast proliferation, collagen deposition and formation of intercellular ground substance. This can be seen as either a sheet of fibrous tissue overlying the lamellar scleral flap (Figure 11.8), or as sheets of fibrous tissue forming an "encapsulated bleb" (Figure 11.9). With increased resistance comes an increase in IOP required to force fluid out of the eye. Too high a pressure, and the operation is deemed to have failed.

Antiproliferative drugs applied at the time of surgery,[21–25] and, if required, given by subconjunctival injection in the immediate postoperative period,[26,27] can delay or inhibit this fibroblast response, minimising the development of resistance.

At the present time the two most commonly used drugs are 5-fluorouracil (5FU) and mitomycin. Although 5FU was originally given by subconjunctival injection, both 5FU and mitomycin are now given at the time of surgery. An absorbent sponge, approximately 7 × 3 × 5 mm size, is soaked in the appropriate drug. This sponge is placed between the episclera and sclera (before dissection of the scleral flap) and left in position for a timed period. After removal the treated area is washed copiously with at least 20 ml balanced salt solution. Care needs to be taken in handling these cytotoxic drugs; a separate trolley should be used, with separate instruments, and a no-touch technique used by the surgeon. The

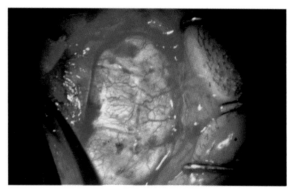

Figure 11.8 Revision of unsuccessful drainage bleb, conjunctiva reflected to reveal fibrous tissue covering the scleral flap.

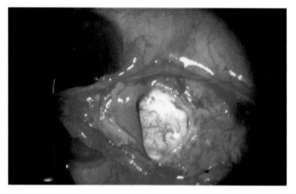

Figure 11.9 Revision of drainage bleb, incision into an encapsulated bleb revealing a thick fibrous tissue wall.

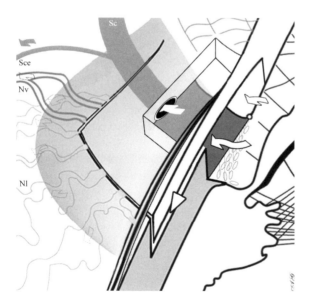

Figure 11.7 Suggested aqueous exit route after viscocanalostomy. **Sc**, Schlemm's canal; **Sce**, drainage channels from Schlemm's canal; **Nv**, aqueous veins; **Nl**, neolymphatics.

assistant needs to take precautions against spillage and wear suitably protective gloves, and if needed, eyeglasses.

For each case the surgeon chooses the drug, the concentration, and duration of application after assessment of the risk of scar tissue formation. Although there are no absolute rules, a scale for increasing antifibroblast action can be seen as follows:

- Subconjunctival 5 FU 25 mg/ml for 5 mins
- Subconjunctival 5 FU 50 mg/ml for 5 mins
- Subconjunctival mitomycin 0.1–0.5 mg/ml for 3–5 mins.

Additional "top ups" of postoperative 5 FU can be injected subconjunctivally, if despite treatment, excess healing is seemed to be occurring. Risk factors for failure because of excessive healing are set out in Table 11.1.

5FU produces a temporary "switching off" of the fibroblasts, so that its duration of action could be anticipated to last for 4–6 weeks, enough to cope with the immediate healing response, but not a persistent one. Mitomycin kills the cells, therefore has a more lasting effect.[28,29]

Excessive healing, which could need subconjunctival injections ("top ups") of 5FU, would be suspected with the development of persistent vascular dilation on and around the bleb,

retraction of a suture line and straightening up of conjunctival vessels, as well as increasing IOP. Vascular engorgement around an avascular drainage bleb is shown in Figure 11.10.

Excessive tissue loss seen after the use of mitomycin is avoided if the duration of application is kept to a minimum[30] (3 instead of 5 minutes), the sponge size is large and its placement is posterior to the site of the scleral flap ("posterior placement" is easier on either side of the superior rectus insertion, thus avoiding the perforating anterior ciliary vessels). Late dissolution of the scleral flap with resulting over drainage and hypotony will be avoided when the sponge is placed posterior to the outline of the flap.

Antimetabolites have proved to be a major advance in the inhibition of wound healing. To date their use remains rather non-specific, leading to many complications. This is of particular relevance with post-filtration cataract formation. In a south Indian study, eyes treated with mitomycin were found to be more likely to develop cataract after trabeculectomy, than those treated with placebo.[31] With better preoperative assessment of risk, combined with newer drugs better able to target specific steps in the wound healing response, it is likely that the postoperative Target IOP level will be easier to achieve in the future.[28]

Table 11.1 Risk factors for failure in fistulising surgery

1) Inherent fibroblast response
   Youth
   Atopy
   Black Races
2) Prior fibroblast activation
   Conjunctival Surgery
   Chronic glaucoma medication
   Chronic Blepharitis
3) Altered aqueous composition
   Prior intraocular surgery
   Subsequent intraocular (usually cataract) surgery
   Chronic uveitis

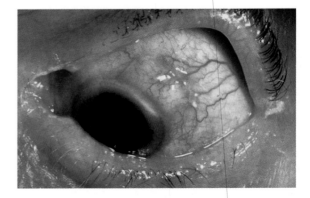

Figure 11.10 Failing drainage bleb. Large dilated blood vessels around a small bleb.

Tubes and plates in refractory glaucoma

Despite the advances in fistulising surgery and antimetabolite use, there remains a sub-group of eyes for which fistulising surgery is technically impossible, or inadvisable. The first group largely comprises those eyes that have already undergone repeated glaucoma surgery leaving extensive scarring of the limbal conjunctiva – it is no longer acceptable to undertake fistulising surgery in the inferior 180° of the limbus, for there is an unacceptably high risk of postoperative endophthalmitis.[32] The second group is those eyes for which fistulising surgery is not advisable. The composition of this group is of interest and falls into three categories: firstly, eyes where ocular decompression creates unacceptable risk, either from ocular decompression such as Sturge–Weber Syndrome, because of bleeding into the suprachoroidal space, and aniridia, because of the risk from lens corneal contact; secondly, eyes where internal closure of the fistula is very likely, such as the iridocorneal endothelial (ICE) syndrome, because of spread of the aberrant endothelial cells over the inside of the bleb; and thirdly, eyes where tear quality deficiency increases the risk of postoperative infection, such as atopy. The absolute indication for tube surgery must, however, be left to the surgeon when faced with an individual case.

Tube surgery involves the placement of a non-allergenic silicone tube into the anterior chamber (at the limbus), or the vitreous cavity (via the pars plana). The small cross sectional diameter of the tube allows insertion into the eye through a small entry site thus minimising ocular decompression. Fluid passes down the tube to a plate or sump and is absorbed through the fibrous tissue capsule around the plate.[33] There needs to be a rate retarding device, such as a valve (Krupin, Ahmed) stent[34] or external (vicryl) tie to limit aqueous egress over the first 4 weeks while a fibrous tissue capsule develops around the plate (Figure 11.11).[35] The long-

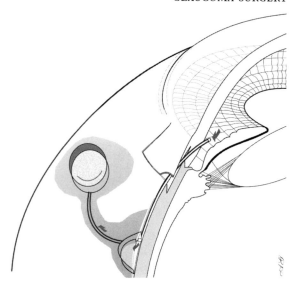

Figure 11.11 A double plate Molteno tube. The arrows show aqueous exit route to the fibrous tissue capsule covering the first plate and then continuing on to the second plate

term success of the operation depends upon fluid flowing across the fibrous tissue capsule that develops around the plate. The hydraulic resistance to flow probably increases with time, so that the larger surface area plates may well offer some advantages.[36]

The tube is separated from the conjunctiva at the limbus by a lamellar scleral flap, donor sclera, fascia lata or other explanted tissue, to prevent late conjunctival erosion. The plates are anchored over the equator between the rectus muscles. There is no ideal design of tube. Molteno,[37] Krupin,[38] Ahmed[39] and Baerveldt[40] are the devices currently used. Because indications for implantation are following repeated glaucoma surgery, the healing response will be aggressive. In these circumstances antimetabolites should be applied to the under-surface of the conjunctiva overlying the plate(s).[41–43]

The major complications of tube surgery occur early as a result of ocular hypotony from bulk outflow and late from erosion, failure, and corneal tube contact. Slightly surprisingly, infection is an unusual complication (Table 11.2).

Table 11.2 Complications of tube surgery

A) Early – due to bulk outflow
Flat anterior chamber/tube endothelial contact
Choroidal effusions/suprachoroidal haemorrhage
B) Late
Corneal endothelial decomposition from tube contact
  (especially in diabetic eyes. Remember "eye-rubbing"
  in children)
Tube extrusion from the anterior chamber – particularly
  with eye growth in children
Tube occlusion – especially with coexistent iritis
Conjunctival erosion – at suture lines over the tube
Loss of IOP control – fibrosis around the plate

The results of glaucoma surgery

A successful result for glaucoma treatment has by consensus been a reduction of IOP to normal, or to a target pressure. The reduction is seen as a proxy for the true outcome of treatment that should be the halting of progression. Target pressures today are set at levels that are most likely to halt progression.[44] For the purposes of this discussion, results will be confined to the effect of surgery on IOP.

The trabeculectomy operation has a good record of successfully reducing IOP.[45] The results are best if the surgery was for primary open angle glaucoma in a Caucasian patient who has not been on medical treatment for too long a time,[2,46] i.e. there were no "risk factors" for failure. Depending on the level of pressure chosen as a criterion for successful surgery, the reported success rates are 80–90%, with a survival rate at five years around 70%, without any added medical treatment.[47,48] Should the IOP after surgery fail to achieve the desired target pressure, additional reduction can usually be achieved by the addition of anti-glaucoma medications, so that together, medical and surgical treatment can achieve IOP levels not reached by medical treatment alone. This has become of increasing importance with recognition of the low target pressures required to halt progressive visual field loss in high tension[44] and normal tension glaucoma.[49] Non-perforating surgery may have a similar effect to conventional fistulising surgery on reducing IOP. However, the published studies to date are mid-term[50–52] (Sourdille P. Personal Communication, March 1999), and have not had the benefit of peroperative anti-metabolites. Only further studies will show whether this type of surgery produces the same degree of long-term IOP control.

The different approaches for combined glaucoma and cataract surgery have been shown to achieve good reductions of IOP and, in the opinion of many surgeons, are the approach of choice for these two ocular conditions. The exact approach will depend upon individual preferences. To date there does not appear to be a great deal of difference between them in terms of IOP results.

Complications of glaucoma surgery

Complications are the Achilles' heel of glaucoma surgery. An essential part of the skill of the ophthalmic surgeon is to be able to prevent, and where necessary, to treat complications. There is concern that the widespread use of antimetabolites has increased their incidence. Non-perforating surgery may be less likely to produce many of the problems arising after fistulising surgery. The complications may be said to be "early" ("peroperative", days or weeks post-surgery), or "late" (months or years post-surgery) (Table 11.3). Many of these complications are associated with shallowing of the anterior chamber and causes for this have been set out in Table 11.4.

Table 11.3 Complications seen after glaucoma surgery

Early
  • Haemorrhages
  • Inflammation
  • Hypotony and shallow anterior chamber
  • Uveal effusion
  • Malignant glaucoma
  • "Wipe-out"
Late
  • Lens opacities and cataract
  • Long-lasting hypotony and maculopathy
  • Hypertension
Endophthalmitis
Loss of vision

Table 11.4   Shallowing of the anterior chamber after fistulising surgery

Cause	Features	Treatment
1) Soft eye		
Over drainage		
a) external	Seidel	surgical repair if masive leak
b) internal	effusions	await resolution
	(empty b-scan)	drain if affecting central VA
		await resolution
Underproduction no bleb	no effusions	
	epiciliary membrane	VR membrane peel
2) Hard eye		
Bleeding	choroidal mass	leave
	(b-scan with echoes)	drain for pain/v. high IOP
Misdirection	lens iris diaphragm forward	cycloplegics/vitrectomy/
	prominant ciliary processes CCAG	lens extn+post capsulotomy

Early complications

Haemorrhage

Bleeding into the anterior chamber may be a primary event, occurring at the time of surgery, or a secondary haemorrhage developing days later from a previously damaged blood vessel. The usual origin is in blood vessels lying at the root of the iris and cut at the time of the iridectomy. The risk of bleeding can be minimised by performing the iridectomy radically and/or away from the iris root. In eyes at high risk of bleeding the risk can be lessened by intraocular tamponade with a viscoelastic.

Inflammation

An aqueous flare and cells, together with heightened and prolonged episcleral congestion indicate postoperative anterior chamber inflammation. This inflammation will be associated with an increased fibroblast response in the episclera, increasing the risk of "early failure" after surgery. Eyes with pre-existing inflammatory eye disease prior to surgery, or a poor blood aqueous barrier, are all prone to this response. Once recognised it needs be suppressed with increased dosage of topical steroids.

Early ocular hypotony and shallow anterior chamber

Excess (bulk) outflow of aqueous from the anterior chamber in the immediate postoperative period will lead to hypotony and shallowing of the anterior chamber. The hypotony may well be complicated in eyes with unhealthy choroidal vasculature (because of advanced glaucoma, systemic cardiovascular disease or choroidal disease), and is caused by an exudation of hyperosmolar fluid into the suprachoroidal space. In severe cases rupture of a choroidal blood vessel will lead to a suprachoroidal haemorrhage. The hyperosmolar fluid promotes non-conventional outflow of aqueous with further shallowing of the anterior chamber and maintenance of the hypotony. The process will continue until a) the cause of the bulk outflow through the trabeculectomy is halted, and b) the osmololality of the suprachoroidal fluid falls below intravascular levels and it is absorbed. Unfortunately choroidal effusions divert aqueous away from the trabeculectomy and are associated with episcleral congestion. These two combine to promote wound healing around the fistula, so that by the time the effusion absorbs, the trabeculectomy flap is scarred tightly shut.

It is essential to recognise the possibility of this complication. The scleral flap should be seen at the end of the operation to provide resistance to fluid outflow by the force required to inject balanced salt solution into the anterior chamber. The IOP at the end of the operation should be well within the normal range (as assessed by digital or applanation tonometry).

If doubt persists after these manoeuvres, the anterior chamber can be reflated with a visco-elastic at the end of surgery.

Should ocular hypotony with shallowing of the anterior chamber develop in the immediate postoperative period, the eye needs to be checked for aqueous leaks. Massive leaks (continuous fluid trail from the limbus to the lower eyelid margin) need immediate repair. Small leaks will heal spontaneously. Shallowing of the anterior chamber is associated with the formation of choroidal effusion. Fluid in the suprachoroidal space leads to anterior rotation of the ciliary body on scleral spur with forward movement of the lens–iris diaphragm. Only massive effusions that cause visual loss should be drained. The anterior chamber should only be reformed if the lens comes into contact with the cornea, otherwise spontaneous reformation can be awaited. Scarring of the bleb should be minimised during the period of minimal drainage with intensive topical steroids and subconjunctival injections of 5FU.

Ocular hypertension

The use of releasable sutures and laser suture-lysis has allowed the surgeon to err on the side of "tightly sewn" flaps, often followed by increased IOP at the time of the first dressing. Massage, suture release, and "needling" (whereby a narrow gauge needle is insinuated beneath the lamellar scleral flap to separate any blood clot) will all allow free aqueous flow at this time. Progressive fibrosis can then increase resistance to flow with rising IOP. This needs to be corrected with fibroblast inhibitors such as topical steroids and subconjunctival 5FU.

Suprachoroidal haemorrhage

This is a rare peroperative complication of fistulising surgery. Eyes predisposed are those with high myopia, high preoperative IOP, and eyes that have undergone previous vitrectomy or intracapsular surgery. Characteristically the anterior chamber shallows after the eye has been opened and decompressed. The IOP may well increase depending on the volume of blood that enters the suprachoroidal space. Immediate treatment involves closure of the wound with tight suture closure, so that increasing IOP can tamponade the affected blood vessel. Subsequent treatment depends on the degree of pain and hypertension. In about one third of cases, either of these two problems is sufficient to warrant further surgery to drain the blood. Most cases can be left to resolve spontaneously.[53]

Malignant glaucoma

Malignant glaucoma, also called ciliary block glaucoma and aqueous misdirection syndrome, is characterised by a shallow anterior chamber associated with raised IOP in the presence of a patent iridectomy. The term malignant was used originally to describe the fact that topical pilocarpine seemed to worsen the condition. In this condition aqueous fluid passes posteriorly into the posterior segment, rather than anteriorly into the posterior chamber. This misdirection is secondary to obstruction at the site of the tips of the ciliary processes, and their close proximity to the lens equator. Eyes predisposed to this are typically eyes with small anterior segments, usually seen and undergoing treatment for chronic angle closure glaucoma.[54]

Aqueous misdirection is seen in the postoperative period, typically days rather than weeks, less commonly months later. The lens iris diaphragm moves forwards, the angle of the anterior chamber narrows and the sclerostomy fails.

Treatment is by giving topical cycloplegic drugs. Atropine 1% 2–4 times a day may be required. It may need to be continued for weeks, occasionally months or years. Should this fail, then remedial surgery designed to remove the obstruction is required. This can be localised aspiration of the anterior vitreous, i.e. that closest to the suspensory ligament (difficult to achieve in the phakic eye), or lens removal, together with a posterior capsulotomy. The former approach succeeds by removing the direct cause of the block, the latter by bypassing it.[54]

"Wipe-out"

A rare complication of filtration surgery is the loss of central field in the immediate postoperative period. The phenomenon "wipe-out" seems to occur most often when there is visual loss splitting fixation. The cause is unknown but is probably caused by sudden vascular insufficiency in an already compromised eye. Patients who complain of sudden visual loss in this way should be investigated for other causes, such as macular haemorrhage and oedema, before concluding that the patient has suffered visual loss in this way.[55–57]

Late complications

Lens opacities and cataract

Lens opacities and cataract may develop as a direct result of earlier complications, such as anterior capsular opacities after lens corneal touch, or posterior opacities with long-term steroid use. More often there appears to be an increase in the rate of developing sclerosis of the lens at a rate faster than would be expected from ageing effect alone. The cause of this is unclear, whether it can be a complication of the glaucoma, medical treatment, the surgery, or antimetabolites (see above). The development is sufficiently frequent to ensure that many elderly patients require lens removal one to two years after fistulising surgery.

Hypotony and hypotony "maculopathy"

Ocular hypotension can be said to be an IOP lower than two standard deviations from the mean, and may be physiological. Hypotony, on the other hand, is an IOP low enough to produce ocular morbidity. Late hypotony appears to be a problem associated with dissolution of the conjunctiva overlying the sclerostomy.[58] This is seen after the application of peroperative metabolites,[59] particularly mitomycin C.[60–62] Death of the surface epithelium allows transconjunctival drainage. At first this is restricted to punctate leaks (shown on fluorescein staining as multiple staining areas or

"sweating"). Continuation of the conjunctival degeneration leads to larger leaks with frank hole formation in the conjunctiva. The fluorescein appearances of "sweating" and frank hole formation are shown in Figure 11.12a and b. The rate of flow exceeds the rate of aqueous production and hypotony ensues.

Ocular hypotony induces fluctuations in vision, perhaps because of distortion from eyelid movements. The low IOP causes shortening of the eyeball, which in turn produces radiating perifoveal folds in the retinal pigment epithelium visible on fundoscopy. Persistence is followed by degenerative change in the overlying retina and permanent visual loss. Thus a low IOP without visual symptoms and physical signs of choroidopathy may just be watched, but with symptoms, and particularly with visible

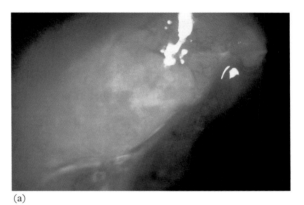

(a)

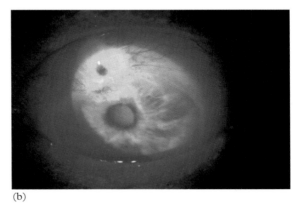

(b)

Figure 11.12 Transconjunctival flow of aqueous (a) "sweating" with puctuate fluoresein staining, and (b) frank leak with dilution of fluorescein by the aqueous stream.

retinal change, it needs to be treated (Figure 11.13).

Treatment is designed to reduce bulk outflow of aqueous, "stem the leak". Should this be due to "sweating" then inflammation in the bleb can be stimulated by the injection of autologous blood.[63,64] Typically there is a frank hole which usually requires repair of the conjunctiva over the sclerostomy.[65] The scleral flap needs be examined at the time of repair to ensure that any defect here is detected and repaired too (Figure 11.14).[66,67]

The failing bleb

After many years of good control some eyes undergo a slow increase in IOP. Histological examination of the drainage blebs in these cases shows layered deposition of collagen interspersed with ground substance. This deposition is the result of slow replication of fibroblasts around the sclerostomy with a progressive increase in resistance in fluid flow across its walls.[68] The fibroblast activity may have been a response to chemical constituents in the aqueous,[69] or a mechanical "stretch" effect of increased surface tension on vessel walls.[70] Any insult such as intraocular surgery (cataract extraction) or inflammation (blebitis) which boosts fibroblast activity, will hasten this process. In theory, long-term topical antiglaucoma drops applied to such eyes to reduce IOP will

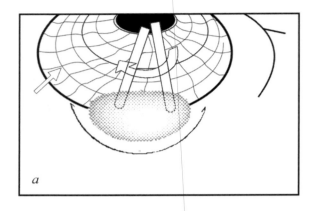

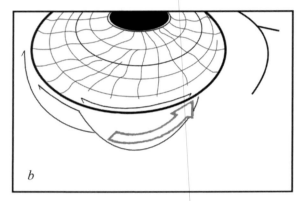

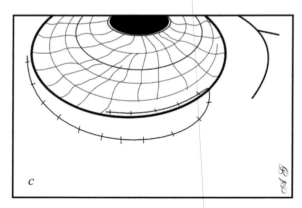

Figure 11.14 Stages in the repair of a degenerate bleb in an eye with chronic hypotony

(a) the small arrow shows the site for an initial praracentesis for injection of viscoelastic to reflate the eye. The oval shaded area shows the site of the dissecting bleb. The large arrow shows the dissection with a blunt spatula of the bleb surface from the underlying cornea, prior to its removal

(b) and (c) shows rotation of full thickness conjunctival flap to cover the defect. Care should be taken to close any scleral defect first.

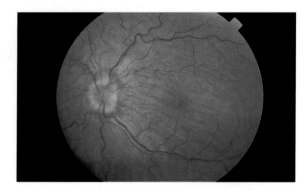

Figure 11.13 Fundus picture showing retinal folds in hypotony choroidopathy.

also stimulate fibroblast activity and hasten the process of "bleb failure".

A proportion of these eyes will require further fistulising surgery. This can be a revision at the same site, or a new operation at an adjacent site. With revision it is usually necessary to apply antimetabolite to the underside of the bleb to inhibit further fibroblast proliferation. Care must be taken not to introduce the drug into the eye through any sclerostomy that might still exist.

Endophthalmitis and "blebitis"

The thin walled avascular bleb is a recognised entry route for opportunist infection into the eye. Risk factors include the following:

- prominent and exposed blebs, ocular trauma, contact lens wear
- abnormal tear quality, reduced lysozyme content (atopes, dry eye states)
- chronic eyelid infection – blepharitis
- lacrimal sac infection – mucoceles
- trabeculectomies sited in the inferior 180° of the limbus.

The timing of the infection appears to depend upon the development of the avascular bleb resulting in reduced resistance to bacterial contamination. As this develops over time, it can be assumed that the risk will increase over time. An overall rate of 1% per year is probably a reasonable estimate.

Blebitis refers to the presence of exudate within the bleb, but without evidence for inflammation within the eye. Endopthalmitis presumes that the infection has penetrated within the eye. In both cases the patient will give a recent history of redness, pain and discharge, followed by visual loss. In these eyes there will be cellular activity within the eye, ranging from a few cells within the anterior chamber to an hypopyon plus vitreous cellular activity. The duration of symptoms is inversely proportional to the virulence of the organism.

The most commonly involved bacteria are *streptococci, haemophillus influenzae* and *staphylococci*.

Treatment should be both topical and systemic (vancomycin 25 mg/ml, cefazoline 50mg/ml or amikacin 50 mg/ml), for blebitis and endophthalmitis, and should be a combination of drugs able to combat gram positive and gram negative organisms. Treatment should be started without waiting for culture results. In addition intravitreal culture and injection of intravitreal (vancomycin 1mg/0.1ml and cephazolin 2mg/0.1 ml or amikacin 0.5 mg/0.1ml) often with dexamethasone 0.5 mg/0.1ml, injected separately at the pars plana through the same 30 G needle).[23]

The low complication rate of non-penetrating surgery

Non-penetrating glaucoma surgery appears to offer a lower risk of complications than conventional fistulising surgery. This is because early postoperative hypotony seems to be uncommon, and late bleb related complications seem to be rare. It remains to be seen if the long term complication rate remains as low.

References

1 Jay JL, Allan D. The benefit of early trabeculectomy versus conventional management in primary open angle glaucoma relative to severity of disease. *Eye* 1989; **3**: 528–35.
2 Migdal C, Gregory W, Hitchings R. Long-term functional outcome after early surgery compared with laser and medicine in open-angle glaucoma. *Ophthalmology* 1994; **101**: 1651–6.
3 Elliott RH. A preliminary note on a new operative procedure for the establishment of a filtering cicatrix in the treatment of glaucoma. *Ophthalmoscope* 1909; 7: 807.
4 Elliott RH. Sclero-corneal trephining in the Operative treatment of glaucoma. 1913. George Pulman & Sons.
5 Scheie HG. Retraction of scleral wound edges as a fistulising procedure for glaucoma. *Am J Ophthalmol* 1958; **45**: 220.
6 Cairns JE. Trabeculectomy. Preliminary report of a new method. *Am J Ophthalmol* 1968; **5**: 673–7.
7 Savage JA, Condon GP, Lytle RA, Simmons RJ. Laser suture lysis after trabeculectomy. *Ophthalmology* 1988; **95**: 1631–8.
8 Kolker AE, Kass MA, Rait JL. Trabeculectomy with releasable sutures. *Trans Am Ophthalmol Soc* 1993; **91**: 131–41.
9 Johnstone MA, Wellington DP, Ziel CJ. A releasable scleral-flap tamponade suture for guarded filtration surgery. *Arch Ophthalmol* 1993; **111**: 398–403.
10 Zimmerman TJ, Kooner KS, Ford VJ, *et al.* Trabeculectomy vs. nonpenetrating trabeculectomy: a retrospec-

tive study of two procedures in phakic patients with glaucoma. *Ophmalmic Surg* 1984; **15**: 734–40.

11 Kozlov VI, Bagrou SN, Anisimoua SY, Osipov AV, Mogilevtsev VV. Non penetrating deep sclerectomy with collagen. *IRTC (Eye Microsurgery)* 1990; 3 RSFSR Ministry of Public Health, Moscow 44–6.

12 Steigmann R. Viscocanalostomy. *Highlights Ophthalmol* 1996; **4**: 67–70.

13 Bechetoille A, Bresson–Dumont H, Urier N. Non penetrating trabeculectomy with aspiration of justacanalicular trabeculum: Six month follow-up in primary open angle glaucoma. *Invest Ophthalmol Vis Sci* 1998; **39**(4): 5473–7.

14 Kershner RM. Nonpenetrating trabeculectomy with placement of a collagen drainage device. *J Cataract Refract Surg* 1995; **21**: 608–11.

15 Chen PP, Budenz DL. The effects of cataract extraction on the visual field of eyes with chronic open-angle glaucoma. *Am J Ophthalmol* 1998; **125**: 325–33.

16 Hurvitz LM. Combined surgery for cataract and glaucoma. *Curr Opinion Ophthal* 1993; **4**: 73–8.

17 Wyse T, Meyer M, Ruderman JM, et al. Combined trabeculectomy and phacoemulsification: a one-site vs a two-site approach. *Am J Ophthalmol* 1998; **125**: 334–9.

18 Wishart PK, Austin MW. Combined cataract extraction and trabeculectomy: phacoemulsification compared with extracapsular technique. *Ophmalic Surg* 1993; **24**: 814–21.

19 Joos KM, Bueche MJ, Palmberg PF, Feuer WJ, Grajewski AL. One-year follow-up results of combined mitomycin C trabeculectomy and extracapsular cataract extraction. *Ophthalmology* 1995; **102**: 76–83.

20 Gianoli F, Mermoud A. (Cataract-glaucoma combined surgery: comparison between phacoemulsification combined with deep sclerectomy, or trabeculectomy) Chirurgie combinee cataracte-glaucome: comparaison entre phacoemulsification associee a une sclerectomie profonde, ou a une trabeculectomie. *Klin Monatsbl Augenheilkd* 1997; **210**: 256–60.

21 Chen CW, Huang HT, Sheu MM. Enhancement of IOP control. Effect of trabeculectomy by local application of an anticancer drug . Act XXV Con Ophth 1986; 1487.

22 Kitazawa Y, Kawase K, Matsushita H, Minobe M. Trabeculectomy with mitomycin: A comparative study with fluorouracil. *Arch Ophthalmol* 1991; **109**: 1693–8.

23 Khaw PT, Sherwood MB, Doyle JW, et al. Intraoperative and post operative treatment with 5–fluorouracil and mitomycin-c: long term effects in vivo on subconjunctival and scleral fibroblasts. *Int Ophthalmol* 1992; **16**: 381–5.

24 Egbert PR, Williams AS, Singh K, Dadzie P, Egbert TB. A prospective trial of intraoperative fluorouracil during trabeculectomy in a black population. *Am J Ophthalmol* 1993; **116**: 612–6.

25 Lanigan L, Sturmer J, Baez KA, Hitchings RA, Khaw PT. Single intraoperative applications of 5-fluorouracil during filtration surgery: early results. *Br J Ophthalmol* 1994; **78**: 33–7.

26 Weinreb RN. Adjusting the dose of 5–fluorouracil after filtration surgery to minimize side effects. *Ophthalmology* 1987; **94**: 564–70.

27 Anonymous. Five-year follow-up of the Fluorouracil Filtering Surgery Study. The Fluorouracil Filtering Surgery Study Group. *Am J Ophthalmol* 1996; **121**: 349–66.

28 Khaw PT, Grierson I, Hitchings RA, Rice NS. 5-fluor-

ouracil and beyond (editorial). *Br J Ophthalmol* 1991; **75**: 577–8.

29 Khaw PT, Doyle JW, Sherwood MB, Grierson I, Schultz G, McGorray S. Prolonged localized tissue effects from 5–minute exposures to fluorouracil and mitomycin C. *Arch Ophthalmol* 1993; **111**: 263–7.

30 Megevand GS, Salmon JF, Scholtz RP, Murray AD. The effect of reducing the exposure time of mitomycin C in glaucoma filtering surgery. *Ophthalmology* 1995; **102**: 84–90.

31 Robin AL, Ramakrishnan R, Krishnadas R, et al. A long-term dose-response study of mitomycin in glaucoma filtration surgery (see comments). *Arch Ophthalmol* 1997; **115**: 969–74.

32 Caronia RM, Liebmann JM, Friedman R, Cohen H, Ritch R. Trabeculectomy at the inferior limbus. *Arch Ophthalmol* 1996; **114**: 387–91.

33 Hitchings RA. Tube implants, their development and role in glaucoma care. In: Al Sayyad F, Spaeth GL, Shields MB, Hitchings RA (eds). The Refractory glaucomas. 1st edn. New York, Tokyo: Igaku-Shion, 1995: 200–26.

34 Sherwood MB, Smith MF. Prevention of early hypotony associated with Molteno implants by a new occluding stent technique. *Ophthalmology* 1993; **100**: 85–90.

35 Lim KS, Allan BD, Lloyd AW, Muir A, Khaw PT. Glaucoma drainage devices; past, present, and future. *Br J Ophthalmol* 1998; **82**: 1083–9.

36 Hitchings RA, Joseph NH, Sherwood MB, Lattimer J, Miller MH. Use of one-piece valved tube and variable surface area explant for glaucoma drainage surgery. *Ophthalmology* 1987; **94**: 1079–84.

37 Price FW Jr, Wellemeyer M. Long-term results of Molteno implants. *Ophmalic Surg* 1995; **26**: 130–5.

38 Krupin T, Kaufman P, Mandell AI, et al. Long-term results of valve implants in filtering surgery for eyes with neovascular glaucoma. *Am J Ophthalmol* 1983; **95**: 775–82.

39 Coleman AL, Hill R, Wilson MR, et al. Initial clinical experience with the Ahmed Glaucoma Valve implant. *Am J Ophthalmol* 1995; **120**: 23–31.

40 Lloyd MA, Baerveldt G, Heuer DK, Minckler DS, Martone JF. Initial clinical experience with the Baerveldt implant in complicated glaucomas. *Ophthalmology* 1994; **101**: 640–50.

41 Susanna R Jr, Nicolela MT, Takahashi WY. Mitomycin C as adjunctive therapy with glaucoma implant surgery. *Ophmalic Surg* 1994; **25**: 458–62.

42 Perkins TW, Cardakli UF, Eisele JR, Kaufman PL, Heatley GA. Adjunctive mitomycin C in Molteno implant surgery. *Ophthalmology* 1995; **102**: 91–7.

43 Perkins TW, Gangnon R, Ladd W, Kaufman PL, Libby CM. Molteno implant with mitomycin C: intermediate-term results. *J Glaucoma* 1998; 7: 86–92.

44 Palmberg P. Epidemiology of POAG and rationale for therapy. *Glaucoma Abstracts* 1989; **6**: 10–23.

45 Jay JL, Murray SB. Characteristics of reduction of IOP after trabeculectomy. *Br J Ophthalmol* 1980; **64**: 432–5.

46 Lavin MJ, Wormald RPL, Migdal CS, Hitchings RA. The influence of prior therapy on the success of trabeculectomy. *Arch Ophthalmol* 1990; **108**: 1543–8.

47 Watson PG, Grierson I. The place of trabeculectomy in the treatment of glaucoma. *Ophthalmology* 1981; **88**: 175–96.

48 Mills KB. Trabeculectomy: a retrospective long-term

follow-up of 444 cases. *Br J Ophthalmol* 1981; **65**: 790–5.

49 Collaborative normal tension glaucoma study group. The effectiveness of intraocular pressure reduction in the treatment of normal-tension glaucoma. *Am J Ophthalmol* 1998; **126**: 498–505.

50 Sanchez E, Schnyder CC, Mermoud A. (Comparative results of deep sclerectomy transformed to trabeculectomy and classical trabeculectomy) Resultats comparatifs de la sclerectomie profonde transformee en trabeculectomie et de la trabeculectomie classique. *Klin Monatsbl Augenheilkd* 1997; **210**: 261–4.

51 Sanchez E, Schnyder CC, Sickenberg M, Chiou AG, Hediguer SE, Mermoud A. Deep sclerectomy: results with and without collagen implant. *Int Ophthalmol* 1996; **20**: 157–62.

52 Demailly P, Lavat P, Kretz G, Jeanteur-Lunel MN. Nonpenetrating deep sclerectomy (NPDS) with or without collagen device (CD) in primary open-angle glaucoma: middle-term retrospective study. *Int Ophthalmol* 1996; **20**: 131–40.

53 Reynolds MG, Haimovici R, Flynn HWJ, Di BC, Byrne SF, Feuer W. Suprachoroidal hemorrhage. Clinical features and results of secondary surgical management (see comments). *Ophthalmology* 1993; **100**: 460–5.

54 Ruben S, Tsai J, Hitchings RA. Malignant glaucoma and its management. *Br J Ophthalmol* 1997; **81**: 163–7.

55 Kolker AE. Visual prognosis in advanced glaucoma: a comparison of medical and surgical therapy for retention of vision in 101 eyes with advanced glaucoma. *Trans Am Ophthalmol Soc* 1977; **75**: 539–55.

56 Henry JC. Snuff Syndrome. *J Glaucoma* 1994; **3**: 92–5.

57 Bayer AU, Erb C, Ferrari F, Knorr M, Thiel HJ. The Tubingen Glaucoma Study. Glaucoma filtering surgery – a retrospective long-term follow-up of 254 eyes with glaucoma. *German J Ophthalmol* 1995; **4**: 289–93.

58 Migdal CS, Hitchings RA. Morbidity following prolonged postoperative hypotony after trabeculectomy. *Ophmalic Surg* 1988; **19**: 865–7.

59 Stamper RL, McMenemy MG, Lieberman MF. Hypotonus maculopathy after trabeculectomy with subconjunctival 5–fluorouracil. *Am J Ophthalmol* 1992; **114**: 544–53.

60 Geijssen HC, Greve EL. Mitomycin, suture-lysis and hypotony. *Int Ophthalmol* 1992; **16**: 371–4.

61 Zacharia PT, Deppermann SR, Schuman JS. Ocular hypotony after trabeculectomy with mitomycin C. *Am J Ophthalmol* 1993; **116**: 314–26.

62 Seah SKL, Prata JA, Minckler DS, Baerveldt G, Lee P, Heuer DK. Hypotony following trabeculectomy. *J Glaucoma* 1995; **4**: 73–9.

63 Wise JB. Treatment of chronic postfiltration hypotony by intrableb injection of autologous blood. *Arch Ophthalmol* 1994; **111**: 827–30.

64 Leen MM, Moster MR, Katz LJ, Terebuh AK, Schmidt CM, Spaeth GL. Management of overfiltering and leaking blebs with autologous blood injection. *Arch Ophthalmol* 1995; **113**: 1050–5.

65 Duker JS, Schuman JS. Successful surgical treatment of hypotony maculopathy following trabeculectomy with topical mitomycin C. *Ophmalic Surg* 1994; **25**: 463–5.

66 Schwartz GF, Robin AL, Wilson RP, Suan EP, Pheasant TR, Prensky JG. Resuturing the scleral flap leads to resolution of hypotony maculopathy. *J Glaucoma* 1996; **5**: 246–51.

67 Haynes WL, Alward WA. Rapid visual recovery and long term intraocular pressure control after donor scleral patch grafting for trabeculectomy induced hypotony maculopathy. *J Glaucoma* 1995; **4**: 200–1.

68 Hitchings RA, Grierson I. Clinicopathological correlation in eyes with failed fistulising surgery. *Trans Ophthalmol Soc UK* 1983; **103**: 84–8.

69 Joseph JP, Grierson I, Hitchings RA. Chemotactic activity of aqueous humor. A cause of failure of trabeculectomies? *Arch Ophthalmol* 1989; **107**: 69–74.

70 Riser B, Cortes P, Zhao X, Bernstein J, Dumler F, Nairns R. Intraglomerular pressure and mesangial stretching stimulates extracellular matrix formation in rats. *J Clin Invest* 1992; **90**: 1932–43.

12 Cost of treatment: international treatment patterns, prescribing habits and costs

G KOBELT

Treatment patterns for chronic disease will inevitably vary from country to country. This variation is the result of both the availability of treatments, and the expertise and inclinations of the physician. The result can be quite startling differences in approach to the same disease. This chapter looks at some of the differences that can be found in the management of chronic glaucoma, and pays particular attention to the resulting differences in costs.

Issues in economic studies of glaucoma

Despite the high and growing prevalence of glaucoma, economic assessments have been rather scarce compared to other diseases. One explanation may be that treatment options are relatively limited, and for many of them, rather inexpensive. In addition, the disease affects mainly the elderly population and has, therefore, even when severe, limited consequences in terms of production losses.

The total direct cost of treating the disease is, however, not negligible, and the practising ophthalmologist can no longer ignore the economic challenge of glaucoma management. The demand from society and payers to justify uses of scarce resources, particularly in chronic diseases, is increasing. The resources used for detecting and treating glaucoma, therefore compete with alternative uses of resources, both within and outside the field of ophthalmology.

Two recent studies have estimated the cost of glaucoma treatment, in the UK in 1990,[1] and in Sweden in 1995.[2] Costs in the UK were estimated at £88 million, (US$140 million), and in Sweden at 375 million Swedish kronor (US$ 48 million). Thus, costs per capita are lower in the UK when the commercial exchange rate is used, and there are several likely explanations for this. Direct spending on a disease is influenced by a number of factors, both medical and economic. The most obvious among these factors related to healthcare are the availability of screening programmes, the number of and the access to medical facilities, the number of ophthalmologists, the choice of treatment alternatives, the prevailing treatment strategies or treatment sequences, and the resources used for them. Other important factors are the price of the different resources, the payment system, and the incentive structure within the system. Prices for different resources vary between countries because both the general price level and the relative prices may differ, which in turn will influence the resource use. A complicating factor is that in healthcare market prices are not always available for the resources, and that prices or charges sometimes bear no relation to the true opportunity cost of the resource. Comparisons of the cost of treatment between countries, and even within countries, are therefore rather difficult and provide limited insights. However, if the use of different resources to achieve a similar goal is compared, valuable information on the costs and outcome of different treatment strategies may be gained.

Whenever new treatments are introduced it is necessary to estimate their impact on both outcome and costs, and economic evaluation is a valuable tool to analyse the cost-effectiveness of new treatments. However, a treatment is never cost-effective in itself, but only in a defined indication and in relation to a defined alternative. When many alternatives are available, there will also be a large number of different treatment strategies, and the choice will be between strategies, not individual treatments. Glaucoma is a good example of the need for, and the importance of, investigating the cost-effectiveness of different treatment strategies. Different alternatives are available, surgical interventions as well as pharmaceutical products, and the costs of patient management can vary considerably, depending on the sequence in which they are used. Several new topical agents have recently been introduced, increasing both the need for knowledge about current use of resources, as well as the interest in the potential effects on outcome of these new agents and the changes they will introduce in patient management.

Cost-effectiveness analysis in glaucoma presents a challenge. The ultimate goal of treatment is to avoid disease progression to blindness, by treating elevated intraocular pressure (IOP). The available epidemiology does not provide a definite link and risk-function between elevated IOP and the final outcome. In clinical practice, IOP is used to assess the effectiveness of treatments, but it does not represent an outcome measure that expresses a patient benefit. Thus, analyses are limited to assess the costs of different strategies to manage IOP, while the clinical objective has to be accepted as a given.

Patient management and costs in current clinical practice

Assessments of the effectiveness of different treatments are usually available only from published clinical trials. Such studies will pro-spectively compare alternative individual treatments, but will seldom include sequences of different treatments. Treatments will be assessed for efficacy and safety under strictly controlled conditions and in selected patient groups. While this provides all required information with a high internal validity, it is usually quite different from what happens in normal clinical practice. Treatments will be used in a wider range of patients and in different settings, leading sometimes to quite different results. It is therefore important to observe treatment in normal practice to confirm the outcome and/or speculate on the potential impact on changes in therapy. Clearly this is a time-consuming and costly exercise and prospective observation may not always be possible. Retrospective chart analyses provide an alternative for data collection, although one has to accept that some of the information will be incomplete and some of the data imprecise. The clinician will likely rely more on the controlled data, while the payer will be focusing more on the real clinical practice. The truth may lie somewhere in between, and it is therefore interesting to combine the two.

A recent chart review in nine different countries on three continents provides interesting insight into prevailing treatment patterns and resulting costs in a broadly defined group of patients.[2–6] The study included patients with recently diagnosed primary open angle glaucoma or ocular hypertension who had started treatment with standard β-blocker monotherapy (Table 12.1). In all countries a retrospective analysis of individual patient charts was performed in a number of representative sites, using the same data collection protocol and method. At baseline, patient demographics and data on diagnosis, and relevant co-morbidity were collected. Details on all resource utilisation, therapy changes and reasons for them, as well as the development of IOP in both eyes, was retrospectively followed for two years after treatment initiation. Standard costs for each resource were determined in each country and

Table 12.1 Study Population: a country by country comparison

	Australia	Canada	France	Germany	Netherlands	Spain	Sweden	UK	USA
Total sample	203	243	225	200	200	242	218	208	264
Females	102	140	117	115	115	142	120	102	174
Males	101	103	108	85	85	100	98	106	90
Mean age (years)	64.3	63.9	60.7	63.7	66.8	64.5	69	67.8	68.3
Ethnic Origin: Caucasian	115	226	217	200	200	242	213	186	73
Black	2	11	7	–	–	–	2		30
Other	1	5	1	–	–	–	2		6
Diagnosis (baseline)									
POAG Simplex	190	174	177	142	175	175	122	164	187
Ocular hypertension	8	58	40	44	25	27	12	38	72
Exfoliation glaucoma	5	5	7	9	–	36	84	3	5
Pigmented glaucoma		6	1	5	–	4	–	3	–
VFD in study eye									
None, or minor	115	148	95	49	113	115	96	112	166
Moderate	51	47	75	111	66	89	68	52	48
Severe	37	22	55	40	21	38	51	34	15
ONH in study eye									
None or minor excavation	57	133	90	65	77	115	88	117	105
Moderate excavation	68	77	65	120	86	90	87	60	105
Severe excavation	78	29	70	15	37	37	43	31	27
IOP in study eye									
at baseline (mm Hg)	25.9	28.8	23.9	31.2	25.5	26.6	31.5	28.6	25.5

an average cost of treatment per patient for the period calculated.

The results of this analysis, which covers treatment practices between 1992–1996, are interesting in several ways. Clearly, goals of treatment are similar, but the means to reach them vary substantially both between and within countries.

From a medical point of view, the goal of treatment appears to be to lower IOP to a target level of around 18 mm Hg. However, the criteria for initiating therapy are very different, as are the sequences of different second- and third-line treatments following β-blockers. These variations can to some extent be explained by the variations in financing and organisation of the healthcare system. The point of entry into the system, a university clinic, a surgical centre or an office-based medical ophthalmologist, will influence the choice of treatment. For the most part the variations between different hospitals and different practitioners remain unexplained. From an economic point of view, total cost per patient as well as costs of the individual resources are very different in different countries. However, costs in all

countries are consistently correlated with the initial level of IOP, the initial treatment success and the subsequent number of treatment changes. This result is surprisingly stable across countries despite the differences in both the types and quantities of resources used and the prices. It indicates a strong rationality in the treatment, in so far as costs are related to the severity of the disease as well as to the effectiveness of the initial treatment.

Similarities and differences in goals of treatment

The following summaries will look at results from this study across countries, pointing to similarities and differences, while focusing on medical parameters and resource use that appear to drive the costs.

IOP is consistently recorded on patient charts as the one parameter that can be influenced with treatment, and all recordings were collected to estimate treatment effect. The effect was analysed as the change in IOP after initiation of treatment and at the end of two years (Table 12.2). IOP levels differed considerably at

Table 12.2 IOP Development

IOP in mm Hg at baseline, after two weeks treatment (first) and at the end of the 2 year follow-up (last), and the reductions, in percent of baseline IOP after two weeks treatment and at the end of the 2 year follow-up in nine different countries. Success (%) reports the number of patients, in per cent of all patients, that were still controlled on the initial treatment after 2 years

Country	IOP Baseline	IOP First	Red (%)	IOP Last	Red (%)	Success (%)
Australia	25.9	21.1	4.8	18.6	7.4	43.8
Canada	28.8	21.1	7.7	19.4	9.4	63.4
France	23.9	19.8	4.1	17.5	6.4	58.2
Germany	31.2	21.8	9.4	18.8	12.4	46.0
The Netherlands	25.5	20.1	5.4	18.4	7.1	56.0
Spain	26.6	22.4	4.2	18.3	8.3	30.2
Sweden	31.5	21.2	10.3	18.8	12.7	42.2
UK	28.6	20.7	7.9	19.0	9.6	73.1
USA	25.5	19.4	6.1	18.4	7.1	53.0
Mean	27.5	20.8	6.7	18.6	8.9	51.8

baseline, with the highest levels seen in Sweden (31.5 mm Hg) and the lowest levels in France (23.9 mm Hg) and a mean of 27.5 mm Hg. The first IOP measure after initiation of treatment showed a much narrower range (19.4–22.4 mm Hg), a mean reduction of 6.7 mm Hg. In all countries, after two years the mean IOP was 18 mm Hg (17.5–19.4 mm Hg), regardless of baseline IOP levels. This is higher than the 14–16 mm Hg seen in normal subjects of this age group, indicating that normal IOP levels could not be reached with treatments available at the time of the study.

In addition to the initial effect on IOP, the success of the first line treatment could be estimated as the proportion of patients remaining on their first monotherapy at the end of the two year period. However, there was again a large variation in this proportion between the countries, ranging from 30% in Spain to 73% in the UK, with a mean of 52% (Table 12.2).

Interestingly, the proportion of patients maintained on initial treatment did not seem correlated with the magnitude of the initial effect on IOP, but influenced more by treatment preferences in the different countries. On the other hand, the initial treatment effect had a very strong negative correlation with the mean treatment costs over two years. This would be expected, as an unsatisfactory treatment effect

will lead to one or more changes in therapy around which the patients will be more closely monitored, with more visits and tests. Multiple changes clearly increase the cost, and in all countries costs were positively correlated with the number of changes, while the number of changes was positively correlated with IOP at baseline and negatively correlated with the initial effect on IOP (Table 12.3).

Variations in treatment

Costs are influenced in a very consistent way in all countries by the effectiveness of the initial treatment and by the number of treatment changes, regardless of the differences in baseline diagnosis, resource utilisation pattern, or costs for the individual resources or services. While one would expect considerable variation in the cost of the resources, it is rather surprising to see the large differences in resource utilisation. In a field where basically only three types of treatments are used, (medication, argon laser trabeculoplasty (ALT) and trabeculectomy), and where these are the same products and the same procedures across the countries, one would have expected fewer differences. Considering also that the effect after two years is about the same, regardless of everything else, one could clearly raise the question

109

Table 12.3 Predictors of treatment changes

Log{Odds of likeliness of Therapy Switch from β-blockers in a subgroup} =
Intercept + $\beta_1 \cdot$ IOP baseline + $\beta_2 \cdot$ IOP reduction + $\beta_3 \cdot$ Female + $\beta_4 \cdot$ Age + $\beta_5 \cdot$ POAG + $\beta_6 \cdot$ Exfoliation glaucoma + $\beta_7 \cdot$ Pigmentary glaucoma + $\beta_8 \cdot$ Moderate VF defect + $\beta_9 \cdot$ Severe VF defect + $\beta_{10} \cdot$ Moderate ONH damage + $\beta_{11} \cdot$ Severe ONH damage + Error

Explanatory variable	Benchmark	Adjusted Odds Ratio[a] of Explanatory variable group versus Benchmark group on the Likeliness of Therapy Switch from β-blockers during the 2-year period								
		Australia N = 201	Canada N = 214	UK N = 198	Spain N = 242	France N = 223	Germany N = 200	Netherlands N = 200	Sweden N = 211	USA N = 198
IOP baseline	Per 1 mm Hg	1.250***	1.372***	1.368***	1.434***	1.316***	1.204***	1.194***	1.266***	1.193***
IOP baseline	Per 5 mm Hg	3.047***	4.866***	4.806***	6.056***	3.954***	2.528***	2.429***	3.250***	
IOP reduction	Per 1 mm Hg	0.772***	0.720***	0.808***	0.800***	0.804***	0.788***	0.890***	0.801***	0.890***
IOP reduction	Per 5 mm Hg	0.275***	0.194***	0.345***	0.327***	0.336***	0.304***	0.560***	0.329***	
Female	Male	0.721	1.125	0.916	0.949	0.780	0.638	0.918	1.568	2.256**
Age	Per 1 year	1.031*	1.030*	1.001	1.032**	1.004	1.036**	1.007	0.994	1.009
Age	Per 10 years	1.362*	1.339*	1.005	1.372**	1.042	1.424**	1.072	0.942	
POAG	OH	4.568	1.402	18.201***	2.236	1.873	0.000	3.023*	9.445*	1.353
Exfoliation glaucoma	OH	999.000	7.707	26.337	2.315	0.778	0.000		16.883**	3.149
Pigmentary glaucoma	OH		1.334*	18.340*	1.031	999.000	0.157			
VF defect moderate	None/minor	2.952***	1.140	1.184	1.495	1.858	999.000	1.013	0.547	1.240
VF defect severe	None/minor	2.036	1.622	1.444	0.794	4.807***	999.000	3.004*	1.828	7.856**
ONH damage moderate	None/minor	0.714	1.935	0.842	0.798	0.919	1.015	1.899	1.307	1.585
ONH damage severe	None/minor	2.541**	3.866	2.435	4.080	1.620	0.963	2.060	0.677	1.782

a ***, **, * significant at the 1%, 5%, 10% level

How to read Table 12.3 (Example, Australia):
– a patient is 1.250 times more likely to change therapy for every 1 mm increased baseline IOP, and 3.047 times more likely for every 5 mm increased baseline IOP
– a patient is 0.772 times less likely to change therapy for every additional 1 mm of initial treatment effect, 0.275 times less likely for every 5 mm
– a patient with POAG is 4.568 times more likely to change therapy than a patient with OH
– a patient is 2.952 times more likely to change therapy with moderate VFD, 2.036 with severe VFD, than a patient with no or mild VFD

whether standardisation and treatment guidelines would not be useful.

The choice of the second line treatment varied considerably between countries. Overall, medical therapy with either a different monotherapy or addition of a second drug to the β-blocker was the preferred option in most countries, but the choice of drugs was very different. Exceptions to this were the Netherlands and the UK. In the Netherlands, ALT was most frequently used as second line intervention, with patients remaining on β-blockers. In the UK, ALT and trabeculectomy were used in the same proportion, and more frequently than medical therapy. Table 12.4 gives the details of second line therapy choices in the different countries.

Surgical interventions differed not only in the place in the treatment sequence, but also very much in their overall use. While almost no trabeculectomies were performed in Australia, Canada and Germany, these were very frequent in France, Spain and the UK. The frequency of ALT was even more variable, with the most intensive use not only in Spain and Sweden, but also in France, Germany and the Netherlands. One could speculate as to the reasons for this. In Sweden and Spain, part of the explanation might be the high proportion of exfoliation glaucoma identified, while in France, Germany and the Netherlands the

place of treatment, i.e. a large proportion of office-based ophthalmologists, might contribute to the explanation. Similarly, the point of treatment and the organisation of the payment for services might explain partly the huge variation in the mean number of visits per patient. Another reason for this could be found in the customs of the different countries relating to physician visits per capita. Figures 12.1, 12.2 illustrate the differences in resource consumption, for surgical interventions and for physician visits and diagnostic tests.

Not surprisingly, inpatient treatment also was very different. National clinical practices in respect to hospitalisation are known to differ, and as expected was most frequent in France, Spain and the UK. Sweden had a very high number as well, but this was due to one centre where all patients were hospitalised at diagnosis, a practice that has since been abandoned. Both the frequency of hospital admissions and the length of stay have steadily decreased over the past decade in all countries, and the number of hospital days in this sample is likely to be higher than what it would be today.

As mentioned earlier, standard costs or tariffs vary considerably due to price levels and payment systems, and total costs per patient would therefore be different even if treatment patterns were the same. In addition, it is reasonable to

Table 12.4 Preferred second line therapy after β-blockers

Country	N	Patients with no change (% of total)	Patients with change (% of total)	Patients with change (% of patients with changes)				
				Mono- or Combination Therapy	ALT	Surgery TRAB	Surgery ALT + TRAB	Stop treatment
Total Cohort	1990		963 (48%) 13	539 (56%)	216 (23%)	51 (5%)	267 (28%)	157 (16%)
Australia	203	89 (44%)	114 (56%)	87 (77%)	15 (13%)	0 (0%)	15 (13%)	10 (10%)
Canada	243	154 63%)	89 (47%)	40 (45%)	32 (36%)	2 (2%)	34 (38%)	15 (17%)
Germany	200	92 (46%)	108 (54%)	96 (88%)	9 (8%)	2 (2%)	11 (11%)	1 (1%)
France	225	131 (58%)	94 (42%)	50 (53%)	23 (25%)	8 (9%)	31 (33%)	12 (13%)
Netherlands	200	112 (56%)	88 (44%)	35 (40%)	35 (40%)	4 (5%)	39 (45%)	14 (15%)
Spain	242	73 (30%)	169 (70%)	82 (49%)	53 (32%)	13 (8%)	66 (40%)	18 (11%)
Sweden	218	92 (42%)	126 (58%)	49 (38%)	27 (23%)	1 (1%)	28 (24%)	49 (38%)
UK	208	152 (73%)	56 (57%)	22 (39%)	14 (25%)	15 (27%)	29 (52%)	5 (9%)
USA	253	134 (53%)	119 (47%)	72 (60%)	8 (7%)	6 (5%)	14 (12%)	33 (28%)

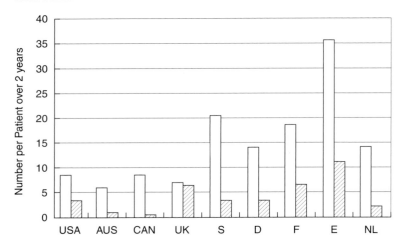

Figure 12.1 Mean number of surgical interventions per patient over 2 years (total number of interventions in the cohort divided by the number of patients). □, ALT; ▨, TRAB.

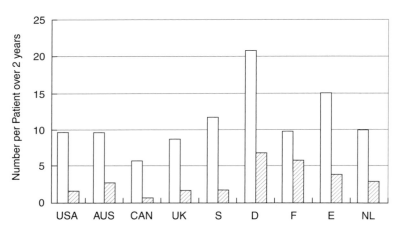

Figure 12.2 Mean number of medical visits and diagnostic tests per patient over 2 years. □, Visits; ▨, Tests.

assume that prices will influence consumption. A comparison based on costs must, therefore, be used with caution. For illustrative purposes, total costs per patient are indicated in Figure 12.3 using the commercial exchange rate of June 1998.

Modelling in the future

In the absence of a clear relation between IOP and blindness, the only relevant economic evaluation at the introduction of new treatments for glaucoma is an estimate of the cost. A model integrating clinical data for several new

glaucoma medications, and the patient management data from the above observations, has been proposed.[7] The model indicates that there might be savings if a new and effective treatment reduces the need for switching therapy and for surgery. An earlier cost-effectiveness study at the time of the introduction of β blockers showed significant substitution possibilities between improved medical therapy and surgery.[8] However, it appears that there is further potential for cost reductions, although it is not yet known whether this will be short term only, by delaying switches and surgical procedures, or whether some of these costs can be avoided.

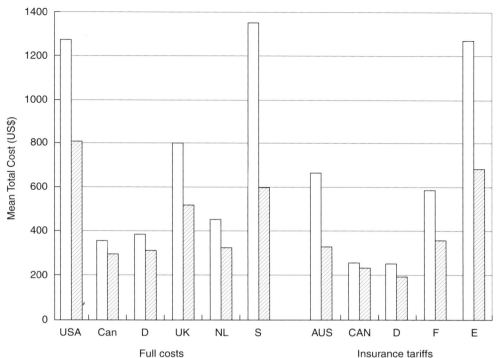

Figure 12.3 Mean cost per patient over 2 years, calculated as full social opportunity cost or as charges. □, Year 1; ▨, Year 2.

There are few economic or patient management studies in glaucoma, despite a high prevalence of the disease. The goal of treatment is to manage IOP towards a target level in order to preserve vision, and all treatments available reduce IOP. However, the exact link between IOP and blindness is not known, and economic evaluations are therefore limited to the cost of managing the disease. The cost of treatment is influenced not only by the price of a treatment, but also by its effectiveness to achieve the desired control. Treatment choices must be based on both in order to provide efficient healthcare.

The cost of treatment is further influenced by the sequence in which different treatments are chosen and by the prevailing treatment patterns in a given setting. Access to different types of healthcare facilities, different points of entry into the health care system, different organisation and payment of services, will all lead to variations in resource consumption, as will pre-

ferences and beliefs of both patients and physicians. Comparison of the cost of treatment is therefore fraught with difficulties and has to be used with caution. It is important to observe current practice, as it will provide valuable information. Sometimes, what we do is different from what we think we do, and certainly clinical practice is very different from controlled clinical trials. In view of the general quest for an efficient provision of healthcare, be it in order to use scarce resources in the best way, or in order to standardise treatments and develop treatment guidelines, the first step is to observe current reality.

References

1 Coyle A, Drummond M. The economic burden of glaucoma in the UK – The need for a far-sighted policy. *Pharmaco Economics* 1995; 7 (6): 484–9.
2 Gerdtham UG, Hågå A, Karlsson G, Kobelt G, Jönsson B. Observational costing study in open angle primary glaucoma in Sweden and the USA. EFI Research Paper No.6566 (Stockholm School of Economics) 1996.
3 Gerdtham UG, Williamson T, Hågå A, Kobelt G,

Jönsson B. Observational costing study in open angle primary glaucoma; results for Canada. EFI Research Paper No.6569 (Stockholm School of Economics) 1997.

4 Kobelt G, Gerdtham UG, Alm A. (1998) Cost of treating primary open angle glaucoma and ocular hypertension. *J Glaucoma* 7: 95–104.

5 Kobelt G, Jönsson L, Gerdtham UG, Krieglstein G. Direct costs of glaucoma management following initiation of medical therapy. *Graefe's Arch Ophthalmol* 1998 (in press).

6 Kobelt G. in Jönsson B, Krieglstein G (eds). Primary Open Angle Glaucoma – Differences in International Treatment Patterns and Cost. *Isis Medical Media* Oxford, UK. 1998.

7 Kobelt G, Jönsson L. Modelling cost and cost-effectiveness of new treatments for glaucoma. *Int J Medical Tech Assess* (accepted for publication) 1998; **15**: 1.

8 AD Little Inc. Use of β-Blockers in the Treatment of Glaucoma: A cost-benefit study. PMA Cost-Effectiveness of Pharmaceuticals, Report 8. 1984.

13 The detection of visual field progression

A C VISWANATHAN

The detection and quantification of change in visual fields is one of the most important and problematic areas of glaucoma management. An early, accurate measure of whether a field series shows progressive damage is essential: significant deterioration is likely to prompt a change in treatment, whereas confirmed stability provides more convincing reassurance than lowered intraocular pressure (IOP) alone that therapy is successful.

Measurement of change

Automated versus manual perimetry

The benefit of manual perimetry is that an experienced examiner can perform fast, flexible testing for a variety of visual field abnormalities in subjects who might not be able to produce reliable tests under the more demanding conditions imposed by an automated perimeter. It was used when assessing cross-sectional prevalence of visual field damage in a large, population based study to deduce the overall rate of progression in open-angle glaucoma.[1]

However, the versatility of manual perimetry may also limit its effectiveness, since it is a source of both variation and bias. The examiner may neglect areas of the visual field which are not thought to be important. The pattern of visual field abnormalities may be "forced" to comply with preconceived ideas. The result of the test is highly dependent upon the level of training of the examiner. Furthermore, manual perimetry gives poorly reproducible results in the central field and at the edges of gradually deepening scotomas such as those found in glaucoma. For these reasons, when quantifiable, reproducible results are required, automated perimetry is used. The combination of automated perimetry with static testing has the advantages that it is operator independent and yields numerical data relating to the spatial coordinates of the test locations and sensitivities at those locations: these data are amenable to sophisticated statistical analysis, unlike the results of manual perimetry.

Full threshold versus suprathreshold strategies

Full threshold strategies provide more detailed information than suprathreshold strategies since they indicate the depth of scotomas rather than merely their presence or absence. Thus, although suprathreshold testing is appropriate when a rapid distinction between normality and abnormality is required, full thresholding is better for the long-term follow-up of patients whose visual fields are known to be abnormal and may be slowly deteriorating.

Clinical judgement versus numerical analysis

The most commonly used method of deciding whether a visual field series shows progression or not is for a clinician to inspect the series visually and use clinical judgement to form an opinion. Unfortunately this approach is flawed.

Human observers, even experienced ones, are not able to detect visual field progression reliably using clinical judgement alone.[2] One possible reason for this is that the standard output of most automated perimeters contains no information relating to progression or stability. When clinicians are presented with a visual field series that has been processed to highlight areas of possible deterioration, the level of agreement about progression is greater.[3] Although clinical judgement is by definition at the root of clinical decision making, the simple visual assessment of field series presented as the standard output of an automated perimeter, is an inadequate basis for this judgement. Rather, clinical decisions concerning visual field progression should be based on the results of computerised numerical change analysis of visual field series. The most widespread of these analyses are described below.

Summary measures

One group of methods relies on estimates of change in summary measures of the field. Examples of this approach are seen in regression analysis of the mean defect value,[4] mean deviation,[5] other global measures,[5] measurement of whole-field and quadrantic sensitivity losses,[6] and trend and regression analysis of various estimates of the sensitivity of the whole field or parts of it.[7-9] The Glaucoma Hemifield Test has been used to detect incident field loss among patients with elevated IOP.[10] However, the analysis of summary measures, whether based on the whole field or on clusters of points within it, has been found to be "remarkably poor"[11] and "of little value"[12] in detecting glaucomatous change.

Summaries measures largely, or completely, ignore the detailed spatial information contained within computerised field tests and are insensitive to early localised change.[13] Furthermore, different regions of the visual field may deteriorate at different rates.[9,14,15] Thus, the analysis of summary measures should be

avoided if the early detection of visual field deterioration is required.

Pointwise measures

Techniques that evaluate progression on a point-by-point basis avoid the problems with summary measures described above. They may be divided into two categories: event analysis, and trend analysis.

Event analyses rely on detecting a significant change from an established baseline. For example, the Collaborative Normal-Tension Glaucoma Study Group initially specified an endpoint, based on sensitivity loss, at which patients would be said to have shown unequivocal deterioration. However, the authors noted a surprisingly large number of patients reaching the endpoint. Statistical analysis revealed that the endpoint chosen would be expected to lead to a false diagnosis of progression 57% of the time. In order to correct this, a requirement for progression to be confirmed on multiple repeat tests was introduced.[16] The most recent report from the study group gives the endpoint as "a follow-up visual field was said to show progression relative to baseline if it contained two or more points that had changed by at least 10 dB relative to the average baseline values for these points; these two progressing points had to be adjacent, both could not be peripheral, both could not cross the nasal meridian, and the sensitivity at each deteriorating point had to be less than the minimum of the values of this point in each of the three baseline visual fields". Progression was also deemed to have taken place if at least one of the innermost four points showed at least a 10 dB deterioration relative to its average value at baseline, with a value that was less than its minimum value in each baseline field. Progression was considered to be confirmed when "four of five consecutive follow-up fields showed progression relative to the baseline fields, with at least one non-peripheral progressing point (or the one central point) being common to all four fields".[17] Event analysis is dependent on the baseline and does not give a measure of rate of change (see below).

Trend analyses do not construct a baseline. The behaviour of the visual field is analysed and progression is diagnosed if a significant tendency to deteriorate is detected. When this is done on a pointwise basis the technique of linear regression of sensitivity on time is often used. Test locations are labelled as showing progression if a significant negative regression line is calculated, e.g. individual test locations from glaucoma patients were found to deteriorate significantly at rates of one to five decibels per year[5,18] when visual field testing was performed annually. The effect of the frequency of visual field testing on the ability to detect glaucomatous visual field deterioration is discussed further below.

The differences between event analyses and trend analyses may be further appreciated from a consideration of two commercially available software packages for the Humphrey Field Analyzer: Statpac 2 (Humphrey Instruments Inc, San Leandro, CA, USA), and PROGRESSOR (University College, London, UK).

Statpac 2

The Statpac 2 Glaucoma Change Probability analysis[19] is an event analysis. It is the "native" statistical Glaucoma Change Probability software available as an add-on for the Humphrey Field Analyzer. The programme uses the thresholds from the two most reliable of the first three fields in the series as a baseline. Each subsequent field is compared on a point-by-point basis to this baseline. Test locations are labelled with a black triangle (Figure 13.1) if $p < 0.05$ for the null hypothesis of no glaucomatous change compared to a database of stable glaucoma field series.

PROGRESSOR

PROGRESSOR[20] is a trend analysis. It is a software package which analyses visual field progression using pointwise linear regression of sensitivity on time. The pointwise linear model has been demonstrated to provide a valid framework for detecting and forecasting glaucomatous loss.[21] This technique has been used for several years to investigate glaucomatous visual field change[22,23] and has recently been re-examined.[5] PROGRESSOR produces a cumulative graphical output as shown in Figure 13.2a. Each test location is shown as a bar graph in which each bar represents one test. The length of the bar relates to the depth of the defect (longer bars represent lower sensitivities) and the colour of the bar relates to the p value of the regression slope (Figure 13.2b). Thus, undamaged locations are seen as series of short grey bars, damaged but stable locations are seen as long series of long grey bars, and progressing locations are seen as series of progressively lengthening bars which change colour as the regression slope becomes more significant.

Comparison of event analysis and trend analysis

Both Statpac 2 and PROGRESSOR provide sensitive methods for the detection of glaucomatous visual field deterioration, whether widespread or focal, but each algorithm has its limitations.

Statpac 2 relies on its database of normal values being a representative sample of the population from which the patient under test is drawn. Only data from the two baseline tests and the test under consideration is analysed: data from any intervening tests is ignored. This is of particular concern because the baseline tests are usually amongst the first attempted by the patient, and thus often the least reliable. By its very nature as an event analysis, Statpac 2 may give an indication that change has occurred but gives no information about the rate of change. This measure of rate is a prerequisite if prevention of clinically significant visual damage is to be achieved, since it is through knowledge of the speed of deterioration that the degree of future loss of visual function

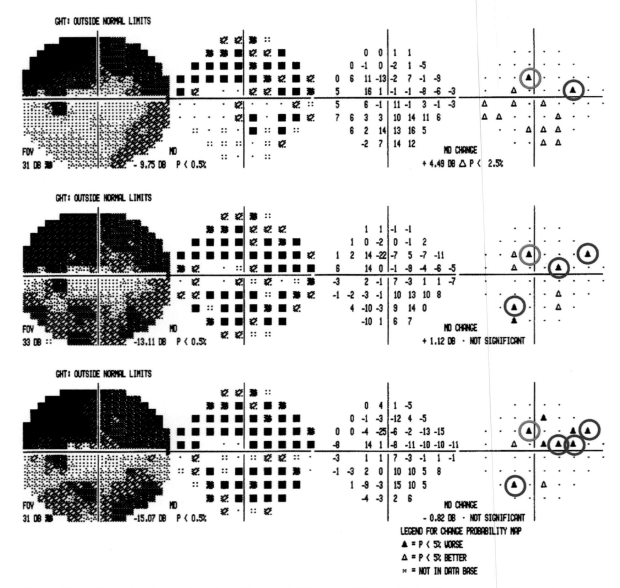

Figure 13.1 Example of a section of the Statpac 2 Glaucoma Change Probability analysis. The test locations circled in blue are labelled as showing significant deterioration in two out of the three fields shown. The test location circled in red is labelled as showing significant deterioration in each of the three consecutive fields.

may be anticipated. If the rate of visual field loss suggests that the patient will be visually disabled within their lifetime, appropriate therapeutic measures may be instituted. Only by assessing rate can outcome be determined.

PROGRESSOR treats individual test locations as statistically independent from one another. This is clearly not the case. Points which are labelled as showing statistically significant deterioration must be interpreted judiciously: statistical significance is not analogous to clinical significance. Owing to its reliance on linear trend analysis, PROGRESSOR might be expected to be relatively insensitive to sudden, stepwise decay, though recent work[24] suggests this is not the case.

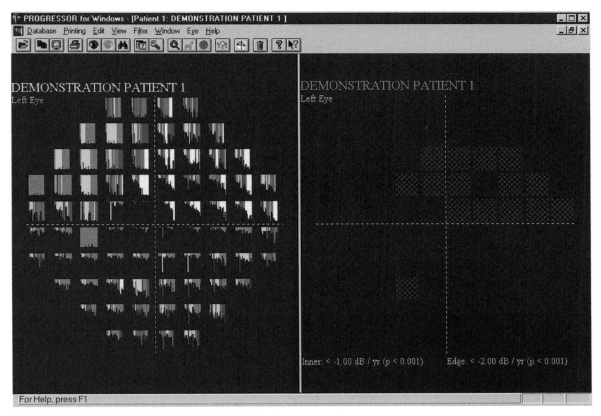

Figure 13.2a   Example of the PROGRESSOR output for the same visual field series as in Figure 13.1. The left pane shows the cumulative graphical output and the right pane shows the test locations which satisfy progression criteria. Note that the pattern of progressing points is similar to that of the circled points in Figure 13.1.

Statpac 2 and PROGRESSOR have been compared directly in their ability to detect visual field deterioration.[25] Both algorithms were applied to a selection of visual field series that demonstrated unequivocal deterioration. The algorithms were compared in their ability to detect progression and in the speed of detection. Although both Statpac 2 and PROGRESSOR detected the deterioration in all the field series, PROGRESSOR was consistently superior in terms of the speed of detection. Other work[26] has examined the level of agreement between pointwise linear regression, and Statpac 2 in glaucoma. The two techniques were found to show good agreement about which test locations were progressing, if these locations were deteriorating at more than five times the normal age-related decline in sensitivity. If the locations deteriorated at a more moderate rate, however, Statpac 2 failed to detect progression which was diagnosed by pointwise linear regression. The authors ascribed this finding to the fact that locations that have lost a moderate degree of sensitivity have more test-retest variability than points with either high or low sensitivity.[27] These moderately depressed points are thus less easily detected by Statpac 2, which relies on a point falling outside the test-retest confidence limits of the baseline before progression is diagnosed. Conversely, the authors found a number of test locations which showed a high degree of fluctuation throughout the visual field series which could not be adequately described by pointwise linear regression. Statpac 2 labelled a proportion of these locations as progressing. Point-wise linear

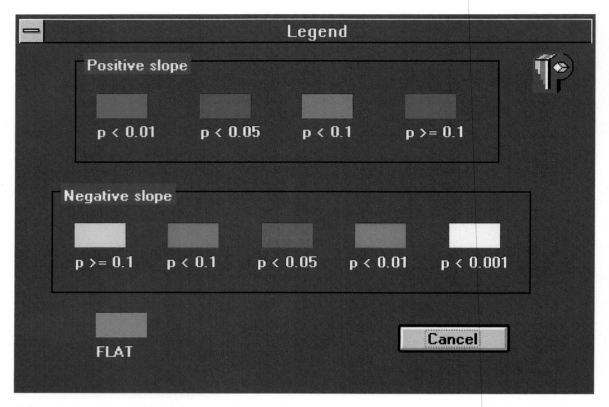

Figure 13.2b   PROGRESSOR legend. This legend relates the colour of a given bar in the PROGRESSOR bar graphs to the p value of the regression slope for that test.

regression and other trend analyses were found to agree more closely with human observers than an event-based glaucoma change analysis.[28]

Errors in measurement

Fluctuation

One of the greatest obstacles to the reliable detection of visual field change in glaucoma is the high level of inherent variability between tests. This is known as long-term fluctuation and is a particular feature of glaucoma.[29] The contribution of long-term fluctuation must always be borne in mind before accepting a single field test as showing definite deterioration compared to the previous tests in a series. In general, confirmatory tests should be sought before decisions about patient management

are made (see "pointwise measures" above). A promising avenue of research is the application of digital image processing techniques, such as those used to process images obtained by magnetic resonance imaging (MRI), to reduce the "noise" in the results of computerised perimetry. These spatial filtering techniques take account of the interdependence of neighbouring retinal test locations and have been shown to improve the repeatability of automated perimetry by a factor of two[30] and to improve the predictability of glaucomatous decay.[31]

New perimetric strategies such as the Swedish Interactive Threshold Algorithm (SITA) have also been demonstrated to reduce variability. The between subject pointwise variability was found to be approximately 10% less for SITA than for conventional full threshold perimetry.[32] Inter-individual variability was also reduced, resulting in narrower confidence intervals for normal variability.[33] This is most likely a result of the shorter test times associated with this algorithm and consequent reduced visual fatigue. Although narrower confidence limits would be expected to lead to earlier, more reliable detection of visual field deterioration, the SITA algorithm also yields higher pointwise light sensitivities than conventional full threshold tests,[33] and there is some evidence that scotoma size is reduced and that early defects may be missed.[34] These differences make it difficult to compare visual fields from SITA with "conventional" Humphrey test results in a visual field series.

Learning effects

Some subjects show a marked increase in sensitivity from the initial test to subsequent tests. This tends to be more marked in the superior and peripheral parts of the field. Other subjects, however, do not show any learning effect and produce reliable tests from the outset. Most learning effects have disappeared after the first two visual field tests,[35] although occasionally learning effects may persist for many years (Figures 13.3, 13.4). If learning effects are suspected, the results of visual field tests should be ignored until a stable baseline is achieved. Inclusion of "pre-learning" fields in a series will delay the recognition of any subsequent deterioration by both event and trend analyses. Factors that can influence these effects are set out in Chapter 6.

Change criteria

The sensitivity and specificity of any method used to detect field change are critically

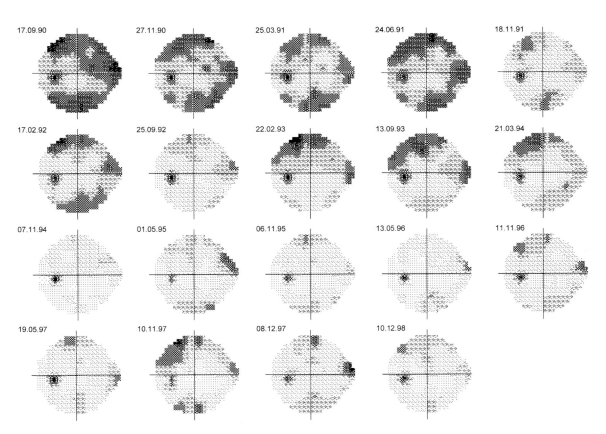

Figure 13.3   A series of visual fields showing the persistence of learning effects over a period of eight years.

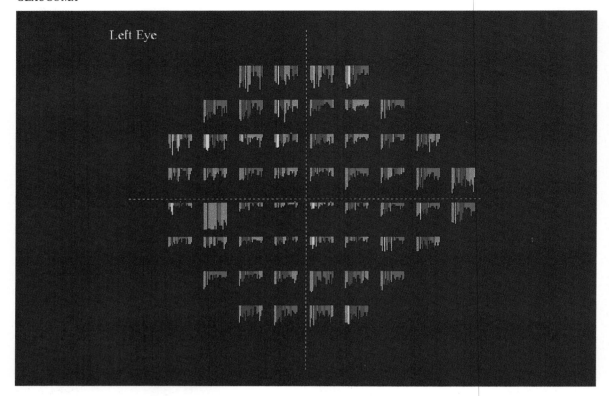

Figure 13.4 PROGRESSOR output for the same visual field series as shown in Figure 13.3. The progressively shortening green bars indicate improvement in sensitivity over time, which in this patient is attributable to learning effects.

dependent on the criteria used to differentiate progression from stability. For example, if an event analysis specifies a pointwise $p < 0.05$ probability criterion for the diagnosis of progression, in a 30–2 test grid consisting of 76 test locations, about four locations in each test would be expected to be labelled as progressing when they are actually stable (false positives). The originators of Statpac 2 suggest the requirement for a location to be repeatedly ascribed a high probability of change over a series of consecutive fields, before progression is diagnosed.[19] Another recommendation is that progression should depend on clusters of neighbouring points being labelled as progressing. These proposals will increase the specificity of the analysis at the expense of sensitivity. The Collaborative Normal-Tension Glaucoma Study Group has recently reported the change criteria described in "pointwise measures" above.[17]

Change criteria used for trend analyses such as pointwise linear regression should specify a slope criterion as well as a probability criterion: a significant regression line should demonstrate a specific minimum level of deterioration before a test location is labelled as progressing. This lessens the risk of false positives. Furthermore, if a slope criterion is not specified, the physiological age-related decline in sensitivity may be falsely labelled as glaucomatous progression.[26]

At present there are no universally accepted progression criteria. It is unlikely that any single set of criteria will be applicable to the wide spectrum of disease seen in glaucoma patients and glaucoma suspects. In terms of practical management of the glaucoma patient, the results produced by any set of progression criteria must be examined within the clinical context.

Frequency of testing

Even sensitive, reliable methods are critically dependent on the frequency with which visual field tests are performed. Progressive visual field loss cannot be detected unless it is adequately sought. When considering how often to measure the visual field of a glaucoma patient several factors need to be taken into account. These factors include: the type of glaucoma, the number and results of previous tests, the age of the patient, recent changes in glaucoma therapy, the availability of perimetric resources, and the ability of the patient to produce reliable tests. Further details are set out in the earlier chapter on visual field testing (see Chapter 6). Reliability is discussed further below. However, one of the commonest and most important reasons for repeatedly measuring visual fields is in order to detect progressive damage as early as possible. A recent study[36] examined whether performing visual field tests once a year rather than three times a year would lead to a clinically significant delay in the detection of progressive glaucoma. The results were striking. Less than half of the progressing locations were detected when visual field tests were analysed only once a year. Furthermore, the "once a year" strategy entailed a delay in recognition of progression of more than one year over a four year study period.

The Collaborative Normal-Tension Glaucoma Study Group has reported that an event type of analysis can be used to diagnose visual field progression in a timely, sensitive and specific way.[16] In this analysis, patients were followed with visual field tests every three months. If the criteria for suspected progression were met, the patient returned within one to four weeks for one or two confirmatory tests. If progression was confirmed in this way on two consecutive series of visits three months apart, true progression was diagnosed. However, this study protocol entailed a high frequency of testing which would have profound resource implications if it were implemented on a routine basis, since it may have involved three tests every three months. The most recent "four-of-five" confirmatory testing protocol reported by the Collaborative Normal-Tension Glaucoma Study Group has been described in "pointwise measures" above.[17]

Artefact

Many factors may cause an apparent worsening of the visual field that is not truly related to progressive glaucoma. The commonest and most troublesome of these is long-term fluctuation (see above), but artefacts affecting the visual field, which are usually more easily remedied than long-term fluctuation, must also be considered.

Pupil size

A reduction in pupil size results in a decrease in threshold values, especially in the peripheral visual field, and in an increase in the variability of threshold measures. These effects are particularly relevant in regard to miotic therapy for glaucoma, e.g. an apparent visual field progression may be found to coincide with the start of a course of pilocarpine drops. If this patient's pupil is dilated with a short-acting topical mydriatic administered before the visual field test (if this is clinically appropriate), the result will be free from the adverse effects of the miotic and a fairer comparison with previous tests may be made.

Refractive error

Uncorrected refractive error causes defocusing of the retinal image of the test stimulus. For example, five dioptres of simulated hypermetropic blur on a Goldmann size III stimulus reduces the central sensitivity by approximately six decibels. Refractive errors > 1.00 dioptre should be corrected. Many perimeters use a testing distance for which a presbyopic correction will also be necessary. Unfortunately, the correction of refractive errors itself poses problems. Many perimeters incorporate a holder for a standard trial lens in order to correct the eye under test, but the small diameter of these lenses may mean that the edge of the lens may encroach upon the visual field and cause a lens rim artefact. This appears as a defect at the edge of the central visual field. It does not usually respect either the horizontal or vertical meridians, but may mimic a nerve fibre bundle defect. Lens rim artefacts are more common in the elderly and in hypermetropes. They may be avoided by ensuring that the patient's eye is as close to the correcting lens as possible and well centred behind the lens. Patients' own spectacles should be used if possible (unless they are bi-, multi-, or vari-focal, or inappropriate to the testing distance) since they give a larger field of view than a trial lens.

Lid/brow artefact

Apparent defects in the superior visual field may result from slight ptosis, prominent eyelashes, dermatochalasis or prominent brows. Incorrect positioning of the patient at the perimeter may be a contributory factor. These artefacts may be extremely difficult to distinguish from incipient arcuate scotomas. If the cause is ptosis, however, the problem is easily solved: if the lid is gently lifted with adhesive tape for the duration of the test, to abolish the ptosis but still allow the patient to blink fully, the artefact disappears.

Media opacities

Opacities in the lens (or posterior capsule following extracapsular cataract surgery) may cause progressive visual field deterioration. Media opacities usually cause a generalised reduction of sensitivity across the whole field (this may be difficult to distinguish from diffuse glaucomatous loss). Occasionally localised lens opacities may cause focal visual field defects but these are rarely as well defined as nerve fibre bundle defects. Examination of the ocular media will reveal any opacities dense enough to affect the visual field.

The Collaborative Normal-Tension Glaucoma Study Group has reported that the data from patients who developed cataract during the trial had to be removed from the analysis before the protective effect of IOP lowering on visual field deterioration in normal-tension glaucoma could be demonstrated.[17] The Group also attempted to control for the effects of cataract on mean deviation by adjusting the individual patient's mean deviation values for the corresponding readings of foveal sensitivity by regression analysis. This was based on the assumption that changes in foveal sensitivity primarily reflect cataract formation rather than the effects of glaucoma. Before these adjustments were made, a significantly different change in mean deviation, from the time of randomisation to the time of IOP stabilisation, was found between the treated and untreated groups. After the adjustments, no difference was found.

Macular disease

Advancing age-related macular degeneration may produce field changes reminiscent of progressive glaucomatous paracentral scotomas but this rarely leads to any clinical confusion, as examination of the macula readily reveals the true source of the visual field damage.

Reliability

Before a field test may be included in any glaucoma change analysis, some account must be taken of its reliability. This involves attention to the factors mentioned above. In addition, automated perimeters calculate reliability indices that are shown on the output display. For example, the Humphrey Field Analyzer calculates fixation losses, false positives, and false negatives. Fixation losses are measured by the Heijl-Krakau technique: once the position of the physiological blind spot has been ascertained, stimuli are presented within this area. Any reported as seen represent inaccurate fixation. False positives are recorded when the machine behaves exactly as if a stimulus were about to be presented, but none is, and the subject reports the (non-existent) stimulus as seen. False negatives are detected when a stimulus known to be above the threshold at a particular location is presented at that location and the subject does not record the stimulus as seen.

Visual fields that have a large proportion of fixation losses, false negatives, or especially false positives, are likely to be unreliable. The Humphrey Field Analyzer displays a "low patient reliability" message to alert the examiner to this. These messages should be interpreted with caution as there is no proven association between machine-generated reliability indices and actual patient reliability. If the machine fails to determine the location of the physiological blind spot correctly, the Heijl-Krakau technique will record a large number of fixation losses even though the subject's fixation is steady. Furthermore, early glaucoma may be associated with an increased proportion of false negatives in some patients. In these cases false negatives are an index of disease rather than poor reliability.

Dynamic range

All perimeters are restricted in the maximum brightness of stimulus possible. Once a test location deteriorates towards a level of sensitivity at which even the brightest stimulus produced by the machine elicits no response, further deterioration cannot be measured, as the sensitivity of the location is beyond the dynamic range of the instrument. If this process occurs during follow-up, then only the measurable portion of the location's behaviour is available for analysis: the data is effectively censored. This may explain the finding that locations that have a low initial sensitivity are rarely detected as deteriorating by glaucoma change algorithms.[15]

Results of treatment

Glaucoma treatment is at present aimed almost exclusively at lowering IOP. This ratio-nale is based on the observation that higher IOP tends to be associated with more severe disease. Cross-sectional studies indicate that an IOP > 16 mm Hg is associated with a higher rate of visual field progression in primary open angle glaucoma (POAG).[37] For this reason 16 mm Hg is often specified as a desirable target pressure in POAG. A large prospective trial (the Early Manifest Glaucoma trial in Malmö) is currently in progress to evaluate the effects of treatment on visual field progression in POAG, but results are not yet available. Similarly, the ongoing Ocular Hypertension Treatment Study has not yet reported on whether topical ocular hypotensive medications prevent or delay the onset of glaucoma in ocular hypertensive patients, though it has stressed the importance of confirmatory retesting when using an event analysis: 88% of follow-up visual fields showing abnormalities based on the Glaucoma Hemifield Test or Corrected Pattern Standard Deviation were not confirmed as abnormal on subsequent retesting.[38]

Longitudinal treatment studies, including visual field analysis, have been conducted in normal-tension glaucoma patients. Although some of these studies use event analysis and some use trend analysis, they consistently indicate that effective lowering of IOP retards progressive visual field damage.[17, 39–42]

References

1 Quigley HA, Tielsch JM, Katz J, Sommer A. Rate of progression in open-angle glaucoma estimated from cross-sectional prevalence of visual field damage (see comments). *Am J Ophthalmol* 1996; **122** (3): 355–63.

2 Werner EB, Bishop KI, Koelle J, Douglas GR, LeBlanc RP, Mills RP, *et al.* A comparison of experienced clinical observers and statistical tests in detection of progressive visual field loss in glaucoma using automated perimetry. *Arch Ophthalmol* 1988; **106** (5): 619–23.

3 Chauhan BC, Drance SM, LeBlanc RP, Lieberman MF, Mills RP, Werner EB. Technique for determining glaucomatous visual field progression by using animation graphics. *Am J Ophthalmol* 1994; **118** (4): 485–91.

4 Weber J, Koll W, Krieglstein GK. Intraocular pressure and visual field decay in chronic glaucoma. *Ger J Ophthalmol* 1993; **2** (3): 165–9.

5 Smith SD, Katz J, Quigley HA. Analysis of progressive change in automated visual fields in glaucoma. *Invest Ophthalmol Vis Sci* 1996; **37** (7): 1419–28.

6 Wegner A, Ugi I, Hofman A. A long-term visual field evaluation of glaucoma patients treated topically with timolol or carteolol. In: Mills RP (ed). *Perimetry Update* 1992/1993. Amsterdam: Kugler & Ghedini, 1993: 143–45.

7 Holmin C, Krakau CE. Regression analysis of the central visual field in chronic glaucoma cases. A follow-up study using automatic perimetry. *Acta Ophthalmol Copenh* 1982; **60** (2): 267–74.

8 Wu D, Schwartz B, Nagin P. Trend analyses of automated visual fields. *Doc Ophthalmol Proc Ser* 1987; (49): 175–89.

9 O'Brien C, Schwartz B, Takamoto T, Wu DC. Intraocular pressure and the rate of visual field loss in chronic open-angle glaucoma. *Am J Ophthalmol* 1991; **111** (4): 491–500.

10 Katz J, Quigley HA, Sommer A. Detection of incident field loss using the glaucoma hemifield test. *Ophthalmology* 1996; **103** (4): 657–63.

11 Chauhan BC, Drance SM, Douglas GR. The use of visual field indices in detecting changes in the visual field in glaucoma. *Invest Ophthalmol Vis Sci* 1990; **31** (3): 512–20.

12 Birch MK, Wishart PK, O'Donnell N. Determining progressive field loss. In: Mills RP, Wall M (eds). *Perimetry Update* 1994/1995. Amsterdam: Kugler & Ghedini, 1995: 31–6.

13 Wild JM, Hussey MK, Flanagan JG, Trope GE. Pointwise topographical and longitudinal modelling of the visual field in glaucoma. *Invest Ophthalmol Vis Sci* 1993; **34** (6): 1907–16.

14 Hoskins HD, Jensvold N, Zaretsky M, Hetherington J. Rate of progression of discrete areas of the visual field. In: Heijl-A (ed). *Perimetry Update* 1988/1989. Amsterdam: Kugler & Ghedini, 1989: 173–76.

15 O'Brien C, Schwartz B. The visual field in chronic open angle glaucoma: the rate of change in different regions of the field. *Eye* 1990; **4** (Pt 4): 557–62.

16 Schulzer M. Errors in the diagnosis of visual field progression in normal-tension glaucoma. *Ophthalmology* 1994; **101** (9): 1589–94.

17 Collaborative Normal-Tension Glaucoma Study Group. The effectiveness of intraocular pressure reduction in the treatment of normal-tension glaucoma. (see comments). *Am J Ophthalmol* 1998; **126** (4): 498–505.

18 Katz J, Gilbert D, Quigley HA, Sommer A. Estimating progression of visual field loss in glaucoma. *Ophthalmology* 1997; **104** (6): 1017–25.

19 Heijl A, Lindgren G, Lindgren A, *et al.* Extended empirical statistical package for evaluation of single and multiple fields in glaucoma: Statpac 2. In: Mills RP, Heijl A (eds). *Perimetry Update* 1990/1991. Amsterdam: Kugler & Ghedini, 1991: 303–15.

20 Fitzke FW, Hitchings RA, Poinoosawmy D, McNaught AI, Crabb DP. Analysis of visual field progression in glaucoma. *Br J Ophthalmol* 1996; (80): 40–8.

21 McNaught AI, Crabb DP, Fitzke FW, Hitchings RA. Modelling series of visual fields to detect progression in normal tension glaucoma. *Graefe's Arch Clin Exp Ophthalmol* 1995; (233): 750–5.

22 Noureddin BN, Poinoosawmy D, Fitzke FW, Hitchings RA. Regression analysis of visual field progression in low tension glaucoma. *Br J Ophthalmol* 1991; **75** (8): 493–5.

23 Poinoosawmy D, Wu J, Fitzke FW, Hitchings RA. Discrimination between progression and non-progression visual field loss in low tension glaucoma using MDT.

In: Mills-RP (ed). *Perimetry Update 1992/1993*. Amsterdam: Kugler & Ghedini 1993: 109–14.

24 Crabb DP, Hitchings RA, Fitzke FW. Detecting gradual and sudden sensitivity loss in series of visual fields. In: Wall M, Heijl A (eds). *Perimetry Update*. Amsterdam/NY: Kugler 1998/1999 (in press).

25 Viswanathan AC, Fitzke FW, Hitchings RA. Early Detection of Visual Field Progression in Glaucoma: A Comparison of PROGRESSOR and Statpac 2. *Br J Ophthalmol* 1997; **81** (12): 1037–42.

26 Wild JM, Hutchings N, Hussey MK, Flanagan JG, Trope GE. Pointwise univariate linear regression of perimetric sensitivity against follow-up time in glaucoma. *Ophthalmology* 1997; **104** (5): 808–15.

27 Heijl A, Lindgren A, Lindgren G. Test-retest variability in glaucomatous visual fields. *Am J Ophthalmol* 1989; **108** (2): 130–5.

28 Nouri-Mahdavi K, Brigatti L, Weitzman M, Caprioli J. Comparison of methods to detect visual field progression in glaucoma (published erratum in *Ophthalmology* Jan 1998; **105** (1): 7) *Ophthalmology* 1997; **104** (8): 1228–36.

29 Flammer J, Drance SM, Zulauf M. Differential light threshold. Short- and long-term fluctuation in patients with glaucoma, normal controls, and patients with suspected glaucoma. *Arch Ophthalmol* 1984; **102** (5): 704–6.

30 Fitzke FW, Crabb DP, McNaught AI, Edgar DF, Hitchings RA. Image processing of computerised visual field data. *Br J Ophthalmol* 1995; **79** (3): 207–12.

31 Crabb DP, McNaught AI, Fitzke FW, Hitchings RA. Spatially enhanced modelling of sensitivity decay in low-tension glaucoma. In: Wall M, Heijl A (eds). *Perimetry Update* Amsterdam/NY: Kugler 1994/1995: 73–81.

32 Pacey IE, Wild JM, Cubbidge RP, Hancock S, Cunliffe IA. The between-subject, between-algorithm variability of normal sensitivity with the SITA Standard and SITA Fast threshold algorithms. *Invest Ophthalmol Vis Sci* 1998; **39** (4): S493.

33 Bengtsson B, Heijl A. Sensitivity to glaucomatous visual field loss in full threshold, SITA Standard and SITA Fast tests. In: Wall M, Heijl A (eds). *Perimetry Update* Amsterdam/NY: Kugler 1998/1999 (in press).

34 Goldberg I. The Swedish Interactive Thresholding Algorithm (SITA) in patients with prior experience with the full threshold Humphrey Field Analyzer. In: Wall M, Heijl A (eds). *Perimetry Update* Amsterdam/NY: Kugler 1998/1999 (in press).

35 Werner EB, Adelson A, Krupin T. Effect of patient experience on the results of automated perimetry in clinically stable glaucoma patients. *Ophthalmology* 1988; **95** (6): 764–7.

36 Viswanathan AC, Hitchings RA, Fitzke FW. How often do patients need visual field tests? *Graefe's Arch Clin Exp Ophthalmol* 1997; **235**: 563–8.

37 Palmberg P. Epidemiology of POAG and rationale for therapy. *Glaucoma Abstracts* 1969; **6**: 10–23.

38 Keltner JL, Johnson CA, Spurr JO, Kass MA, Gordon MO. Confirmation of visual field abnormalities in the Ocular Hypertension Treatment Study (OHTS). *Invest Ophthalmol Vis Sci* 1998; **39** (4): S493.

39 Bhandari A, Crabb DP, Poinoosawmy D, Fitzke FW, Hitchings RA, Noureddin BN. Effect of surgery on visual field progression in normal-tension glaucoma. *Ophthalmology* 1997; **104** (7): 1131–7.

40 Fontana L, Viswanathan AC, Poinoosawmy D, Hitchings RA, Scullica L. Surgery for normal tension glaucoma. Target intraocular pressure and visual field progression. *Acta Ophthalmol Scand Suppl* 1997; **224**: 43–4.

41 Hitchings RA, Wu J, Poinoosawmy D, McNaught A. Surgery for normal tension glaucoma. *Br J Ophthalmol* 1995; **79** (5): 402–6.

42 Koseki N, Araie M, Shirato S, Yamamoto S. Effect of trabeculectomy on visual field performance in central 30 field in progressive normal-tension glaucoma. *Ophthalmology* 1997; **104** (2): 197–201.

14 The identification of progression in cupping of the optic disc

T GARWAY-HEATH

Primary open angle glaucoma (POAG) is a progressive optic neuropathy. The goal of the management of the glaucoma patient is to slow the progression of the neuropathy so that visual loss, sufficient to impair the quality of life of the patient, does not occur within the patient's lifetime.

POAG is characterised by progressive structural changes at the optic nerve head (ONH) and retinal nerve fibre layer (RNFL) and by visual field loss, the major risk factors for which are raised intraocular pressure (IOP) and greater age. In practise, when abnormal features are identified at the optic disc or in the visual field, a judgement has to be made as to whether the abnormalities are likely to represent a progressive condition. If a risk factor for POAG, such as raised IOP, is present, then progression (and POAG) is often assumed. However, in order to make rational treatment decisions it is necessary to identify the rate of disease progression in individual patients. Slowly progressive disease in an elderly patient may require no treatment at all, whereas the same rate of progression in a young patient may require aggressive intervention if significant visual loss in later years is to be prevented.

The ability to detect disease progression, whether structural changes at the optic nerve or functional changes in the visual field, depends on the reproducibility of the method employed. If the method is highly reproducible, then small changes can be detected. In recent years several new instruments, such as the scanning laser ophthalmoscopes, have been introduced for the imaging of the ONH and RNFL. These have been shown to make reproducible measurements, but few clinics have access to such instruments and rely on conventional methods of recording ONH and RNFL structure, such as by drawings and retinal photography.

Chapter 5 (The identification of glaucomatous cupping) looked at features of the glaucomatous optic disc. This chapter assesses the usefulness of methods by which change in the appearance of the optic disc can be identified. It sets out the advantages and limitations of methods ranging from drawings to scanning laser ophthalmoscopy.

Optic disc drawings

Making a drawing of the optic disc and nerve fibre layer from a stereoscopic examination through a dilated pupil, is an important part of the recording of the ONH structure. This is the case whether or not more sophisticated methods of recording, such as photography, are available. The definition of many features of the ONH is on the basis of contour and depth appreciation, e.g. the neuroretinal rim (NRR)/ optic cup edge, cup depth and the relative position of blood vessels and the optic disc surface. Reliable identification of these features is not possible from a photograph, unless stereophotography and stereoviewing are available in the clinic. Even when stereophotography is available, the act of making a drawing ensures a detailed examination of the nerve, and enables the examining clinician to draw attention to important features. These include features that may indicate that acquired change has already occurred, such as focal narrowing of the NRR, bared vessels and asymmetry between the eyes, and features that may indicate future progression, such as optic disc haemorrhages.

When making a drawing, it is important to keep to conventional definitions of ONH structures.[1] The area of the disc is defined as the area within Elschnig's ring, the cup is defined on the basis of contour, not pallor, and the NRR/optic cup border is taken as the level at which the slope of the NRR steepens. As conventions for making drawings are not widely taught, it is important to keep the diagram simple and to clearly label the features that are being represented. The slope of the NRR is often gentle, with an ill-defined border between NRR and cup in some parts of the disc. In these cases it is often helpful to represent the extremes of the possible border position with dashed lines and to label the NRR as sloping. This alerts clinicians when reviewing the case notes for evidence of progression, that apparent differences in interpretation over time may result from difficulty in defining the NRR/cup border.

Assigning a cup:disc ratio is almost universal when clinically assessing the ONH. However, estimations of different observers may vary greatly, and the recording of a cup: disc ratio in the absence of a diagram is of little use.

Pickard first illustrated the value of serial drawings more than 70 years ago.[2] By careful drawing of ONH cupping, he was able to demonstrate progressive changes over time (Figure 14.1). It is unusual, however, for the glaucoma patient to have the luxury of care by a single clinician over an extended period and more often drawings will be made by several different clinicians. The variation between different observers in their evaluation of the ONH and the subsequent drawing is large and confidence to detect real changes is consequently low. For this reason only large changes are likely to be detected reliably.

Optic disc photography

The advantage of photography over drawings of the ONH is obvious, with photography providing a true-to-life image of the ONH. All glaucoma patients, and particularly glaucoma suspects, should have ONH photography, if it is available, at the time of the first visit. This provides as a baseline from which changes can be detected. There are a number of ways in which to photograph the ONH and RNFL and each has advantages and disadvantages.

Colour transparencies

Colour transparencies provide a high resolution permanent record of the ONH appearance. The image in the transparency is small and some form of magnifying and lighting system is needed to view the images.

Monoscopic fundus photography results in a two-dimensional image. It is often difficult to compare the clinical stereoscopic view of the ONH with the photographic monoscopic image, and therefore to detect change. The apparent extent of cupping is often smaller in a monoscopic image, so that when a monoscopic

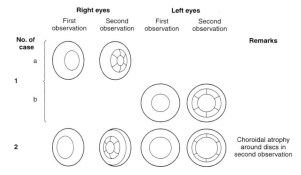

Figure 14.1 A sample of one of the drawings made by Pickard to demonstrate changes in optic disc appearance over time. Reproduced from Pichard R, A method of recording disc alterations and a study of the growth of normal and abnormal disc cups. *Br J Ophthalmology* 1923; 7: 81–91 with permission from the BMJ Publishing Group.

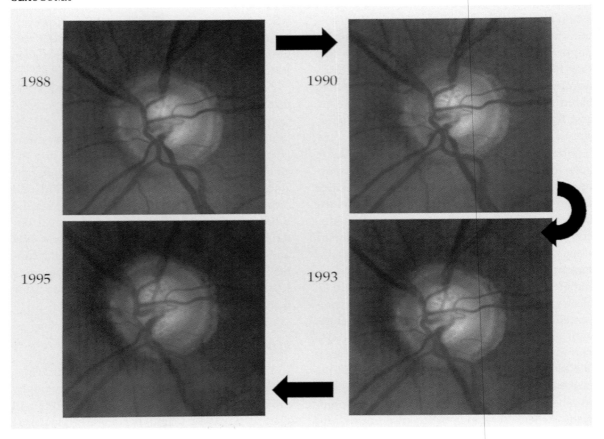

Figure 14.2   Optic nerve head photographs of an ocular hypertensive patient taken over the years 1988 to 1995. These show progressive narrowing of the neuroretinal rim in the superonasal and inferior segments of the optic nerve head, with the development of an inferior retinal nerve fibre defect adjacent to the thinned inferior rim.

photograph is compared with the stereoscopic view at the slit lamp, a false impression of cup enlargement may be gained. It is often easier to compare photograph with photograph, although differences in colour saturation between images, resulting from changes in flash intensity or developing cataract, can give a false impression of change. A series of photographs over the years 1988–1995 of an ocular hypertensive patient is presented in Figure 14.2. Progressive thinning of the superonasal and inferior NRR is seen, with the development of an inferior RNFL defect adjacent to the thinned inferior NRR. Figure 14.3 illustrates the onset over the years 1993–1997 of a corresponding visual field defect by analysis in the PROGRESSOR programme.

Strategies have been developed to maximise change detection from sequential photographs taken over a period of time. The techniques of flicker-chronoscopy[3] and stereochronoscopy enable the detection of very small changes over time. Two ONH photographs taken at different times are placed in a stereoviewer and aligned so that they are precisely superimposed. Illumination of the images is then rapidly switched from one image to the other ("flickered"). Small lateral displacements of ONH structures (over time) produce movement in the flickering image. When the two images are viewed simultaneously small lateral displacements are seen to stand out in relief ("stereo"). These methods of comparing images for change are so sensitive that even the venous pulse can be detected. However, false impressions of change can be

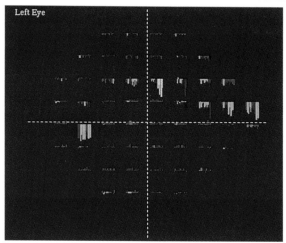

Figure 14.3 Visual field analysis for the patient illustrated in Figure 14.2. Pointwise linear regression of light sensitivity over time by the PROGRESSOR for Windows programme demonstrates the development of an arcuate visual field defect.

generated by magnification differences between the image pairs and by parallax, resulting from inconsistent alignment between the camera and eye. Unfortunately, the methods are time-consuming and require equipment that is not widely available.

Where such aids to the viewing of sequential images are not available, stereoscopic fundus photography, which enables appreciation of depth and contour changes, has advantages over monoscopic photography. The photographic stereoscopic image is more like the clinical stereo-scopic image. This is of value because it has been demonstrated that clinical evaluation of ONH images is more consistent under stereoscopic conditions.[4] As depth and contour clues are being used when comparing sequential stereo-scopic photographs, the clinician is less likely to be misled by apparent colour changes due to variations in fundus illumination.

The value of sequential stereoscopic ONH photography for the detection of progressive change in glaucoma has been demonstrated in a number of studies.[1,5,6] These studies have shown that it is possible to detect progressive morphological change at the ONH by subjective

evaluation, before the onset of visual field defects. The pattern of NRR changes occurring in a group of ocular hypertensive subjects has been described from sequential stereoscopic photographs.[7] The most common pattern of initial change in this study was a diffuse thin-ning of the NRR (43% of those showing change), and then notching of the NRR, with (17%) or without (26%) diffuse thinning. There was a subjective development of pallor, without contour change, in 13%. Diffuse NRR thinning was the major feature of progression in 78%.

Polaroid photography

This has the advantage of producing a magni-fied image that does not require a light-box for viewing. It is not an easy task to compare the small stereoscopic image seen during the clinical exam-ination with the magnified photographic image. Polaroid photography enables the production of a photographic image during a patient's visit. It is therefore possible to compare same-day and previous photographic images for acquired differ-ences in ONH morphology. Polaroid camera attachments are available for both monoscopic and stereoscopic fundus cameras. Polaroid reso-lution is lower than that of transparencies and colours may change over time, so that the photo-graph may not last as long as the patient. The format is also relatively expensive.

Black and white transparencies and prints

It is possible to photograph the RNFL using a wide-angle fundus camera, low-sensitivity, high resolution, black and white film and a blue narrow-band interference filter. Special film development techniques are also required and experience is needed to evaluate the photo-graphs reliably. The RNFL is less visible in lightly pigmented fundi and the fundi of the elderly, especially when lens opacities are pre-sent. However, RNFL photography in patients in whom the RNFL can be seen clearly, is a useful tool to detect the presence,[8] and progres-sion,[9] of glaucomatous changes. Figure 14.4

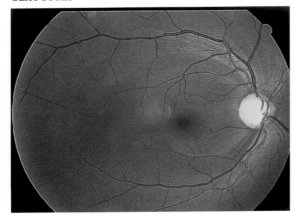

Figure 14.4 Black and white fundus photograph of a glaucoma patient taken with a blue filter demonstrates wedge-shaped defects in the nerve fibre layer.

illustrates a glaucoma patient in whom discrete RNFL defects can be seen clearly.

The evaluation of RNFL photographs is subjective and although semi-quantitative grading protocols have been developed in an attempt to measure RNFL loss in glaucoma, the reproducibility of grading scores is only moderate.[10] The more objective technique of densitometry has been applied to RNFL photographs to quantify changes in glaucoma, and the sources of variation in repeated imaging and analysis have been evaluated.[11] The technique requires specialist photography and image analysis and has not gained widespread usage.

The pattern of progression of RNFL defects in ocular hypertensive patients has been described.[7] Over half of the patients showing change had diffuse thinning of the RNFL and the remainder had either localised (wedge-shaped) loss, or a combination of diffuse and localised loss.

The methods described above are adequate to demonstrate that progression has taken place. The mere presence of progression, however, is not sufficient to make informed treatment decisions. The necessary information is the rate of progression. To determine the rate of progression, quantitative measurements of the ONH structure are required. Various measurement techniques have been developed,

ranging from computer programmes that enable magnification-corrected measurements of ONH photographs, to digital imaging devices and scanning laser ophthalmoscopes (the confocal scanning laser ophthalmoscope and the scanning laser polarimeter).

Magnification-corrected measurements of optic nerve head photographs

Planimetry is the term given to measurements made from photographic images. A number of programmes of varying sophistication are available. The Moorfields planimetry programme enables stereoscopic viewing of digitised stereoscopic ONH photographs on the computer screen. An observer is then able to outline the margin of the ONH and the NRR/optic cup border on the image, using a mouse. The computer programme then calculates the area of the NRR for the whole ONH and for ONH segments, corrects for the magnification due to the optics of the fundus camera and the eye, and relates the results to a normative database. Figure 14.5 is an example of the analysis for a glaucoma patient.

The usefulness of planimetry is limited by the subjective nature of the examination, as it relies on the judgements of individual observers as to the position of ONH and NRR/optic cup borders. The consistency of examinations between different observers is probably not good enough to detect small changes over time, but the repeatability of examinations by single observers has been shown to be high. Despite this, it was calculated that the NRR area had to change by more than 8.2% (between two photographs) for the change to reach the 99% confidence level for intraobserver reproducibility.[12] However, analysis of several photographs in a series over time allows detection of change with greater confidence. It is possible to take a series of such examinations to determine whether there is a progressive change in NRR area.

Airaksinen[13] made planimetric measurements

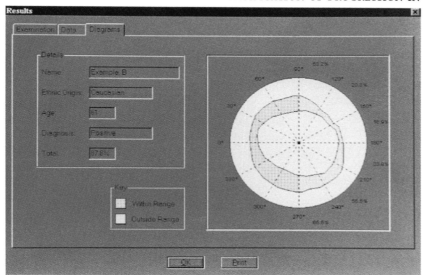

Figure 14.5 Report generated for the planimetric analysis of the optic nerve head photograph of a glaucoma patient. The diagram highlights segments of the nerve head in which the neuroretinal rim area falls outside the normal range.

of a series of normal, ocular hypertensive and glaucomatous eyes over a period of 5–15 years. A statistically significant rate of loss of NRR area was shown in 57% of patients with ocular hypertension and in 79% of those with glaucoma. The patients were divided into groups and a mean rate of loss was calculated for each, so that the NRR area declined at 0.23% per year in normals, 0.47% and 2.75% per year in stable and deteriorating ocular hypertensives, respectively, and by 3.47% per year in patients with deteriorating glaucoma. For individual patients the determination of a rate of NRR change is restricted by the measurement repeatability. If the NRR values are plotted over time, linear regression analysis will provide an estimate of rate of loss and levels of confidence for the rate of loss (which should exceed "0" before the change is accepted as real).

Patterns of loss can also be ascribed to the NRR changes,[13] such as linear, episodic or curvilinear. However, measurement variability (random variations in a parameter) can give rise to spurious patterns and this should be borne in mind when models of change are sought.

Over recent years evidence has accumulated that NRR loss frequently occurs before the onset of recognisable visual field loss by conventional "white-on-white" perimetry, in ocular hypertensive individuals. There is also evidence to suggest that ONH analysis is more sensitive to change in early disease and that visual field analysis is more sensitive in more advanced disease where visual field loss is already established.[12]

Given the limitations of planimetry, digital imaging devices have been developed to make ONH analysis more objective and analyses more repeatable.

Digital optic nerve head imaging

One such device is the Optic Nerve Head Analyzer (Rodenstock Instruments). This instrument projects stripes of light onto the ONH which are deformed according to surface topography, and simultaneously records stereoscopic videographic images. Depth information is gained by performing a cross-correlation of points on the stripes in the two halves of the stereo pair. This function is performed across the whole image to generate a surface topography. An observer outlines the ONH margin, and the software defines the cup edge by identifying the NRR surface within the ONH margin that lies at a set depth below the ONH edge. The definition of the optic cup is thus more objective than planimetric definitions, as the only subjective input is the observer-defined ONH margin. The standard deviation for NRR area measurements from repeated imaging and analyses is, nevertheless, still quite high and has been estimated at 0.117–0.231 mm^2 (about 15% of the mean NRR area).[14] The source of greatest variability was found to be instrument variability (images taken on different occasions) rather than variability arising from the operator input to the analysis. The same study presented the 95% and 99% confidence intervals for real change, calculated from the variability data, as a guide to those wishing to use the instrument to detect change in the clinical setting.

Funk[15] acquired several images over an average of nearly 18 months from 47 ocular hypertensive eyes, and performed linear regression analysis of NRR area over time. Because of the relatively short follow-up, he extrapolated the changes seen to 24 months before analysing for change. By this method 8 of the 47 eyes were determined to have a progressive loss in NRR area. Measurement variability was deemed too great to be able to determine a "progressing" or "stable" status in 38% of eyes.

Scanning laser polarimetry

An example of this form of scanning laser ophthalmoscope is the Nerve Fibre Analyser (NFA or GDx, Laser Diagnostic Technologies Inc). The instrument is a recent development that enables objective measurements of the RNFL to be made. A polarised near infrared (780 nm) laser beam is scanned across the fundus at the optic nerve head and parapapillary retina. The light passes through the RNFL and is partially reflected by deeper structures. The RNFL has properties of birefringence and causes a change in the state of polarisation of the reflected light (retardation). The NFA detection unit quantifies the amount of retardation, which is correlated with RNFL thickness. The RNFL is not the only birefringent structure in the eye, and the NFA includes a compensator unit to correct for retardation arising in the cornea. The measurements of the NFA have been validated histopathologically in eyes with the cornea removed, with 1° of retardation corresponding to 7.4 μm of RNFL thickness.[16] Reproducibility of measurements has been shown to be good, though one study found that while intra-observer variation (image acquisition and analysis) was low, with a coefficient of variation (standard deviation/mean) for RNFL thickness measurements of 4.5–4.9%, the variation between observers was much greater.[17]

The instrument has been used to detect change in measured RNFL parameters in ocular hypertensive subjects.[18] Of 46 subjects followed for three years, eight developed a borderline or abnormal visual field. Of these, one had an abnormal RNFL parameter in the first year, three developed an abnormal parameter in the second year, and three developed an abnormal parameter in the third year. Crossing the threshold from normal to abnormal parameters is taken to indicate that progression has taken place. Longer follow-up of such a group of patients may enable rates of progression to be quantified.

Confocal scanning laser ophthalmoscopy

Scanning laser ophthalmoscopes, such as the Heidelberg Retina Tomograph (HRT, Heidelberg Engineering), are a recent development that enables objective measurements of the ONH to be made. The method of imaging utilises the confocal principle, in which a laser beam is brought to a focus in a given plane at the fundus and reflected light is received at a photodetector unit through an aperture with the focus set at the illuminated retinal plane. In this way only light from the plane of focus is imaged, with resolution subject to the optics of the human eye. A series of "optical sections" of the fundus is recorded by changing the plane of focus in an axial manner, beginning in the vitreous in front of the optic disc and ending behind the lamina cribrosa. In order to construct a topographic representation of the optic disc, the HRT takes a series of 32 consecutive "optical sections". For any given point at the optic disc, a graph can be constructed of the intensity of light reflected at that point, in each of the 32 sections (the axial intensity distribution or "z-profile"). The peak in the z-profile (the optical section giving the most reflected light at that point) approximates to the surface in structures with a single reflecting surface. "Surface" determination is performed by identification of the centre of gravity of the z-profile (which is usually close to the peak) and is repeated at the 65,536 "pixel" locations in the area imaged, and the surface topography is generated from the result. The images are scaled after making corrections for magnification due to the optics of the HRT and the eye.

In order to produce conventional topographic parameters, such as the optic disc, cup and neuroretinal rim areas, and optic cup and neuroretinal rim volumes, it is necessary to define the area of interest. This is done interactively with the examiner outlining the margin of the ONH on the computer screen. The software then defines a "reference plane" which is a plane parallel to, and depressed below, the surface of the retina. Structures lying above the reference plane are defined as neuroretinal rim, and space below the reference plane is defined as optic cup. For follow-up examinations the software has the facility to "export" the defined ONH edge from one image to another. This reduces one source of variability between analyses.

Different approaches to change detection with this instrument have been made using conventional parameters such as NRR area or surface height measurements within the images. Kamal[19] derived 95% confidence intervals for change in NRR area from a group of 21 normal subjects with "mean topography" images acquired one to two years apart. The "mean topography" images are derived from the average of three single topography images taken a few minutes apart in one session. In a longitudinal study 47 of 164 ocular hypertensive eyes showed change in NRR area greater than the upper 95% confidence interval. This approach is useful to demonstrate that change in the ONH has occurred, although it does not provide information on the rate of change.

The repeatability of measurements made on a series of three images taken a few minutes apart has been evaluated in a series of ocular hypertensive and glaucomatous patients presenting with an optic disc haemorrhage.[20] The mean coefficient of variation for NRR measurements was found to be 3.9%. This level of variability is still sufficiently high to limit the ability of the instrument to detect change when two images are compared. The ability to detect change can be improved considerably by acquiring more than one image at a patient's visit and by acquiring images at frequent intervals. This approach was taken to investigate a series of patients with disc haemorrhages for progressive NRR loss.[20] Eight eyes of eight glaucoma patients and seven eyes of six patients with ocular hypertension were followed for an average of 30 months, and had images acquired at an average of 6 monthly intervals, with three images taken at each visit. Progressive loss of NRR was demonstrated in 11 of the 15 eyes. Figure 14.6 illustrates two of the 15 HRT images acquired from one of these eyes, the first taken at the time of the haemorrhage and the second taken 36 months later. Figure 14.7 illustrates the NRR area measurements made from each of the images plotted against time. A progressive reduction in NRR area can be seen clearly. A considerable advantage of this method is that the analysis can provide a figure for the rate of change. The examples illustrated (Figures 14.6, 14.7) demonstrate a loss of inferotemporal NRR of 0.021 mm^2 per year (95% confidence intervals 0.014–0.027 mm^2 per year). Such knowledge of the rate of change can inform treatment decisions and can also provide evidence of the efficacy of treatment interventions. Further work is needed to establish in which patients, and at what stage of disease, frequent imaging is of most benefit for the measurement of progression, but the evidence so far illustrates the promise of the approach.

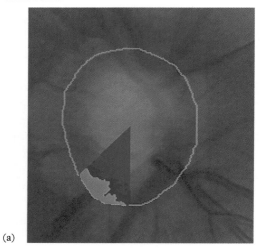

(a)

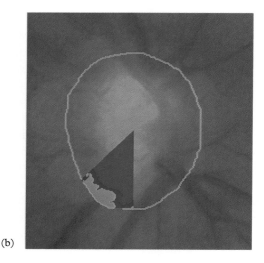

(b)

Figure 14.6 The analyses of topography images (Heidelberg retina tomograph) of a patient with an early glaucomatous visual field defect. Two of a series of 15 are shown, (a) taken at the time of a disc haemorrhage and (b) taken 36 months later. The analysis for the inferotemporal part of the nerve head is illustrated: green and blue represents neuroretinal rim and red represents optic cup.

Chauhan[21] has developed an approach that involves the generation of "confidence interval maps" derived from the variation in surface height measurements between three images taken in the same session. The map consists of an array of 64 × 64 super pixels (reduced from the original 256 × 256 pixels). In this way,

regions of the ONH with high and low between-image variability can be identified. Apparent change over time has to exceed location specific values for variability in order to be considered real change. Figure 14.8 illustrates surface height changes in a glaucomatous eye over a two and a half year period, together with the visual field tests over the same period. The height of a super-pixel is measured from a reference level (the mean height of the "reference ring" in peripapillary retina in the peripheral part of the image), which is assumed to be stable over time. The sensitivity to change of the method is, therefore, likely to be greater when sources of variation in the mean height of the reference ring are controlled, such as careful centring of the ONH in the image frame. The effect of posterior movement of the retinal surface at the reference ring, as a result of thinning of the RNFL, in progressive glaucoma is likely to be small, because of the peripheral location of the reference ring, but may result in underestimation of diffuse changes, relative to localised changes. The method appears to be very sensitive to changes in surface height from one occasion to another.[22]

Apparent change may result from uncontrolled variability in image acquisition and processing or from changes in the prevailing ocular conditions at the time of imaging. In order to identify progressive change, as opposed to

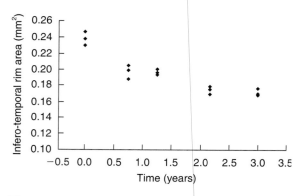

Figure 14.7 Neuroretinal rim area measurements for each of the images in the series for the optic nerve head illustrated in Figure 14.6. Rim area is plotted against time from disc haemorrhage

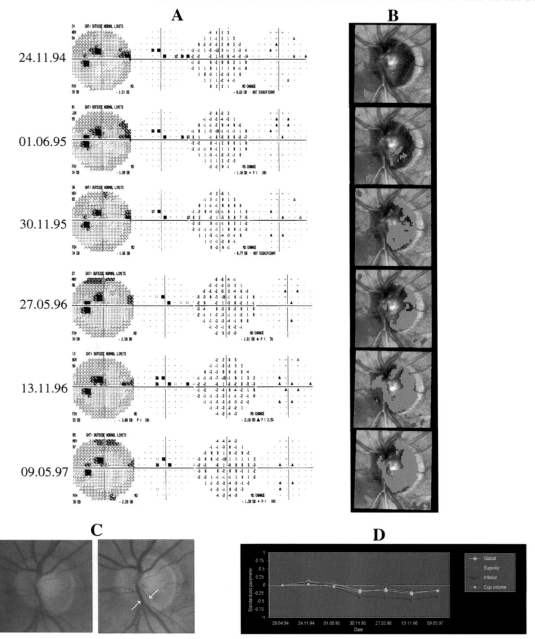

Figure 14.8   Serial scanning laser ophthalmoscope images and visual fields from the left eye of a glaucoma patient. A, the Glaucoma Change Probability analysis does not show visual field progression. B, probability maps derived scanning laser tomograph images (same time points as visual field tests): red pixels indicate significant loss of surface height, green pixels indicate a gain in surface height. C, optic disc photographs taken on 24.11.94 (left) and 09.05.97 (right). D, analysis of standard tomographic parameters over time. Reproduced with permissin from Morrison J, Pollack I. *Glaucoma: The Essentials* published by Thieme.

apparent change, analyses showing change at the same location and greater than that found in normal eyes is required in images from three consecutive imaging sessions. The method has the advantage that change analysis applies to the whole image and is not confined to a region of interest (the ONH), and there is no need for the (subjective) definition of the ONH margin. Methods to quantify and determine rates of change have yet to be developed and the clinical significance of changes detected will need to be evaluated. This approach to change detection is being incorporated into HRT software.

References

1 Sommer A, Pollack I, Maumenee AE. Optic disc parameters and onset of glaucomatous field loss. I. Methods and progressive changes in disc morphology. *Arch Ophthalmol* 1979; **97**: 1444–8.

2 Pickard R. A method of recording disc alterations and a study of the growth of normal and abnormal disc cups. *Br J Ophthalmol* 1923; **7**: 81–91.

3 Bengtsson B, Krakau CE. Flicker comparison of fundus photographs. A technical note. *Acta Ophthalmol* 1979; **57**: 503–6.

4 Varma R, Steinmann WC, Scott IU. Expert agreement in evaluating the optic disc for glaucoma. *Ophthalmology* 1992; **99**: 215–21.

5 Odberg T, Riise D. Early diagnosis of glaucoma. The value of successive stereophotography of the optic disc. *Acta Ophthalmol Copenh* 1985; **63**: 257–63.

6 Pederson JE, Anderson DR. The mode of progressive disc cupping in ocular hypertension and glaucoma. *Arch Ophthalmol* 1980; **98**: 490–5.

7 Tuulonen A, Airaksinen PJ. Initial glaucomatous optic disk and retinal nerve fiber layer abnormalities and their progression. *Am J Ophthalmol* 1991; **111**: 485–90.

8 Quigley HA, Miller NR, George T. Clinical evaluation of nerve fiber layer atrophy as an indicator of glaucomatous optic nerve damage. *Arch Ophthalmol* 1980; **98**: 1564–71.

9 Quigley HA, Katz J, Derick RJ, Gilbert D, Sommer A. An evaluation of optic disc and nerve fiber layer examinations in monitoring progression of early glaucoma damage. *Ophthalmology* 1992; **99**: 19–28.

10 Airaksinen PJ, Drance SM, Douglas GR, Mawson DK, Nieminen H. Diffuse and localised nerve fiber loss in glaucoma. *Am J Ophthalmol* 1984; **98**: 566–71.

11 Eikelboom RH, Cooper RL, Barry CJ. A study of variance in densitometry of retinal nerve fiber layer photographs in normals and glaucoma suspects. *Invest Ophthalmol Vis Sci* 1990; **31**: 2373–83.

12 Zeyen TG, Caprioli J. Progression of disc and field damage in early glaucoma. *Arch Ophthalmol* 1993; **111**: 62–5.

13 Airaksinen PJ, Tuulonen A, Alanko HI. Rate and pattern of neuroretinal rim area decrease in ocular hypertension and glaucoma. *Arch Ophthalmol* 1992; **110**: 206–10.

14 Bishop KI, Werner EB, Krupin T, *et al* . Variability and reproducibility of optic disk topographic measurements with the Rodenstock Optic Nerve Head Analyzer. *Am J Ophthalmol* 1988; **106**: 696–702.

15 Funk J. Early detection of glaucoma by longitudinal monitoring of the optic disc structure. *Graefe's Arch Clin Exp Ophthalmol* 1991; **229**: 57–61.

16 Weinreb RN, Dreher AW, Coleman A, Quigley H, Shaw B, Reiter K. Histopathologic validation of Fourier-ellipsometry measurements of retinal fiber layer thickness. *Arch Ophthalmol* 1990; **108**: 557–60.

17 Hoh ST, Ishikawa H, Greenfield DS, Liebmann JM, Chew SJ, Ritch R. Peripapillary nerve fiber layer thickness measurement reproducibility using scanning laser polarimetry. *J Glaucoma* 1998; **7**: 12–5.

18 Tjon-Fo-Sang MJ, Lemij HG. A 3–year follow up of patients with ocular hypertension with scanning laser polarimetry. *Invest Ophthalmol Vis Sci (ARVO abstracts)* 1998; **39**: S1126.

19 Kamal DS, Viswanathan AC, Garway-Heath D, Hitchings RA, Poinoosawmy D, Bunce C. Detection of optic disc change with the Heidelberg retina tomograph before confirmed visual field change in ocular hypertensives converting to early glaucoma. *Br J Ophthalmol* 1999; **83**: 290–5.

20 Garway-Heath DF, Kamal DS, Fitzke FW, Hitchings RA. Repeated optic disc imaging with the Heidelberg Retina Tomograph detects progressive neuroretinal rim loss in ocular hypertension and glaucoma. *Invest Ophth Vis Sci (ARVO abstracts)* 1998; **39**: S699.

21 Chauhan BC, LeBlanc RP, McCormick TA, Rogers JB. Test-retest variability of topographic measurements with confocal scanning laser tomography in patients with glaucoma and control subjects. *Am J Ophthalmol* 1994; **118**: 9–15.

22 Chauhan BC, Blanchard JW, Hamilton DC, *et al*. Technique for detecting serial topographical changes in the optic disc and peripapillary retina using scanning laser tomography. *Invest Ophthalmol Vis Sci* 2000; **41**: in press.

15 The effect glaucoma has on individuals

I E MURDOCH

Glaucoma is the third most common cause for blindness registration and yet registerable blindness is a relatively rare occurrence in this disease. In order to qualify for registration by the World Health Organization (WHO) criteria, an individual must have an acuity of < 3/60 and/or visual field constriction to < 10° in both eyes.[1] Loss of central visual acuity is typically the last occurrence in advanced glaucoma where progressive deterioration of visual field typifies the advance of optic nerve damage.

Work on blind registration has shown that individuals who are registerable blind by virtue of visual field restriction criteria are underrepresented in the totals registered.[2] The burden of visual handicap from the disease in the community is therefore much larger than blindness registration would suggest.

Burden of disease and its therapy

If the effectiveness of interventions to prevent the progression of glaucoma is to be assessed, it is important to gain a clear assessment of the social burden of handicap from the disease. At present there is only one other significant field-dependent measure of social function and that is the DVLA (Driver and Vehicle Licensing Agency) test for fitness to drive.

Because the disease is insidious in nature and relatively slow in progression, taking five years or more to progress to blindness if untreated,[3] many adaptive processes take place in individuals to cope with any visual handicap. Unlike many diseases, coping strategies that evolve to overcome visual handicap are dysfunctional in glaucoma as they conceal the existence and progression of the disease. It is very difficult to estimate the social burden of the disease. How much less productive is an accountant with 50% visual field loss? How much more care is required for an elderly individual living alone with 50% visual field loss?

Our therapy for the disease is preventive. We are still struggling to quantify exactly how preventive our treatment truly is. The therapies themselves have costs (see Chapter 12). Medical therapies are inconvenient, expensive, almost impossible to use for some patients, and potentially damaging to systemic well being. Laser therapies are variably effective and generally have a limited period of action. Surgery has finite risks, time commitments, and potential unwelcome side effects.

Quality of life

Definitions

In recognition of the above, numerous attempts have been made to assess the quality of life in individuals with glaucoma. Quality of life has been given at least three definitions. Firstly, a value modified by length of time lived, symptoms, functional status, perceptions and opportunity. Secondly, "years of healthy life", a graded scale is defined between full health and death for each year lived. Finally, "an individual's perception of their position in life in the context of the culture and value systems in which they live, and in relation to their goals, expectations and concerns. It is a broad-ranging concept affected in a complex way by a person's physical health, psychological state, level of independence, social relationships, and their relationship to salient features of their environment."[4]

Which question?

In assessing the many and various tools used to assess quality of life, it is important to stand back and address the questions being asked. Are we interested in documenting the problems faced by patients with glaucoma? Are we interested in the patients' perception of the handicap caused by the disease process or its therapy? Are we interested in the effectiveness of interventions on the disease process in social or clinical terms, or from the patients' perspective? Are we interested in the most cost-effective way of reducing the health burden caused by the disease in a particular population? Each of these questions requires a different form of trial or study to assess.

Generic or disease-specific assessment?

Quality of life is the most popular concept in present medical literature for assessing outcomes of disease processes and/or interventions beyond laboratory or examination defined endpoints. In assessing this, the first question that arises is whether a disease specific measure should be used or a more generic measure. Generic health measures focus on basic human values and address two main areas, functional status and wellbeing. Dimensions of health such as sleeping, eating, recreation and the ability to communicate are not usually covered by these assessments.[5] They have, however, the major advantage of being able to provide comparative data across diseases. Disease specific measures have large advantages in terms of responsiveness for ocular disease but are not useful for between disease comparisons.

Objective or subjective?

Another question is whether the assessment should be based upon conventional clinical evidence or upon patient ratings. Conventional clinical evidence may show important changes in the patient's clinical status but it is a poor indicator of how the patient feels and functions in day-to-day activity. Substantial progression of a visual field defect in one eye could be an example of this. The patient may not notice the progression, particularly if the fellow eye is unaffected, but such a change has profound clinical implications.

Cognitive, affective and spiritual domains

An underlying principle of quality of life research in medicine is that medical treatments and diseases apply to "whole persons". The assessment of effects therefore includes an evaluation of individuals' overall functioning. This has been divided into two or three components.[6] Firstly, there is a statement or description of an experience, e.g. the presence or absence of a problem; this is a cognitive process. Secondly, there is a value placed on that experience or event, e.g. the importance of the presence or absence of the problem; this is an affective process. Some authors have added a spiritual domain.

Methods of measurement

Many different assessments have been used for quality of life in individuals with ocular disease. A large number of these have been well summarised by Parrish.[7] Some have been generic, such as the Medical Outcomes Study Short Form-36 (SF36), and the Sickness Impact Profile (SIP). Others have been vision-specific such as the Vision-specified Sickness Impact Profile (VF-14), Visual Activities Questionnaire, and The National Eye Institute Visual Functioning Questionnaire.

Results in ophthalmology research pertinent to glaucoma

Correlation with visual acuity

A majority of investigators have looked at the correlation between measured visual function and the quality of life assessment. Generic assessments generally show a poor correlation (< 0.1–0.3) with any form of measured visual function including acuity. One exception is a report by Scott et al. that shows correlation coefficients of 0.4–0.5 between three generic assessments and visual acuity.[8]

Vision specific assessments generally show a moderate correlation (0.4–0.7) with visual acuity. Mangione notes that, although there is usually a linear relationship between quality of life instrument scores and measured visual acuity, there is a large amount of scatter. This means that many individuals have very low correlation between their perceived and measured function.[5] However, such findings do not necessarily invalidate the tools. They reinforce the fact that visual acuity and quality of life instruments may be measuring different constructs.

Correlation with visual fields

Binocular visual field loss is generally not well identified by quality of life instruments.[9] With much searching, Mills and Drance were able to identify five questions that predicted 48% of the variation in visual field disability indices.[10] Some association between poor vision specific questionnaire scores and severe field loss in the better eye was also reported by Gutierrez et al.[11]

Correlation with other tests of visual function

Contrast sensitivity assessments have been reported to be associated with scores from vision specific assessments in patients with glaucoma[12] and cataract.[13] Glare assessments in patients with cataract do not seem as strongly correlated.[13] Colour vision, binocular single vision and other visual function tests have not been frequently studied in this fashion.

More objective measures and visual function

The use of more objective measures has been less frequently reported. However, in the Beaver Dam study four measures were found to be related: a history of falls, hip fractures, gait time, and visual acuity. Contrast sensitivity was also assessed and showed a less consistent relationship.[14]

Effect of change

Cataract surgery generally offers a significant change in visual function as assessed by objective clinical measurements such as visual acuity or contrast sensitivity. The results on quality of life assessments for even this intervention have, however, been quite variable. A vision specific questionnaire in southern India showed a substantial beneficial effect one year after cataract surgery.[15] This was not the case in Nepal.[16] Improvement in vision from any cause over a one year period, was associated with improved vision specific and generic questionnaire responses in three American cities.[17] In contrast, vision specific scores improved in 80%, but generic scores in only 36% for elderly subjects one year after cataract surgery in Massachusetts. Indeed average scores on seven of eight domains in the generic questionnaire had worsened at 12 months.[18]

Some of this variability in results may be explained by factors external to the patients, such as operative skills. This was the likely explanation in the Nepalese study. There were disappointing effects for visual function assessments as well as the vision specific questionnaire assessments in the pseudophakic patients in this study.[16] Another explanation could be poor choice of questionnaire for the purposes of a longitudinal study. It is possible for instruments to be reliable but unresponsive to change over time if the variance between subjects dwarfs the variance within subjects.[19] Our tools for visual assessment may also be inadequate.

The above explanations are unlikely to explain all of the variability noted in the large literature concerning the outcome of cataract surgery that has been well summarised by Legro.[6]

Factors specific to glaucoma that would be of interest to study

Glaucoma, particularly chronic open angle glaucoma, has some aspects that are particularly challenging from a quality of life perspective. As outlined above, our therapy for the disease is preventive. Dissatisfaction with glaucoma medical therapy (e.g. miosis), glaucoma surgery (e.g. bleb dysaesthesia) and a lack of perceived benefit from therapy, may all play a part in quality of life for individuals with the disease. In addition, the relevance of support groups, patient education and patient counselling may contribute to quality of life.

Problems with quality of life assessments

Deficiencies in the construct within an individual

Psychologists have long been aware that expressed attitude or changes in attitude may bear little or no relation to behaviour.[20] Quality of life variables also bear relation to wider issues. Health is a major component of quality of life, but many more dimensions are required to fully describe health-related quality of life.[21] In a study on visual function status there was a correlation with visual acuity in the best eye.[22] The correlation was not straightforward. Some patients functioned quite well despite a poor visual acuity, and some patients with good acuity only had moderate visual function. It is interesting that after cataract surgery patients felt that their vision had improved. The proportion driving a car after surgery, however, only

rose from 21–34% and those reading a newspaper, from 62–68%.[23] Similarly a change in level of physical function was found one year after cataract surgery. The change was affected by baseline physical function and baseline mental status, and could not be solely explained by change in visual acuity.[24] Successful recovery (defined as being more satisfied, more active, and more efficient following surgery) was positively correlated with the level of activity sustained before surgery, and the ability to learn a new visual-motor co-ordination task.[25] This was confirmed in a second study where postoperative reaching, walking, activity and satisfaction, were positively correlated with scores on several preoperative visual motor tasks.[26] Thus it would seem that much wider aspects of the individual relate to a perception of the impact of treatment on the quality of life.

A large body of work has been done investigating the value of questionnaires in quality of life assessments of individuals with glaucoma.[7] However, the questionnaires have focused on activity related functions. Important aspects of recreation and motivation, or the state of mood of the individual, have not been addressed.[27] It is known that individuals with low vision are frequently depressed.[28,29] In addition, the possibility of altered behaviour patterns to avoid stigmata associated with being visually handicapped[30] has not been addressed.

A further point of relevance to glaucoma is the issue of present versus future incapacity. The work concerning cataract generally relates to present incapacity. Work on glaucoma may often focus on future incapacity which has very different constructs. This may be illustrated with the idea of a forthcoming operation. A patient may accept the relative risks prior to surgery, but when faced with the side effects as an experience, say they would have selected a different management option because of what they had now experienced.[31]

Deficiencies in the construct beyond the individual

Beyond the above considerations there are even more factors that relate to individuals' overall quality of life. In particular, social circumstances such as income, family support and political environment (wars, oppression), are important.

Disability adjusted life years (DALYs)

A problem with any measure of quality of life is that it is based around the subjective perception of wellbeing and wholeness, which in true terms are immeasurable. For this reason the World Bank developed an entirely new system for the World development report 1993: Investing in Health.[32]

Construct

Overall, disease in society causes a given burden in terms of decreased productivity and/or increased dependency. There is a finite pot of money and resource that can be given to tackling the problem. Many of the questions being asked boil down to how to best allocate these finite resources to produce maximum benefit in term of decreased burden.

Assessment of the burden of disease may be considered to have at least four important objectives: [33]

- to aid in setting health service (both curative and preventive) priorities
- to aid in setting health research priorities
- to aid in identifying disadvantaged groups and targeting of health interventions
- to provide a comparable measure of output for intervention, programme and sector evaluation and planning.

DALYs use a standard "expected-life lost" that is based on a model life table and the value of time lived at different ages. It is captured using a function that reflects the dependence of the young and the elderly on adults. The time lived with a disability is made comparable with the time lost due to premature mortality by defining six classes of disability severity. In other words, the concept of the DALY centres on an ideal population in which every individual has perfect health for the entirety of their ideal (best available population) life-span. If a male has an expected life-span of 80 years and dies aged 40 then he scores 40 DALYs for his country. Should the male contract a disease at the age of 40 which decreases his productivity by half (makes him half-dead) for the remainder of his 80 year life-span, he scores $40/2 = 20$ DALYs for his country. If he is a quarter-dead at 40 and lives until 80, then he accrues $40/4 = 10$ DALYs. Thus an overall burden of disease is arrived at for a given population against which the cost-effectiveness of interventions can be assessed.

Application

When applied to the leading causes of blindness in the world this method of analysis gives some very encouraging results. Out of over 50 interventions assessed by the World Bank, cataract surgery was a highly cost-effective intervention. The cost per DALY saved ranged from US$15 to just over US$30. This has been confirmed by work in Nepal where the cost per DALY saved was only US$5.[34] There is no work to date investigating glaucoma interventions in this fashion.

The therapies of onchocerciasis, vitamin A supplementation and traditional interventions for trachoma, have also been shown to be highly cost effective. It is time that the cost-effectiveness of glaucoma and other ophthalmic disease interventions is addressed to enable ophthalmology programmes to receive the place they deserve in health programmes.

References

1 WHO methods of assessment of avoidable blindness. WHO offset publication no.54 1980.
2 Bunce K, Wormald R. *Br J Ophthalmol* c.1997.

3 Jay JL, Murdoch JR. The rate of visual field loss in untreated primary open angle glaucoma *Br J Ophthalmol* 1993; **77**: 176–8.

4 Patrick D. What is quality of life in vision research and clinical practice? pp 5–16 in Encounters in glaucoma research 3 – How to ascertain progression and outcome. Anderson DR, Drance SM (eds). Kugler 1996.

5 Mangione CM. Comparing generic and disease-specific measurements. pp 23–35 in Encounters in glaucoma research 3 – How to ascertain progression and outcome. Anderson DR, Drance SM (eds) Kugler 1996.

6 Legro MW. Quality of life and cataracts. *Ophthalmic Surg* 1991; **22**: 431–43.

7 Parish RK. Visual impairment, visual functioning, and quality of life assessments in patients with glaucoma. *Trans Am Ophth Soc* 1996; **94**: 919–1028.

8 Scott IU, Schien OD, West S, Bandeen-Roche K, Enger C, Folstein MF. Functional status and quality of life measurement among ophthalmic patients. *Arch Ophthalmol* 1994; **112**: 329–35.

9 Herwood MB, Garcia-Siekavizza A, Meltzer MI, Hebert A, Burns AF, McGorray S. Glaucoma's impact on quality of life and its relation to clinical indicators – A pilot study. *Ophthalmology* 1998; **105**: 561–6.

10 Mills RP, Drance SM. Esterman disability rating in severe glaucoma. *Ophthalmology* 1986; **93**: 371–8.

11 Gutierrez P, Wilson R, Johnson C, *et al.* Influence of glaucomatous visual field loss on health-related quality of life. *Arch Ophthalmol* 1997; **115**: 777–84.

12 Ross JE, Bron AJ, Clarke DD. Contrast sensitivity and visual disability in chronic simple glaucoma. *Br J Ophthalmol* 1984; **68**: 821–7.

13 Elliott DB, Hurst MA, Weatherill J. Comparing clinical tests of visual function in cataract with the patient's perceived visual disability. *Eye* 1990; **4**: 712–7.

14 Klein BE, Klein R, Lee KE, Cruickshanks KJ. Performance-based and self-assessed measures of visual function as related to history of falls, hip fractures, and measured gait time. The Beaver Dam Eye Study. *Ophthalmology* 1998; **105**: 160–4.

15 Fletcher AE, Ellwein LB, Selvaraj S, Vijaykumar V, Rahmathullah, Thulasiraj RD. Measurements of visual function and quality of life in patients with cataracts in Southern India – Report of instrument development. *Arch Ophthalmol* 1997; **115**: 767–74.

16 Okharel GP, Selvaraj S, Ellwein LB. Visual functioning and quality of life outcomes among cataract operated and unoperated blind populations in Nepal. *Br J Ophthalmol* 1998; **82**: 606–10.

17 Brenner MH, Curbow B, Javitt JC, Legro MW, Sommer A. Vision change and quality of life in the elderly. *Arch Ophthalmol* 1993; **111**: 680–5.

18 Mangione CM, Phillips RS, Lawrence MG, Seddon JM, Orav J, Goldman L. Improved visual function and attenuation of declines in health-related quality of life after cataract extraction. *Arch Ophthalmol* 1994; **112**: 1419–25.

19 Guyatt G, Walter S, Norman G. Measuring change over time: assessing the usefulness of evaluative instruments. *J Chronic Diseases* 1987; **40**: 171–8.

20 Kirk-Smith M, McKenna H. Psychological concerns in questionnaire research. *Nursing Times – Research* 1998; **3**: 203–13.

21 Wiklund I, Karlberg J. Evaluation of quality of life in clinical trials – Selecting quality of life measures. *Controlled Clin Trials* 1991; **12**: 204S–16S.

22 Bernth-Petersen P. Visual functioning in cataract patients – Methods of measuring and results. *Acta Ophthalmol* 1981; **59**: 198–205.

23 Applegate WB, Miller ST, Elam JT, Freeman JM, Wood TO, Gettlefinger TC. Impact of cataract surgery with lens implantation on vision and physical function in elderly patients *JAMA* 1987; **257**: 1064–6.

24 Elam JT, Graney MJ, Applegate WB, et al. Functional outcome one year following cataract surgery in elderly persons. *J Geriontol* 1988; **43**: 122–6.

25 Murphy SB, Donderi DC. Predicting the success of cataract surgery. *J Behavioural Med* 1980; **3**: 1–14.

26 Donderi DC, Murphy SB. Predicting activity and satisfaction following cataract surgery. *J Behavioural Med* 1983; **6**: 313–28.

27 Owen J, Herse P. Low vision and surfing. *Opt Vis Science* 1996; **73**: 558–61.

28 Shmuely-Dulitzki Y, Rovner BW. Screening for depression in older persons with low vision. Somatic symptoms and the Geriatric Depression Scale. *Am J Geriat Psychiatry* 1997; **5**: 216–20.

29 Fagerstrom R. Correlation between depression and vision in aged patients before and after cataract operations. *Psycholog Reps* 1994; **75**: 115–25.

30 Lane SD, Mikhail BI, Reizian A, Courtright P, Marx R, Dawson CR. Sociocultural aspects of blindness in an Egyptian delta hamlet: visual impairment vs visual disability. *Med Anthropol* 1993; **15**: 245–60.

31 Anderson DR. Discussion in: Mangione CM. Comparing generic and disease-specific measurements. pp 31–2 in Encounters in glaucoma research 3 – How to ascertain progression and outcome. Anderson DR, Drance SM (eds). Kugler 1996.

32 Investing in health. World Bank Development Report 1993 and World Development Indicators, World Bank, 1993.

33 Murray CJL. Quantifying the burden of disease: the technical basis for disability-adjusted life years. Bull. *WHO* 1994; **72**: 429–45.

34 Marseille E. Cost–effectiveness of cataract surgery in a public health eye care programme in Nepal. Bull. *WHO* 1996; **74**: 319–24.

16 Primary angle closure: classification and clinical features

P J FOSTER, G J JOHNSON

Primary angle closure glaucoma (PACG) is a scarce condition in the Caucasoid people of Europe and North America, from where much current medical dogma originates. The condition is typically recognised in an acute symptomatic phase and accounts for a relatively small proportion of ocular morbidity in the population. As a consequence PACG has not received the same level of attention in recent years as primary open angle glaucoma (POAG). However, the recognition that the number of people with PACG worldwide probably exceeds POAG, emphasises the importance of this condition in areas with a large non-European population.[1]

The growing emphasis on characteristic progressive end-organ damage ("glaucomatous" optic neuropathy) as a hallmark of POAG has given the classification of this condition a more logical scientific foundation. In the following description primary angle closure (PAC) is considered a distinct anterior segment disease that imbues the sufferer with an increased risk of glaucomatous optic neuropathy, but does not by itself constitute glaucoma.

Definition

The clinical feature *sine qua non* of PAC is significant obstruction of the functional trabecular meshwork (TM) by the peripheral iris, in the absence of a secondary pathological process. People with trabecular obstruction and glaucomatous damage to the optic nerve have PACG.

This approach represents a departure from convention under which individuals with a narrow drainage angle, and either raised IOP or peripheral anterior synechiae, were said to have primary angle closure "glaucoma". Therefore in this scheme, persons suffering an acute symptomatic rise in IOP would not be considered to have glaucoma unless they showed evidence of optic nerve damage. This may be difficult to accept until one considers that 60–75% of persons suffering an acute symptomatic episode of angle closure, recover without optic disc or visual field damage.[2,3] A longitudinal study of 129 patients at risk of angle closure (121 white subjects, mean follow-up 2.7 years, maximum 6 years) found that 6% experienced an episode of acute symptomatic angle closure, and a further 13% developed asymptomatic appositional or synechial angle closure. No comment is made regarding the development of a functional visual deficit, although it seems likely that this occurred in very few subjects.[4] If one intends the term glaucoma to signify a disease characterised by an irreversible defect in visual function, then most persons suffering symptomatic episodes of raised pressure or asymptomatic narrow drainage angles, do not have it. They have PAC.

That elevation of the intraocular pressure (IOP) has retained such prominence as a criterion for diagnosis of PAC, is probably a reflection that (in Europeans) most cases are recognised in the "acute" phase. The contention that raised IOP is a major risk factor for the development of glaucomatous optic neuropathy and that risk is proportional to the degree of pressure elevation and its duration, has not been superseded.[5,6] This theory was developed after clinical observation, largely of patients with POAG, and validated in experimental models. Extrapolation to angle closure glaucoma does not seem erroneous. Accepting that IOP is a risk factor and not the disease consolidates the view that the term "glaucoma" should be reserved for characteristic optic neuropathy combined with a specific functional deficit.

The traditional classification of angle closure, based on symptomatology (acute, sub-acute and chronic), is of limited use and may lead to a misplaced sense of security. This is illustrated by a reliable report from South Africa of individuals with chronic angle closure (with white eyes and clear corneas) with IOPs as high as 72 mm Hg.[7] There is no proven association between symptoms and the development of a visual deficit. Among the populations of East Asia the majority of angle closure is asymptomatic.[8,9] Furthermore, symptomatic classification does not specifically identify the underlying mechanism of angle closure as it should if it is to guide a logical strategy of management. Being a mechanical process, closure of the angle is probably best classified according to physical signs.

Classification

Primary angle closure suspect

An eye in which appositional contact between the peripheral iris and posterior TM is considered possible.

Primary angle closure

Non-ischaemic: An eye with an occludable drainage angle and features suggesting trabecular dysfunction, such as peripheral anterior synechiae, elevated IOP, or excessive pigment deposition on the trabecular surface. The optic disc and visual field are normal.

Ischaemic: The presence of iris whorling, stromal atrophy or glaukomflecken, signifies

previous "acute" PAC. However, as these are areas of ischaemic necrosis we suggest that "ischaemic PAC" is the correct description. Differentiating between non-ischaemic and ischaemic PAC is supported by experimental evidence that the iris and ciliary body are the ocular tissues most sensitive to pressure-induced ischaemia.[10] Damage to the optic nerve only occurs at higher pressures, and therefore anterior segment ischaemic sequelae indicate that nerve ischaemia may have occurred, but do not confirm it.

Primary angle closure "glaucoma"

Glaucomatous optic atrophy, with a characteristic visual field defect in the presence of an occludable drainage angle or signs of PAC.

Mechanisms

The classifications outlined above give a framework for staging the severity of ocular disease from an anatomical predisposition through non-ischaemic and ischaemic anterior segment disease to optic neuropathy with visual loss. Management is then determined by the mechanism responsible for narrowing of the iridotrabecular angle and the severity of damage. There are two currently recognised mechanisms of "primary" closure of the angle:

1. Pupil-block: probably the underlying mechanism in most cases
2. Peripheral iris crowding: this has two currently recognised forms: a) a bulky iris that is thrown into circumferential folds ("prominent last iris roll" type), b) anteriorly rotated ciliary processes that fold the peripheral iris forward toward the trabecular surface ("plateau iris" type).

For further discussion of mechanism see Chapter 17.

Assessment of the drainage angle

Visualisation of the angle by gonioscopy is of paramount importance in managing PAC. The indirect gonioscopy lenses which give an inverted image reflected in a mirror, are established as the most convenient for regular clinical usage. In particular the Goldmann (one and two mirror) and Zeiss (four mirror) models are probably the most useful in regular practice.

The Goldmann lens has the advantage of giving a clear view even for a relatively inexperienced observer, and being stable on the eye once inserted. The lens is "steeper than K", and hence requires a coupling medium. The need for a viscous medium such as hypromellose 2% can be overcome with practice, and hypromellose 0.5% or normal saline substituted. This reduces the subsequent blurring of vision which results from disturbance of the ocular surface. The Zeiss lens being "flatter than K" does not require a coupling medium, and having four mirrors gives a rapid means of inspecting all four quadrants of the angle-recess.

Pressure gonioscopy was first described in 1957 as a method of evaluating the extent of peripheral anterior synechiae in the operating theatre.[11] Indentation of the central cornea forces aqueous into the periphery of the anterior chamber. On the premise that appositional angle closure is reversible and that due to synechiae is not, this technique has found wide usage in evaluation of cases of angle closure, and in determining their prognosis and management. Although originally described using the Zeiss lens,[12] it is equally feasible using the Goldmann lens (Figure 16.1). The latter has the added advantage of causing less folds in Descemet's membrane which may obscure a clear view. When examining the superior angle, the mirror is positioned inferiorly and the subject instructed to look toward the mirror, i.e. down. The lens is held with the forefinger on the upper rim and the thumb on the lower rim. Gentle forward pressure with the thumb will indent the central cornea and, as a result of the increased aqueous pressure, the peripheral iris will be reflected away from the TM and

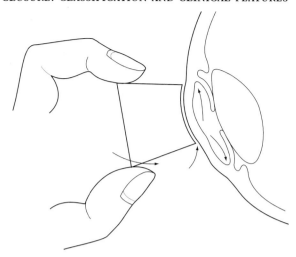

Figure 16.1   Pressure gonioscopy
Pressure gonioscopy is invaluable for differentiating peripheral anterior synechiae from appositional angle closure. Either a Zeiss-style four mirror lens or a Goldmann-style lens may be used. When using the Goldmann lens (above), the patient should look toward the mirror. The edge of the lens lying across the central cornea is then indented with pressure by either the thumb or forefinger. This forces aqueous into the periphery of the anterior chamber, opening areas of appositional angle closure

expose areas of permanent synechial closure. This technique is termed "manipulative" gonioscopy, as opposed to "indentation" gonioscopy (the term given to the examination using the Zeiss lens). The Zeiss lens is unsurpassable for rapid confirmation that an angle is normal and open, and is more effective for pressure gonioscopy when there is a high pressure gradient between anterior and posterior chambers, or in the presence of a very thick iris. However, for detailed examination of difficult subjects with a narrow angle, the Goldmann two mirror lens is probably the superior instrument. Both lenses should be available when assessing glaucoma patients.

The single most important structure to identify when performing gonioscopy is Schwalbe's line. This can be located confidently at the termination of the peripheral corneal wedge, and is usually seen as a slight bump (Figure 16.2). Lying immediately posterior to this point

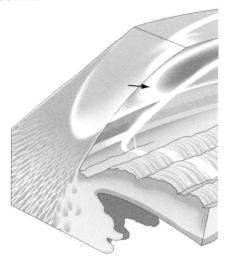

Figure 16.2 The "corneal wedge"
When a fine slit beam thrown obliquely across the peripheral iris, TM and endothelial surface of the cornea is viewed at high magnification ($\times$ 16 or 25), two reflections from the cornea are seen (one each from the inner and outer surfaces). These converge at the junction of clear cornea and opaque sclera to form the "corneal wedge". Schwalbe's line lies at the apex of the wedge, and the TM immediately behind

is the TM. It is believed that the posterior half of the TM is responsible for the majority of aqueous drainage via the trabecular route. When assessing the degree of functional obstruction to drainage, apposition of the iris and posterior TM is of greatest relevance. During gonioscopic examination it is important to avoid high levels of illumination. This may cause pupil constriction and deceptive widening of the angle. The room illumination should be minimal. We use high magnification (ideally

$\times$ 25 to $\times$ 40), a 1–2 mm spot size reduced to a narrow slit, with a medium power setting on the slit lamp transformer (4.5 V). The beam should be horizontally offset when examining the superior and inferior angles, and vertically offset (with a horizontally orientated beam) when examining the nasal and temporal angles. This helps to create a visible corneal wedge and avoids troublesome reflection from the lens. Care should be taken to avoid shining the beam into the pupil, or inadvertent pressure with the gonioscope. Both may cause a significant change in configuration of the angle, which may take several minutes to reverse.

There are two widely used (but often confused) schemes for classifying and recording the gonioscopic appearance of the drainage angle, described by Scheie[13] and Shaffer.[14] Scheie's scheme describes the angle structures that are visible, and the degree of pigmentation in the angle (Table 16.1). The angle width is graded "O" for wide open with the ciliary body being visible, and IV representing a state where no angle structures are visible. Pigmentation is graded "none" to IV. In contrast, the Shaffer system attempts to describe the angular width of the iridocorneal recess, and uses Arabic numerals in the reverse order, "0" meaning an angle of 0° and "4" indicating 30–45°. It is difficult to accurately assess this angle and in practice most ophthalmologists use a combination of these two schemes, but usually record the findings according to Shaffer's convention.

Table 16.1 A comparison of the Scheie[13] & Shaffer[14] gonioscopic grading schemes

Scheie Grade	Description	Risk of Closure	Shaffer Grade	Angle width	Description
O	Wide open	Impossible	4	35–45°	Wide open
I	Slightly narrowed	Impossible	3	20–35°	Wide open
II	Angle apex not visible	Possible	2	20°	Narrow
III	Posterior half of trabeculum not visible	Probable	1	10°	Extremely Narrow
IV	No structures seen	Closed	0	0°	Closed

* The two schemes are presented as approximately equivalent. This is a generalisation, but is valid in most circumstances

Spaeth described a more detailed grading scheme which considers three features of the angle configuration.[15] Angular width is estimated as that between a tangent to the peripheral third of the iris and the surface of the TM (Figure 16.3). The level of insertion of the iris is graded A to E representing "A"nterior to TM, "B"ehind Schwalbe's line, s"C"leral spur, "D"eep into the ciliary body, and "E"xtremely deep (Figure 16.4). Using these grades, a further refinement to this scheme records the point of appositional contact between the iris and TM in brackets, before the actual insertion of the iris. Thus, an angle in which an apparent iris insertion of grade B, and is found to on pressure gonioscopy to be "D", would be recorded as "(B)D". The profile of the iris in the sagittal plane is graded as either "s" steep or convex, "r" regular or flat, and "q" queer or concave Figure 16.5). The Spaeth system is ideally suited to research purposes, especially in regions where angle closure is prevalent, however it is probably too cumbersome for use in routine clinical practice.

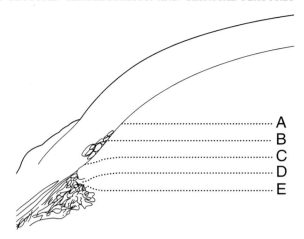

Figure 16.4   Spaeth's iris insertion grades
Five categories of iris insertion: anterior to Schwalbe's line (A), behind Schwalbe's (B), sCleral spur (C), deep (anterior ciliary body) (D), extremely deep (E) (more posterior insertion into ciliary body)

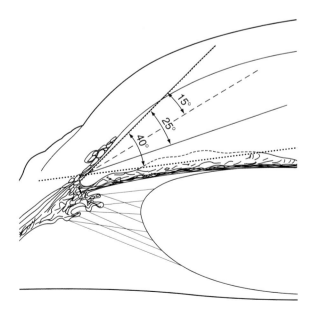

Figure 16.3   Spaeth's irido-trabecular angle construct
Spaeth's grading of the angular width of anterior chamber recess. An imaginary line is extended from the surface of the TM crossed by a tangent drawn from the peripheral third of the iris[15]

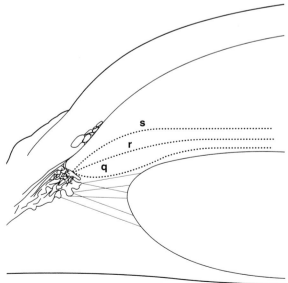

Figure 16.5   Spaeth's iris profile grades
Spaeth described three categories of peripheral iris profile, steep (s), regular (r) and queer (q)[15]

When is an angle "occludable"?

The objective of examining the drainage angle is to determine whether closure is possible and whether there is any evidence that this is occurring. In epidemiological research an occludable angle has been defined as one in which the view of the posterior, usually pigmented, TM is obscured throughout 270° or more of its circumference, without indentation or manipulation of the gonioscope.[7,9,16] This definition has found wide usage more for the purpose of allowing comparison between studies. However, to use this definition in clinical practice would be a gross over-simplification. Wider angles may become occluded, and narrow angles may never become occluded. Gonioscopy should be a dynamic process of accumulating evidence supporting the belief that closure of the angle is possible. Other signs should be elicited to give an indication of the presence of clinically significant angle closure (Table 16.2). Peripheral anterior synechiae are the most important signs to identify (Figure 16.6). They are always pathological. Iris processes are a feature of the normal angle, and although normally few in number and usually fine and lacy, they may be numerous and extend anteriorly for a large circumference of the angle (Figure 16.7).

Pigmentation on the TM may give clues to the presence and clinical course of closure of the angle. In subjects with brown irises, iris pigment may be deposited on either Schwalbe's line (in an interrupted linear pattern) or the surface of the TM (in round or irregular geographical blotches) when there is closure of the angle. Occasionally, patchy adhesions may be seen to divide when performing pressure

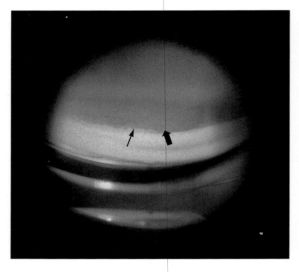

Figure 16.6 A gonio-photograph showing trabecular meshwork (small arrow) and broad peripheral anterior synechiae extending to Schwalbe's line (large arrow)

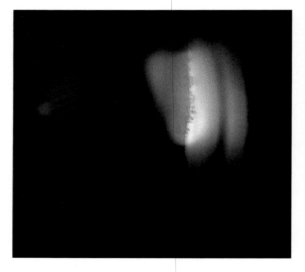

Figure 16.7 A gonio-photograph showing trabecular meshwork partially covered with numerous dendriform iris process

Table 16.2 A comparison of peripheral anterior synechiae with iris processes

	Peripheral synechiae	Iris processes
Distortion of iris contour	Yes	No
Cross-sectional profile	Raised	Flat, or slightly raised
Shape	Saw-tooth (if narrow), Blunt & rounded (if wide)	Lacy, branching
Width	Broader at base than apex	Individually very narrow, but may coalesce into broad sheets

gonioscopy. A fine dusting of pigment on the surface of the inferior and nasal TM is a normal finding in persons over the age of 30, although deposition of pigment on the superior TM may indicate intermittent closure of the angle.[17] An irregular granular pigmentation of the meshwork is believed to be a sign of significant ischaemic damage to the trabeculum. By alternately opening and closing the beam, a dangerously narrow angle may be seen to close and open, demonstrating the potential for closure of the angle (the "on-off" sign).

Although dynamic gonioscopy is held to be the cornerstone of an examination to confirm angle closure, it should be remembered that the static picture is not always representative of the true *in vivo* configuration. The act of placing a gonioscope on the eye will inevitably cause some distortion of the angle configuration if the lens is ill-fitting or if there is inadvertent pressure. This distortion may be caused either by the observer or the upper lid of the subject (especially if the palpebral fissure is small). Excessive tilting of the lens in an attempt to see over the apex of a very convex iris may also cause indentation of the cornea, leading to artefactual widening of the angle. These factors have also been suggested as one explanation of why the superior angle usually appears to be the narrowest quadrant.[18]

Visual fields and optic disc in angle closure glaucoma

Descriptions of the characteristics of visual field loss in PACG are scarce and contradictory (probably as a result of inconsistency in nomenclature). One description of subjects with primary and secondary angle closure found that most (9/11) subjects with chronic disease had visual field loss in a nerve fibre bundle pattern. Conversely, 11/18 subjects who had suffered an acute symptomatic attack of angle closure had no impairment of the visual field. The remaining 7/18 showed typical nerve fibre bundle visual field loss.[2]

Another study of 25 cases of acute unilateral angle closure described a "significant" field defect in over half this group, usually characterised by constriction of the upper field (not felt to be typically "glaucomatous" in nature). Ten of these 25 subjects did exhibit a blue-yellow dyschromatopsia.[19] A Japanese study of 110 subjects with acute (42) and chronic (68) angle closure using Goldmann kinetic perimetry concluded that the pattern of visual field loss in PACG was similar to that in POAG.[20] This is supported by a study of 107 subjects in Singapore, using automated perimetry (POAG: 58, PACG: 49). Early visual field loss showed a propensity to affect the upper visual field in both forms of glaucoma, with the lower field lagging behind in severity until end-stage disease.[21]

Although there are no quantitative descriptions of the pattern of optic neuropathy in angle closure glaucoma, the latter report would suggest that (in "chronic" asymptomatic PACG) the pattern of optic neuropathy is similar to that seen in cases of POAG. Typically, the inferotemporal of the neuroretinal rim is susceptible to early damage.[22] Qualitative descriptions of the appearance of the optic nerve in eyes suffering a symptomatic episode of angle closure suggest that a flat pale disc is often seen. This is probably an indication of ischaemic infarction of the optic disc. In the absence of a prolonged rise in pressure, the lamina cribrosa does not become posteriorly bowed, and hence the cupping of the disc does not develop.

References

1 Quigley HA. Number of people with glaucoma worldwide. *Br J Ophthalmol* 1996; **80**: 389–93.
2 Douglas GR, Drance SM, Schulzer M. The visual field and nerve head in angle closure glaucoma. A comparison of the effects of acute and chronic angle closure. *Arch Ophthalmol* 1975; **93**: 409–11.
3 Dhillon B, Chew PT, Lim ASM. Field loss in primary angle closure glaucoma. *Asia-Pac J Ophthalmol* 1990; **2**: 85–7.
4 Wilensky JT, Kaufman PL, Frohlichstein D, *et al.* Follow-up of angle closure glaucoma suspects. *Am J Ophthalmol* 1993; **115**: 338–46.

5 Pohjanpelta P, Plava J. Ocular hypertension and glaucomatous optic nerve damage. *Acta Ophthalmol* 1974; **52**: 194–200.

6 Davanger M, Ringvold A, Bilka S. The probability of having glaucoma at different IOP levels. *Acta Ophthalmol* 1991; **69**: 565–8.

7 Salmon JF, Mermoud A, Ivey A, Swanevelder SA, Hoffman M. The prevalence of primary angle closure glaucoma and open angle glaucoma in Mamre, Western Cape, S Africa. *Arch Ophthalmol* 1993; **111**: 1263–9.

8 Congdon N, Quigley HA, Hung PT, Wang TH, Ho TC. Screening techniques for angle closure glaucoma in rural Taiwan. *Acta Ophthalmol* 1996; **74**: 113–9.

9 Foster PJ, Baasanhu J, Alsbirk PH, Munkhbayar D, Uranchimeg D, Johnson GJ. Glaucoma in Mongolia – A population-based survey in Hövsgöl Province, N Mongolia. *Arch Ophthalmol* 1996; **114**: 1235–41.

10 Anderson DR, Davis EB. Sensitivities of ocular tissues to acute pressure-induced ischaemia. *Arch Ophthalmol* 1975; **93**: 267–74.

11 Shaffer RN. Operating room gonioscopy in angle closure glaucoma surgery. *Trans Am Ophthalmol Soc* 1957; **55**: 59–66.

12 Forbes M. Gonioscopy with Corneal Indentation. A Method for Distinguishing Between Appositional Closure and Synechial Closure. *Arch Ophthalmol* 1966; **76**: 488–92.

13 Scheie HG. Width and pigmentation of the angle of the anterior chamber. A system of grading by gonioscopy. *Arch Ophthalmol* 1957; **58**: 510–2.

14 Becker B, Shaffer RN. Diagnosis and therapy of the glaucomas. St Louis: CV Mosby 1965.

15 Spaeth GL. The normal development of the human anterior chamber angle: a new system of descriptive grading. *Trans Ophthalmol Soc UK* 1971; **91**: 709–39.

16 Arkell SM, Lightman DA, Sommer A, Taylor HR, Korshin OM, Tielsch JM. The prevalence of glaucoma among Eskimos of Northwest Alaska. *Arch Ophthalmol* 1987; **105**: 482–5.

17 Desjardins D, Parrish RK II. Inversion of anterior chamber pigment as a possible prognostic sign in narrow angles. *Am J Ophthalmol* 1985; **100**: 480–1.

18 Hoskins HD. Interpretive gonioscopy in glaucoma. *Invest Ophthalmol* 1972; **11**: 97–102.

19 McNaught EI, Rennie A, McClure E, Chisholm IA. Pattern of Visual damage after acute angle-closure glaucoma. *Trans Ophthalmol Soc UK* 1974; **94**: 406–15.

20 Horie T, Kitazawa Y, Nosé H. Visual field changes in primary angle closure glaucoma. *Jpn J Ophthalmol* 1975; **19**: 108–15.

21 Seah SKL, Foster PJ, Devereux JG, Oen F, Chew PT, Khaw PT. The spatial distribution and severity of visual field defects in Asians with primary open-angle glaucoma and primary angle closure glaucoma. Krieglstein GK (ed). *Glaucoma Update VI.* Heidelberg, Springer in press.

22 Jonas JB, Fernandez MC, Sturmer J. Pattern of glaucomatous neuroretinal rim loss. *Ophthalmology* 1993; **100**: 63–8.

17 Primary angle closure: epidemiology and mechanism

P J FOSTER, G J JOHNSON

Epidemiology

Prevalence

Ethnicity

A person's ethnic background is one of the major factors determining their susceptibility to primary angle closure (PAC). Population surveys show that PAC is more common among people of Asian descent than those from Europe. Among people aged 40 years and over, the prevalence of PAC (the number of cases present at one point in time) ranges from 0.09% in Europeans,[1] to 1.4% in East Asians,[2,3] to 2.6% in Alaskan Inuit.[4] The most thoroughly studied ethnic group has been the Inuit of Greenland[5] among whom the prevalence reaches 5.0%. The Inuit are believed to share a common ancestry with the Sino-Mongoloid people of north-east Asia. This contention is supported by different strands of evidence including patterns of transfer in molecule polymorphism, rates of rhesus antigen expression, mitochondrial DNA and the correlation of these data with linguistic evolution.[6] Reliable data from the Indian subcontinent are scarce, although available figures suggest there may be approximately equal numbers of people afflicted by primary open angle glaucoma (POAG) and PAC. Among most East Asian populations there is typically a 3:1 excess of PAC, compared with POAG.

Africa is home to the most genetically diverse populations on earth, making generalisations about the likely pattern of PAC impossible. A clinic-based study found the rate of primary angle closure (gonioscopically verified closure of the angle with raised intraocular pressure [IOP]) was equal among the black and white populations of Johannesburg. Among the white population 66% of cases were symptomatic, whereas only 31.5% of the black patients reported symptoms.[7] In Cape Town, South Africa, a population with diverse genetic origin was found to have a 3:2 excess of PAC:POAG (prevalence 2.3% and 1.5% respectively in the population aged 40 years and over). This latter report highlighted that the majority of cases of PAC were chronic, and often had remarkably high IOP despite clear corneas and white conjunctivae.[8]

Sex and age

Female sex is recognised as a major predisposing factor toward development of PAC. The prevalence of occludable drainage angles, PAC (an occludable angle with either peripheral anterior synechiae or an IOP above the statistical norm), and PACG (an occludable angle with glaucomatous optic neuropathy and visual field loss), all tend to be higher in women than men.[2,4,8-10] The manifestations of ocular damage resulting from primary closure of the drainage angle are rare before the age of 40 years. After this the prevalence of disease increases.

Incidence

While prevalence is the standard measure of population morbidity at a specific time, events that are of short duration are more effectively quantified by calculating incidence (the number of new cases occurring over specified period). The acute symptomatic form of PAC is one such event. Incidence figures (given as cases/ 100 000 persons/year for the population aged 30 years and over) range from 4.7% in Finland to 15.5% in Singapore. As with prevalence, incidence increases with advancing age and shows that an excess of females are afflicted (Figure 17.1).[11-14]

Anatomical associations

Although a detailed comparison of the prevalence and incidence figures above is complicated by variation in diagnostic criteria between reports, and differing age structures of the populations concerned (countries with more older people will have more cases because of increasing prevalence with age), it does begin to give some indication of the factors that may determine an individual's susceptibility to PAC. A shallow anterior chamber has long been recognised as a factor that predisposes toward angle closure.[15] The depth of the anterior chamber reduces with age and tends to be shallower in women

than men.[16-18] Ethnic groups that have a high prevalence of PAC have shallower anterior chambers (Figures 17.2, 17.3).[18]

Alsbirk suggested that a shallow anterior chamber confers a significant survival advantage for populations living cold climates (e.g. Northern China, Mongolia, Alaska and Greenland). It was suggested the rich vascular supply of the iris in close proximity with the cornea may significantly raise the temperature of the ocular surface, and prevent the cornea from freezing in the winter temperatures of $-50°$ to $-60°C$ that occur in these regions. The narrow palpebral fissure typical of East Asians would offer a similar advantage.

The depth of the anterior chamber is determined by the position of the lens within the globe, which in turn determines the width of the drainage angle. Although the relationship is not a simple geometric one, we examined anterior chamber depth (using an optical pachymeter) and gonioscopic configuration (assessed in four quadrants, using Shaffer's grading scheme) in 942 Mongolians aged 40–87 years. We found that 74% of variation in the width of the drainage angle could be explained solely on the basis of variation in anterior chamber depth (Foster, Baasanhu, Johnson, 1995; unpublished). Lowe used an index of relative lens position:

$$\text{Relative lens position} = \frac{\text{anterior chamber depth} + \frac{1}{2} \text{ (lens thickness)}}{\text{axial length}}$$

to examine the influence of the thickness of the lens, and its position within the globe in a group 80 normal subjects and 61 patients with primary angle closure, in a clinic practice. He concluded that the depth of the anterior chamber was 1.0 mm shallower in the group with PAC compared with normal subjects. It was suggested that 66% of this difference could be explained by a relatively anteriorly positioned lens, and 33% was attributable to the lens being thicker than normal. Among the same group of patients, eyes with PAC had a significantly shorter axial length than normal

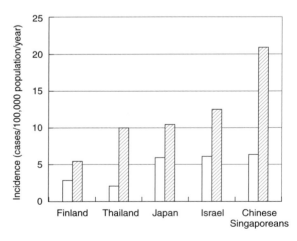

Figure 17.1 Annual incidence of acute angle closure in five nations
☐ men; ▨ women. Figures are given as cases/ 100 000/year in the population aged 30 years and over[11-14]

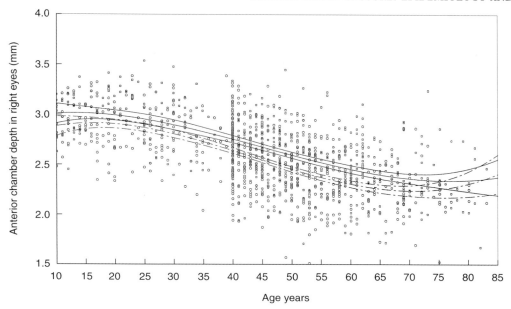

Figure 17.2   Anterior chamber depth variation with age
Regression lines represent population mean anterior chamber depth (in mm) against age (years) for men (solid lines) and women (broken lines). The outer lines represent the 95% confidence intervals for the mean figures

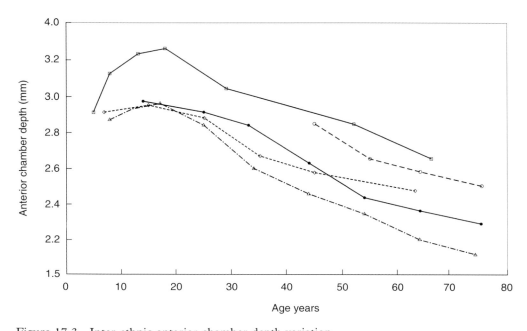

Figure 17.3   Inter-ethnic anterior chamber depth variation
Population mean anterior chamber depth (in mm) against age (in years) in Belgians (squares), Japanese (open circles), Mongols (solid circles), Chinese (diamonds) and Inuit (triangles). Populations with a higher prevalence of angle closure have shallower anterior chambers

eyes. Furthermore, normal eyes showed an inverse relationship between axial length and lens thickness. This finding was not reproduced in eyes with PAC. It was concluded that less co-ordinated development of the intraocular anatomy was a feature of eyes with PAC.[19]

Refractive status, anterior chamber depth, lens thickness and axial length are usually associated. Anterior chambers are shallower in hypermetropes than in myopes.[20,17] Angle closure is typically associated with a hypermetropic refractive state. Increasing living standards and higher educational attainment in Asian and Inuit populations seem to have been paralleled by an increasing prevalence of myopia.[21,22] In Singapore half the male Chinese population aged 15–25 years is myopic. Among those with a university education, this figure rises to 66%.[21] This raises the question of whether the high rate of PAC previously encountered in these populations is destined to decline. This extrapolation would appear logical, although it has been emphasised that PAC may occur in eyes of any refraction and any axial length.[19] Only prospective data will provide the answer.

Screening

These anatomical characteristics of the anterior segment in eyes with PAC may make screening a viable proposition. The aim of screening is to detect disease in an early pre-symptomatic phase in order give treatment that will slow or arrest its progression. Congdon gave a superlative review of the public health aspects of screening for PAC.[23] In the context of routine clinical practice, screening for PAC means assessing all patients aged 30 years and over to determine the potential for angle closure, in order to identify those who require a gonioscopic examination. Screening tests should be quick, simple and reliable. The two most widely used screening tests are the side flashlight test and assessment of limbal chamber depth (the "van Herick" test). The former uses a pen-torch held at the lateral canthus to shine a narrow beam of light across the anterior chamber. A shadow will be cast on the nasal aspect of the iris in an eye with a shallow anterior chamber by the anteriorly situated iris and lens. The performance of this test was assessed in a Canadian clinic practice. Sensitivity and specificity figures of 89% and 88% respectively were reported. The subjects who were not correctly identified had plateau iris configuration.[24] In another clinic-based study in India, sensitivity and specificity were respectively calculated to be 45% and 83% (using a half iris shadow), and 86% and 71% (using a third of the iris in shadow).[25] It is our opinion that this test only achieves optimal performance in the hands of experts.

Estimation of limbal chamber depth, by comparison with the thickness of the peripheral cornea (the van Herick test), is carried out at a slitlamp, with a very thin bright beam falling perpendicularly on the most peripheral part of the temporal clear cornea. The optical cross-section of the limbal chamber is viewed at high magnification ($\times$ 16, or $\times$ 25) from the nasal aspect. The findings, expressed as a fraction of peripheral corneal thickness, are indicative of the gonioscopic configuration.[26] For Greenland Inuit, this technique gave a sensitivity of 91% and a specificity of 53% for detection of subjects with anterior chamber depth 2.0 mm (Figure 17.4).[27] In India these figures were 62% and 89% for detection of angles judged to be occludable on gonioscopic examination.[25]

For hospital-based practice where there is convenient access to the definitive diagnostic test (gonioscopy), both the sidelight test and the limbal chamber depth test should be used to give the highest possible sensitivity (giving a low number of false negative tests) at the expense of specificity (resulting in more false positive tests). By using the flashlight test to detect eyes with one third of the iris in shadow, or the van Herick test to detect a limbal chamber depth less than or equal to one quarter of the peripheral corneal thickness, very few occludable drainage angles would be overlooked. The technique of limbal chamber depth

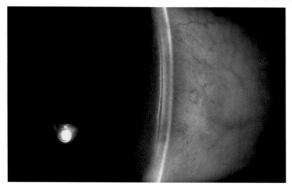

Figure 17.4   Assessment of the depth of the limbal chamber by the van Herick technique
If the limbal chamber depth is ≤ 1/4 of the peripheral corneal thickness, there is a significant chance that gonioscopy will demonstrate an occludable angle

estimation probably produces more consistent and reliable results for the less experienced observer than the side flashlight test.

Mechanism

The final common pathway in the development of primary angle closure is the formation of irreversible synechial adhesions between the peripheral iris and the uveal surface of the trabecular meshwork (TM). In most cases this is probably preceded by intermittent appositional contact. In order to plan management, the mechanism responsible for closure of the angle must be identified. Classification according the following scheme will guide the appropriate choice of therapy, although it is likely that in many cases more than one mechanism is at work.

Pupil-block

This is the underlying mechanism in the majority of cases of primary angle closure, at least in Europeans and East Asians. During a population-based survey of glaucoma in Mongolia, 64 subjects with gonioscopically occludable drainage angles were detected. Of these, 43 (67%) had a steep iris profile, 16 (25%) had a regular iris profile, and only 5 (8%) had an angulated "plateau" iris profile.[2]

A steeply convex iris suggests a pressure differential exists between anterior and posterior chambers. In such patients with narrow drainage angles, iridotomy will result in a marked flattening of iris contour (Figures 17.6 and 17.7).[28] This report emphasised that the axial depth of the anterior chamber did not change. Therefore in steady-state conditions there is a pressure gradient across the iris. The relative block to aqueous flow at the pupil probably results from combined action of the sphincter and dilator pupillae muscles, giving a small resultant force perpendicular to the lens surface (Figure 17.5). This force is greater in eyes with shallower anterior chambers.[29] A rise in poster-

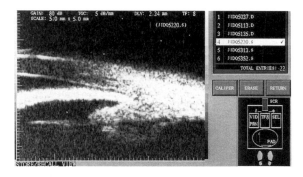

Figure 17.5   Ultrasound biomicroscopic (UBM) view of a temporal drainage angle
A 56 year old Chinese woman with relative pupil-block (before laser) showing an anteriorly convex iris configuration. (Courtesy of Dr Steve Seah & Dr Joe Devereux, Singapore National Eye Centre)

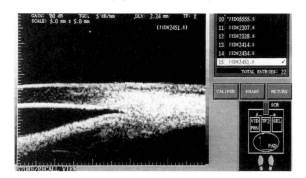

Figure 17.6   UBM view of the drainage angle in the same patient as Figure 17.5 after laser peripheral iridotomy showing a less convex iris configuration and a wider angle. (Courtesy of Dr Steve Seah & Dr Joe Devereux, Singapore National Eye Centre)

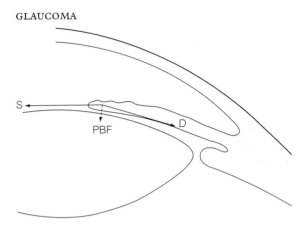

Figure 17.7 A schematic diagram of pupil-blocking forces
Vector D represents the force of the dilator muscle, and vector S the force from the sphincter muscle. PBF is the resultant pupil-blocking force

ior chamber pressure occurs as aqueous production continues. The peripheral iris bows forward, coming into contact with TM. There is some evidence that individuals with PAC may have a generalised autonomic dysfunction, in some cases possibly due to diabetes,[30,31] offering one possible explanation for poor co-ordination of iris muscle function. This is an attractive explanation for the catastrophic pressure rise which is characteristic of the acute symptomatic form of PAC. However, it is not entirely satisfactory when considering "relative" pupil-block in the majority of cases with the chronic asymptomatic disease.

Peripheral iris crowding of the angle

This category accounts for almost all other cases of primary angle closure, given our current understanding of the condition. In contradistinction to pupil block PAC, peripheral iris crowding is a purely anatomical abnormality that may be divided into two categories:

Mass effect

In eyes with a low volume anterior chamber, the iris occupies a larger proportion of the available space. This is even more pronounced in eyes with dark brown, thick irises. As the pupil

dilates, the iris may be thrown into circumferential folds that come into contact with TM. These eyes typically have a relatively anterior iris insertion, e.g. at the level of the scleral spur. These characteristics have previously been described as a "prominent last iris roll". It is difficult to exclude a component of pupilblock in the mechanism of cases such as this.

Plateau iris

Plateau iris configuration is the term given to the gonioscopic appearance of the iris root rising from the anterior surface of the ciliary body and then angulating sharply away from the corneoscleral coat toward the visual axis. Typically these eyes have a relatively deep anterior chamber. The advent of ultrasound biomicroscopy demonstrated the anatomical basis of this condition. The peripheral iris is draped over anteriorly-rotated ciliary processes, causing the angulated iris configuration (Figure 17.8).[32] The ciliolenticular space is often very narrow in these cases. Varying degrees of plateau configuration are seen in the population, both in terms of the height of the plateau and the point of insertion of the iris. In cases where the iris inserts into the apex of the ciliary body, a wide "gutter" can be seen between the face of the TM and the peripheral iris (Figure 17.9).

The term "plateau iris syndrome" refers to cases of primary angle closure with a plateau iris

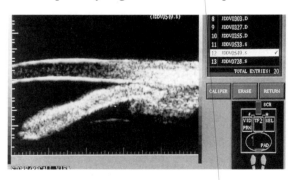

Figure 17.8 Plateau iris configuration seen with the UBM
There is a narrow cleft between the iris and TM (thin arrow). The ciliary body is rotated anteriorly (thick arrow). The ciliolenticular space appears crowded

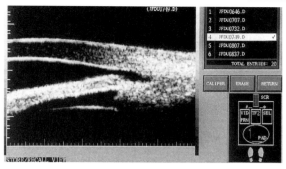

Figure 17.9 Plateau configuration seen with the UBM The iris inserts near the apex of the ciliary body creating a wide gutter-like recess

configuration that has a patent iridotomy, but subsequently suffer spontaneous or mydriatic-induced rises in IOP associated with gonioscopically-confirmed angle closure.

Ciliolenticular block

The dynamics of the ciliolenticular space are not well understood. Cases of primary ciliolenticular block are rare and are believed to occur as a result of misdirection of aqueous into the posterior segment. This probably occurs as a consequence of a crowded ciliolenticular space being further compromised by constriction of the ciliary ring and anterior movement of the lens. This may result from the use of strong miotics in the management of angle closure. A progressing asymmetrical shallowing of the axial anterior chamber is the hallmark of this condition. This feature differentiates ciliolenticular block from pupil-block and iris-crowding forms of PACG. Marked asymmetry in depth of the axial anterior chamber is rare in the latter two forms of angle closure, unless there is gross anisometropia. It is important to realise that the abnormality in ciliolenticular block lies at the ciliary ring (in the initial stages) and in the vitreous cavity (in advanced cases), and it is toward these regions that management must be directed.

"Creeping" angle closure

In some cases of PACG peripheral anterior synechiae are said to "creep" progressively in an anterior direction across the ciliary face, as well as in a circumferential direction. This pattern was originally described in East Asians, but may occur in other ethnic groups. The recognition of this pattern still requires classification under one of the three mechanisms listed above to determine the appropriate management.

Precipitating factors

Environmental agents

Primary angle closure has a definite predilection for those with particular anatomical traits such as shallow anterior chambers. Why many individuals with narrow drainage angles never develop disturbed ocular physiology, or visually destructive sequelae, remains unanswered. The question of external factors precipitating the closure of the angle has long been a popular concept. Numerous drugs that influence the sympathetic nervous system have been implicated in the onset of symptomatic PAC. These include nebulised bronchodilators, tricyclic antidepressants, nasal decongestant agents and anticholinergic agents used to treat Parkinsonism or reduce gut motility. Other agents which have the potential to relax smooth muscle (including glyceryl trinitrate and benzodiazepine anxiolytics) and diuretics (which cause transient shallowing of the anterior chamber, including acetazolamide) also have the potential to cause angle closure. The fact that many of these drugs are based on organic compounds such as belladonna alkaloid derivatives, raises the question of whether the plant-derived traditional medicines so widespread in Chinese culture, may have a role in the onset of some cases of PAC. The association between these agents and the development of symptoms only serves to emphasise that the internal milieu of the eye has been disturbed. It is likely that in the majority of cases these changes are asymptomatic.

Climatic conditions have also been linked with symptomatic PAC. Typically the peak onset of symptoms occurs with extremes of temperature or during the prolonged dark of Arctic winters. Pharmacological agents, water drinking, low light conditions, and prone posture, have all been suggested as clinic-based provocative manoeuvres to induce a rise in IOP confirming the suspicion that an angle may be occludable. While a positive test result is a firm indication that an abnormality exists, a negative finding is of little help and does not indicate the absence of disease. For this reason, and others, provocative testing in the management of PAC has been described as "inaccurate, dangerous and time-consuming".[33] Management is more reliably determined on the basis of the history and a careful clinical examination.

Dilation of the pupil

Whether it is safe to dilate the pupil of individuals with gonioscopically occludable angles is an important question for ophthalmic clinical practice. Drawing on the experience of two large population-based eye disease studies in which subjects received mydriatics, it seems that the risk of inducing an acute IOP rise is very low. In Baltimore USA, the eyes of 4,870 people aged 40 years and over (of European and African heritage) were dilated. None suffered a symptomatic rise in IOP.[34] In the Netherlands 6,760 subjects' pupils were dilated with tropicamide 0.5% and phenylephrine 5%, and then treated with thymoxamine 0.5%. Two (0.03%) of these individuals developed symptomatic PAC in one eye, due to angle closure.[35] One could argue that dilating the pupil and precipitating symptomatic PAC, is a service to the individual, providing a warning is given to re-attend immediately if symptoms supervene. Intuitively, these people are likely to be on the brink of developing PAC, and instructions to re-attend immediately will probably result in more expeditious definitive treatment than if the event was to occur de novo. Of more concern is the possibility of a significant asymptomatic

IOP rise occurring 2–6 hours later as the mydriasis wears off.

Should a rise in IOP be detected, the angle must be re-examined gonioscopically. Only in this way can one attribute the rise in pressure to closure of the angle instead of pigment shedding or dysfunction of a TM previously damaged by ischaemia.

References

1 Hollows FC, Graham PA. Intraocular pressure, glaucoma and glaucoma suspects in a defined population. Br J Ophthalmol 1966; 50: 570–86.
2 Foster PJ, Baasanhu J, Alsbirk PH, Munkhbayar D, Uranchimeg D, Johnson GJ. Glaucoma in Mongolia – A population-based survey in Hövsgöl Province, Northern Mongolia. Arch Ophthalmol 1996; 114: 1235–41.
3 Hu Z, Zhao ZL, Dong FT. An epidemiological investigation of glaucoma in Beijing Shun-yi county. (Chinese) Chung-Hua Yen Ko Tsa Chih (Chinese J Ophthalmol) 1989; 25: 115–8.
4 Arkell SM, Lightman DA, Sommer A, Taylor HR, Korshin OM, Tielsch JM. The prevalence of glaucoma among Eskimos of Northwest Alaska. Arch Ophthalmol 1987; 105: 482–5.
5 Clemmesen V, Alsbirk PH. Primary angle-closure glaucoma (a.c.g.) in Greenland. Acta Ophthalmol 1971; 49: 47–58.
6 Cavalli-Sforza LL. Genes, Peoples and Languages. Sci American 1991; 72–8.
7 Luntz MH. Primary angle-closure glaucoma in urbanised South African, Caucasoid and Negroid communities. Br J Ophthalmol 1973; 57: 445–6.
8 Salmon JF, Mermoud A, Ivey A, Swanevelder SA, Hoffman M. The prevalence of primary angle closure glaucoma and open angle glaucoma in Mamre, Western Cape, South Africa. Arch Ophthalmol 1993; 111: 1263–9.
9 Alsbirk PH. Primary angle-closure glaucoma. Oculometry, epidemiology, and genetics in a high risk population. Acta Ophthalmol 1976; 54: 5–31.
10 Shiose Y, Kitazawa Y, Tsukuhara S, et al. Epidemiology of glaucoma in Japan – A nationwide glaucoma survey. Jpn J Ophthalmol 1991; 35: 133–55.
11 Teikari J, Raivio I, Nurminen M. Incidence of acute glaucoma in Finland from 1973 to 1982. Graefe's Arch Clin Exp Ophthalmol 1987; 225: 357–60.
12 Fujita K, Negishi K, Fujiki K, Kohyama K, Konsomboon S. Epidemiology of acute angle-closure glaucoma. Report I. Jpn J Clin Ophthalmol 1996; 37: 625–9.
13 David R, Tessler Z, Yassur Y. Epidemiology of acute angle-closure glaucoma: incidence and seasonal variations. Ophthalmologica 1985; 191: 4–7.
14 Seah SKL, Foster PJ, Chew PT, et al. Incidence of acute primary angle-closure glaucoma in Singapore. An island-wide Survey. Arch Ophthalmol 1997; 115: 1436–40.
15 Törnquist R. Shallow anterior chamber in acute angle-closure. A clinical and genetic study. Acta Ophthalmol 1953; 31 (Suppl. 39): 1–74.
16 Alsbirk PH. Anterior chamber depth in Greenland Eskimos. I. A population study of variation with age and sex. Acta Ophthalmol 1974; 52: 551–64.

17 Okabe I, Taniguchi T, Yamamoto T, Kitazawa Y. Age-related changes of the anterior chamber width. *J Glaucoma* 1992; **1**: 100–7.

18 Foster PJ, Alsbirk PH, Baasanhu J, Munkhbayar D, Uranchimeg D, Johnson GJ. Anterior chamber depth in Mongolians. Variation with age, sex and method of measurement. *Am J Ophthalmol* 1997; **124**: 53–60.

19 Lowe RF. Causes of shallow anterior chamber in primary angle closure glaucoma. Ultrasonic biometry of normal and angle-closure eyes. *Am J Ophthalmol* 1969; **67**: 87–93.

20 Weekers R, Delmarcelle Y, Collignon J, Luyckx J. Mesure optique de la profondeur de la chambre anterieure application cliniques. *Doc Ophthalmol* 1973; **34**: 413–34.

21 Au Eong KG, Tay TH, Lim MK. Race, culture and myopia in 110,236 young Singaporean males. *Singapore Med J* 1993; **34**: 29–32.

22 Johnson GJ. Myopia in arctic regions. A survey. *Acta Ophthalmol (Suppl.)* 1988; **185**: 13–8.

23 Congdon N, Wang F, Tielsch JM. Issues in the epidemiology and population-based screening of primary angle-closure glaucoma. *Surv Ophthalmol* 1992; **36**: 411–23.

24 Vargas E, Drance SM. Anterior chamber depth in angle-closure glaucoma. Clinical methods of depth determination in people with and without the disease. *Arch Ophthalmol* 1973; **90**: 438–9.

25 Thomas R, George T, Braganza A, Muliyil J. The flashlight test and van Herick's test are poor predictors for occludable angles. *Aust NZ J Ophthalmol* 1996; **24**: 251–256.

26 van Herick W, Shaffer RN, Schwartz A. Estimation of the width of the angle of anterior chambers: incidence and significance of the narrow angle. *Am J Ophthalmol* 1969; **68**: 626–9.

27 Alsbirk PH. Limbal and axial chamber depth variations. A population study in Eskimos. *Acta Ophthalmol* 1986; **64**: 593–600.

28 Jin JC, Anderson DR. The effect of iridotomy on iris contour. *Am J Ophthalmol* 1990; **110**: 260–3.

29 Kondo T, Miura M. A method of measuring pupil-blocking force in the human eye. *Graefe's Arch Clin Exp Ophthalmol* 1987; **225**: 361–4.

30 Clark CV, Mapstone R. The prevalence of diabetes in the family history of patients with primary glaucoma. *Doc Ophthalmol* 1986; **62**: 161–3.

31 Kumar R, Ahuja VM. Glaucoma and concomitant status of the autonomic nervous system. *Indian J Physiol & Pharmacol* 1998; **42**: 90–4.

32 Pavlin CJ, Ritch R, Foster FS. Ultrasound biomicroscopy in plateau iris syndrome. *Am J Ophthalmol* 1992; **113**: 390–5.

33 Lowe RF. Clinical trials of angle closure glaucoma. *Aust NZ J Ophthalmol* 1988; **16**: 245.

34 Lowe RF. Primary angle-closure glaucoma. A review of provocative tests. *Br J Ophthalmol* 1967; 51: 727–732.

35 Patel KH, Javitt JC, Tielsch JM, *et al.* Incidence of acute angle-closure glaucoma after pharmacologic mydriasis (see comments). *Am J Ophthalmol* 1995; **120**: 709–17.

36 Wolfs RCW, Grobbee DE, Hofman A, de Jong PTVM. Risk of acute angle-closure glaucoma after diagnostic mydriasis in non-selected subjects: The Rotterdam Study. *Invest Ophthalmol Vis Sci* 1997; **38**: 2683–7.

18 Primary angle closure: management and prognosis

P J FOSTER, P T K CHEW

Cases of primary angle closure (PAC) encountered in hospital practice characteristically present with a symptomatic rise in intraocular pressure (IOP) or advanced optic disc damage and visual field loss. The management of these cases must be tailored to the individual case. However, there are three basic precepts: 1) immediate control of symptoms and raised IOP, 2) modification of angle configuration, preventing further closure, and 3) detection and control of continuing optic disc and visual field damage.

Management techniques

Immediate control of symptoms and intraocular pressure

For patients presenting with symptomatic PAC, alleviating discomfort and ensuring the systemic wellbeing of the patient must be the first priority. Symptomatic relief is invariably afforded by a reduction in IOP. Furthermore, by extrapolation from data on POAG, raised IOP is the major modifiable risk factor for visual loss from glaucomatous optic neuropathy. The risk of visual loss is proportional to the height of the IOP, and probably the duration for which the IOP is elevated. Experimental data on primates suggests that an IOP around 50–55 mm Hg (15 mm Hg below perfusion pressure[1]) sustained for eight hours, results in patchy necrosis of the iris and ciliary body, while an IOP around 65 mm Hg would cause ischaemic changes in the optic nerve head.[2]

The following regime applies for both pupil-block and peripheral iris crowding mechanisms.

Medical therapy

An unreactive pupil in the presence of complete angle closure suggests there is anterior segment ischaemia. This is an indication for intravenous acetazolamide, which will have an onset of action at around 15 minutes, peaking at 30 minutes. The oral route of administration may be used, but does not reach maximal efficacy until around two hours. Vomiting is another indication for use of intravenous therapy. Applanation tonometry on an oedematous cornea will give a significant underestimate of true IOP at higher pressures.[3] Deciding management policy solely on the basis of tonometry may be confounded by this measurement error. However the finding of a fall in the IOP following treatment is probably a reliable sign of improvement.

Pilocarpine is the second line agent. High dose regimes, e.g. every five minutes, should be used with caution as there is a theoretical risk of pilocarpine toxicity mimicking the features of persistently raised IOP, although, it has been calculated that a dose of 100 mg of pilocarpine would be necessary to reach toxic levels. Paradoxical shallowing of the anterior chamber aggravating angle closure, is another potential complication. Therefore pilocarpine 2% is probably sufficient for individuals with blue/green or hazel irises. Anecdotal reports suggest the dose/response relationship is different for patients with dark brown eyes, meaning that the 4% preparation is probably indicated for Asians. A topical steroid preparation should also be used to reduce the inflammatory reaction that may accompany a symptomatic episode. Table 18.1 summarises medical therapy of symptomatic primary angle closure.

Clinical studies of the immediate management of raised pressure in PAC have shown:

- No difference in IOP reduction between an intensive regime compared with single doses of pilocarpine given at one and six hours after presentation (20 patients, non-randomised).[4]
- Similar success rates using pilocarpine 2% and 4% (22/26 and 21/24 cases respectively). Timolol within one hour followed by pilocarpine at three hours was said to be equally effective, although the results were not conclusive (non-randomised).[5]
- Ocusert Pilo®, a slow release "insert" preparation, (pilocarpine 40 micrograms) has been shown to be as effective as topical pilocarpine in reducing the IOP over a two hour period.[6]
- Aqueous suppressants (topical β-blockers or α_2-adrenoceptor agonists) should also be used. The choice of the agent from either of these classes of drug is not supported by solid evidence. The suggested neuroprotective effect of brimonidine[7] has theoretical advantages for the management of eyes with extremely high IOPs in which a rapidly progressive cycle of ischaemic neuronal death and secondary apoptosis is probably occurring. However this concept is based on experimental data derived from nerves subjected to

crush injury. It is likely that this model does not accurately reproduce the events occurring during symptomatic PAC.

Supportive therapy and analgesia

Many patients with PAC are elderly females of small stature, often with other medical problems including polypharmacy. This makes electrolyte disturbance, particularly hypokalaemia, a significant risk. Vomiting and the use of acetazolamide may cause or rapidly exacerbate this disturbance. This may potentiate the systemic hypotensive effect of β-blockers, further increasing the risk of circulatory disturbances. Assessment of serum potassium should be considered. The use of intravenous hyperosmotics such as mannitol, can further aggravate circulatory problems, especially in small patients. The 20% preparation is probably most appropriate, used at a dosage of 1g/Kg, although laser iridoplasty (below) is probably a more suitable choice of treatment. Analgesia and antiemetics should be used as required.

This is the one area in which the traditional classification of PAC into symptomatic and asymptomatic types is useful. The symptomatic form has the potential to cause significant systemic disturbance. Considering solely the potential for visual loss, it is not known whether patients presenting with symptomatic PAC are at higher risk than people with asymptomatic disease in the long-term. However the potential for inadequately treated symptomatic PAC to cause blindness should not be underestimated.

Laser and physical treatment

In symptomatic patients, if topical and intravenous medical therapy do not reduce the IOP within three to four hours, additional measures are indicated.

Laser Iridoplasty This is an effective method of managing medically unresponsive PAC that would otherwise require surgical intervention. The aim is to apply low power contraction burns to the iris stroma either

Table 18.1 Immediate therapy for symptomatic primary angle closure

---

1. Acetazolamide (250–500mg) IV stat, then 125 to 250mg q.i.d. P.O. until symptoms subside.
2. Topical pilocarpine 2% stat, then q.i.d.
3. Analgesics and antiemetics as required.
4. Topical β-blocker or α_2-agonist stat, then regularly.
5. Topical steroids prednisolone acetate, 1% q.i.d).

Contra-indications and hypersensitivity to drugs should be excluded prior to starting treatment

---

peripherally or at the sphincter. An Abraham's lens (with a + 66 D section) should be used. The power setting is varied according to the colour and thickness of the iris (Table 18.2). Starting at 100 mW, power is increased until stromal contraction is seen. If pigment is liberated, the power should be reduced. For iridoplasty (Figure 18.1), about ten burns are applied as peripherally as possible in each quadrant in areas which have been found to open with compression gonioscopy (or the inferior quadrant if this is not possible). The aim of sector pupilloplasty (Figure 18.2) is to induce a localised constriction of the sphincter,

Table 18.2 Treatment parameters for iridoplasty and pupilloplasty

Light irides
Iridoplasty – Spot size: 500 μm, duration: 0.5 s, 200–1000 mW power
Sector pupilloplasty – Spot size: 200 μm, duration: 0.5 s, 200–500 mW power

Dark irides
Iridoplasty – Spot size: 100 μm, duration: 0.2 s, 200–600 mW power
Sector pupilloplasty – Spot size: 50 μm, duration: 0.2 s, 100–400 mW power
(power should be increased according to the clarity of the cornea)

causing peaking of the pupil and breaking the pupil block. Both techniques may be used together.[8] Once iridoplasty is successful, iridotomy should be performed without delay.

If corneal oedema obscures a clear view, topical glycerin may be used to temporarily clear the cornea. Topical pilocarpine or an α_2-antagonist are appropriate as premedication. The possibility of a post-laser IOP spike should be remembered. Topical steroids (prednisolone 1% q.i.d.) should be used for five to seven days.

Corneal indentation The use of a cotton bud or the rim of a gonioscope to indent the central cornea probably relieves total pupil block by equalising the pressure differential across the iris, and forces aqueous into the peripheral anterior chamber. This exposes the trabecular meshwork (TM) and increases the hydrostatic pressure driving aqueous out of the eye.[9] The technique works well in the thin relatively flexible irides of Europeans, but the thicker irides of Asians are frequently more difficult to reflect away from the TM, rendering the technique of less use in persons with dark brown eyes.

Modification of angle configuration
Laser peripheral iridotomy (PI)

Laser iridotomy is the technique of choice for managing PAC due to pupil-block. It is very difficult to confirm that any case of PAC does not have a pupil-block component, and hence

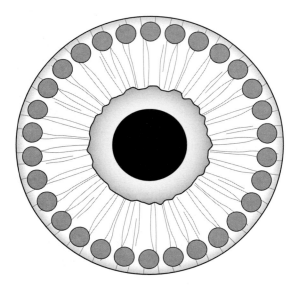

Figure 18.1 Argon laser iridoplasty
Showing peripherally located stromal contraction laser burns, approximately 10 per quadrant.

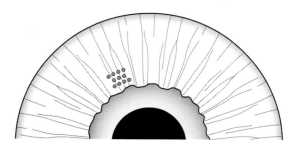

Figure 18.2 Argon laser pupilloplasty
Showing stromal contraction burns located over the sphincter adjacent to the pupil.

iridotomy is indicated in *every* case unless there is a compelling reason not to attempt this. It is widely agreed that laser PI is indicated in patients with any gonioscopic evidence of PAC, e.g. peripheral anterior synechiae or pigment smearing on the TM,[10] and in eyes with occludable drainage angles and raised IOP. The natural history of untreated symptomatic PAC often involves sectorial infarction of the iris. The loss of sphincter tone in this region will alleviate the pupil-block, and theoretically obviates the need for a PI. However, omission of an iridotomy in such an eye that suffered a further episode of angle closure would be difficult to defend.

Although the technique of iridotomy was developed using argon lasers, their use has largely been superceded by Nd:YAG lasers, which allow easier penetration of blue irises and use substantially less energy.[11] Pre-treatment with pilocarpine 2% to stretch the iris, and either apraclonidine (0.5% topical) or acetazolamide (500mg by month) as prophylaxis against post-laser IOP spikes, should be given. Apraclonidine has a theoretical advantage that, as a vaso-constrictor, it may reduce bleeding from the iridotomy. The iridotomy should be sited in the superior quadrant, under the top lid where it cannot cause diplopia (but not at 12 o'clock where gas bubbles may obscure the view). To create an iridotomy without damaging lens or cornea, it is necessary to reach a compromise. The more peripheral the location, the greater the separation between iris and lens, but the smaller the irido-corneal gap. In practice, the exact location is often dictated by the presence of a crypt where the iris is thinnest. In patients with a thick iris stroma, gentle forward pressure with the Abraham's contact lens will show thinner areas to bulge forwards. Once a suitable thin area has been identified, the beam should be focused *within* the iris stroma and aimed away from the posterior pole. We find that one to three single pulses of around 1–2 mJ are often sufficient in blue-eyed patients. For persons with dark brown irises, 10–12 mJ is an appropriate power for the first few shots. Final per-

foration can usually be achieved with lower powers of 2–3 mJ. At higher powers the patient should be warned that the laser shot may be felt. It has been calculated that an iridotomy should be at least 200μm in diameter to effectively prevent pupil-block.[12]

In patients with dark irises or a thick iris stroma, total YAG laser energy of 150 mJ may be needed. Often a plume of dispersed pigment may obscure a clear view of the iridotomy site, necessitating a second treatment session. Haemorrhage will sometimes obscure a clear view, but this can be halted with slight forward pressure with the lens. The use of a sequential argon/Nd:YAG technique avoids these problems. Between 20 and 80 argon burns (700–1200 mW power, 0.1 s duration, 50μm spot size) will produce a "crater" in the iris stroma, which can then be easily perforated using Nd:YAG shots of 1–2 mJ. If charring of the iris begins to occur, the power and duration of the shots should be reduced.[13] Although perforation can usually be achieved at the first treatment session, use of the argon laser increases total laser energy by a factor of 10 to 100.

A topical steroid such as prednisolone acetate 1% should be used hourly on the day of treatment and four times daily for one week thereafter. Complications among a group of 200 patients treated with Nd:YAG laser included: IOP rise > 10 mm Hg (30%), haemorrhage (20%), iritis (11%), posterior synechiae (7%), and corneal changes (4%).[14] Cataract is considered a potential long-term complication although one study found visual acuity was the same or improved in 85% of eyes at an average of 1.8 years after treatment. Cataract progression was responsible for eyes with decreased acuity; the rate of progression was the same as that in similarly aged persons treated by surgical iridectomy.[15]

Surgical iridectomy

Given current evidence, the sole indication for surgical iridectomy is probably the lack of access to a laser. A prospective randomised comparison of laser iridotomy and surgical iridectomy for symptomatic PAC in Europeans, found control of IOP and postoperative VA to be equivalent; 15/21 (70%) and 19/27 (72%) respectively, had an IOP < 21 mm Hg after three years follow-up. Four patients with unsatisfactory medical control of IOP, and one with nerve damage and field loss, were excluded from the study randomisation.[16] The risk of complications from intraocular surgery such as endophthalmitis and iris prolapse do not seem justified when a closed surgical technique is available. The technique may be of use in eyes in which a symptomatic rise in IOP cannot be controlled by medical or laser therapy, especially those in whom corneal oedema is a persistent problem.

Laser iridoplasty or topical pilocarpine

If, after laser iridotomy, peripheral iris-crowding is believed to be a significant contributing factor in closure of the angle, argon laser iridoplasty or topical pilocarpine should be considered. These are intended to draw the peripheral iris away from the face of the TM. Laser iridoplasty is usually considered a temporising measure and probably begins to lose its effect around one to two years after treatment, although it may be repeated several times. Topical pilocarpine 1–2% has a similar effect but has attendant complications of brow-ache, dimming of vision, and accelerated formation of lens opacities.

After the angle configuration has been modified, these patients should be kept under regular review to monitor the status of the optic disc and visual field.

Management and visual prognosis of glaucomatous optic neuropathy in primary angle closure

When symptoms have settled and short-term IOP control has been achieved, a full glaucoma work-up should be carried out. A detailed gonioscopic examination of both eyes, visual field assessment and recording of the optic disc status, preferably by stereophotography, are essential to plan appropriate long-term management. If glaucomatous optic neuropathy is detected, the therapeutic options are as follows:

Laser peripheral iridotomy

Laser peripheral iridotomy is the treatment of choice for people with glaucomatous optic neuropathy in PAC. A detailed study of 140 eyes of 104 people with PAC in Japan, treated by argon laser iridotomy found:[17]

- Prior to treatment 73/109 (67%) of eyes had a cup: disc ratio of 0.7
- The cup: disc ratio enlarged in 31 (28%) and was unchanged in 64 (59%), mean follow-up 1.7 and 2.7 years (in two groups).
- Visual fields defects were minimal or absent in 96/118 (81%), moderate in 19/118 (16%) and advanced in 3/118 (3%). The defects progressed in only 3 patients (all with initially mild changes).
- IOP < 21 mm Hg (with or without medication) after PI was achieved in 94%.
- IOP control was more likely to be successful if there was < 180° PAS. There was no significant change in the amount of PAS during the follow-up period.
- Loss of visual acuity by more than 3 lines occurred in 19%, due to progression of lens opacities.

A retrospective analysis of 57 Singaporeans with symptomatic PAC found that more than 24 hours delay in presentation, or the need for a laser iridoplasty to achieve short-term pressure control, was associated with worse pressure control after laser iridotomy (mean follow-up period 20 months).[18] Another retrospective study in South Africa of 52 asymptomatic patients (78 eyes) followed for a mean period of 22 months[19] found:

- IOP was controlled (≤ 21 mm Hg) without medication in 9%, and with medication in 51% of eyes.

Table 18.3 Long-term intraocular pressure control* in primary angle closure by laser peripheral iridotomy and topical medication

Location	Eyes (Patients)	Acute/fellow/ chronic eyes	Successful without Rx	Successful with Rx	Follow-up	Design
Israel[21]	53 (34)	20/15/18	15/15/0	16/15/?	2 years	Case series
Baltimore (US)[22]	98 (54)	28/20/50	50 total	21/20/46	Mean: 4.4 years	Case series
Chicago (US)[20]	19 (16)	0/0/19	0	12	Mean: 1.3 years	Case series
South Africa[19]	78 (52)	0/0/78	7	40	Mean: 1.8 years	Case series
Scotland[16]	27 (27)	27/0/0	19	23	3 years	RCT**

* Defined as IOP ≤ 21 mm Hg
** RCT: randomised clinical trial

- Trabeculectomy was required in 29% of eyes.
- Risk factors for needing trabeculectomy were: IOP on presentation ≥ 35 mm Hg, 3 quadrants of synechial angle closure, and cup: disc ratio of > 0.6.
- 36% of these eyes with these risk factors for needing trabeculectomy were controlled by PI with or without medication.

The likelihood that a non-invasive procedure will control IOP and arrest progression of optic neuropathy justifies the use of laser PI as first line treatment in all but the most severe cases.[15,20]

Medical therapy

If satisfactory pressure control cannot be achieved with a PI alone, topical medical therapy should be used in a similar manner as for POAG. A target pressure should be set according to the degree of nerve damage and field loss. If the iris contour has been satisfactorily changed by iridotomy (implying that pupil-block was the predominant mechanism), then a β-blocker or prostaglandin analogue would be our first choice. If the iris profile has not changed after the PI (suggesting peripheral iris crowding is the predominant mechanism), pilocarpine 1–2% is a more appropriate choice. An α_2-agonist is an appropriate second-line therapy.

Trabeculectomy

Trabeculectomy is indicated in cases of PAC with glaucoma that cannot be controlled by laser iridotomy and medication. There is often concern that malignant (ciliolenticular block) "glaucoma" may complicate trabeculectomy in cases with PAC, although published data and anecdotal experience do not support this. One study in the UK of 309 eyes, found identical complication rates in the POAG and angle closure groups. Shallow anterior chambers were seen in 22/126 POAG, 24/112 asymptomatic PAC, and 8/71 symptomatic PAC (17%, 21% and 11% respectively). Surgery was most successful in achieving IOP control (< 21 mm Hg with medication, follow-up 7 years) in symptomatic PAC (93%), then POAG (87%), with least success in asymptomatic PAC (80%).[23]

Despite the finding that eyes with PAC do not seem to suffer especially high rates of malignant glaucoma, cases of this problematic complication do nonetheless occur. The condition may be recognised by progressive asymmetrical axial shallowing of the anterior chamber. It is believed the disorder stems from misdirection of aqueous flow by closure of the ciliolenticular space. Dilating the ciliary ring is probably the best preventive measure, the agents of choice being either cyclopentolate or homatropine.

Primary trabeculectomy is an option for cases of PAC in which immediate pressure control cannot be achieved. Patients with very advanced PAS, optic nerve damage, and visual field loss, are often considered for primary trabeculectomy. We favour a trial of laser iridotomy in these people, although if synechial angle closure for more than 180 is identified after laser treatment, the patient should be considered at high risk of needing a trabeculectomy to achieve control.

Lens extraction

Because the position of the lens determines the iris profile, and therefore the angle configuration, lens extraction is a logical choice for surgical management of raised IOP in cases of PAC with visual impairment due to cataract. Extracapsular cataract extraction was used in the management of PAC in 21 eyes of 20 patients (2 with raised IOP alone, 5 symptomatic, and 14 asymptomatic). In 14 cases lens extraction was performed in place of filtering surgery, where peripheral iridectomy or previous filtering surgery had failed. The findings of this study[24] were:

- Mean IOP reduced from 31–16 mm Hg after surgery.
- 16/21 eyes did not require further medication (follow-up: 6–42 months).
- IOP was reduced even if there were extensive previous PAS.
- In 6 patients with previous failed filtering surgery, lens extraction gave a median IOP reduction of 17.5 mm Hg (range 5–30).

A second study examining the IOP control achieved by cataract extraction in 17 patients (19 eyes: 9 symptomatic and 10 asymptomatic)[25] found:

- Pressure < 22 mm Hg without medication was achieved in 68%.
- IOP with medication was < 22 mm Hg in 94%.
- In 9 eyes with a cup: disc ratio 0.7, median IOP after surgery 17.5 (range: 14–21) mm Hg, on a median of 0 medications (0–2).

The authors of both studies concluded that combined cataract extraction and trabeculectomy may not be necessary in PACG.

Antimetabolites and drainage implants

We are not aware of any peer-reviewed publications dealing specifically with the use of antimetabolites or drainage implants in PACG. Their use is probably justified along similar lines to those in reports dealing with a wider spectrum of glaucoma cases.

Neuro-protection

The theory that the primary pathological insult in glaucomatous optic neuropathy is followed by a secondary neurodegenerative process, probably mediated by a neurotransmitter, such as glutamate and free radicals triggering apoptotic cell death, suggests that it may be possible to prevent some neuronal damage occurring after a period of elevated IOP. Blockade of the self-perpetuating neurochemical cascade by antagonists targeted on the N-methyl-D-aspartate (NMDA) glutamate receptor subgroup, using agents such as MK 801, has given promising experimental results.[26] There are no agents currently on the market with a proven neuroprotective capacity for glaucoma therapy.

Management of the asymptomatic narrow angle

In a multi-centre study of 129 asymptomatic patients with anterior chamber depth < 2 mm, or drainage angles that were potentially occludable, only 6% developed signs or symptoms consistent with PAC over a mean period of 2.7 years (maximum follow-up 6 years).[27] It would therefore appear that an individual's risk of developing visually threatening sequelae is low on a year-to-year basis. However, it is now accepted practice to perform a laser iridotomy on patients with early gonioscopic evidence of angle closure,[10] reflecting the perceived (although unproven) high benefit/risk ratio for this procedure. This view is probably justified when one considers the potential for late-presentation or misdiagnosis under non-ophthalmological care, and the low incidence of sight-threatening complications of laser iridotomy.

The management of an eye contralateral to one that had an episode of symptomatic PAC is open to less conjecture. Follow-up of 200 such "fellow" eyes found 113 were managed by

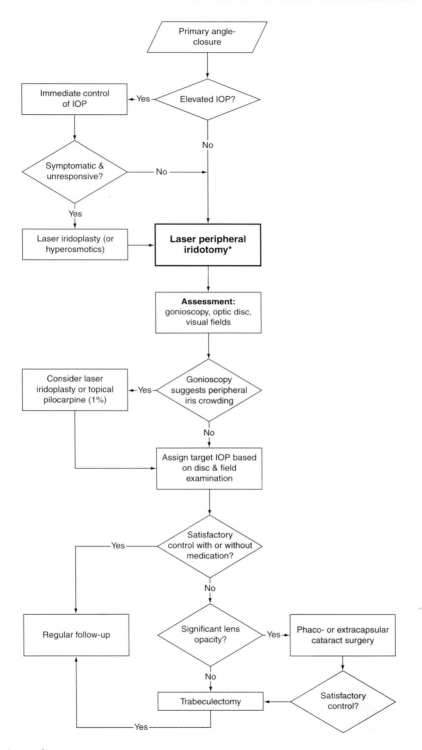

Figure 18.3 Flowchart of management strategy.

observation or with topical pilocarpine. Of this number 58 developed symptomatic PAC (half within a five year period), 26 of the 58 were using topical pilocarpine.[28] In a further 250 patients with PAC, 72 did not have prophylactic peripheral iridectomy. Forty three developed PAC (33 symptomatic, 10 asymptomatic or unknown), 33 of these were affected within 6 years.[29] This is overwhelming evidence in favour of prophylactic peripheral iridotomy by laser, or surgical iridectomy if no laser is available.

References

1 Alm A, Bill A. Ocular circulation. In: Moses RA, Hart WM, (eds). *Adler's physiology of the eye.* St Louis: CV Mosby 1987: 183–203.

2 Anderson DR, Davis EB. Sensitivities of ocular tissues to acute pressure-induced ischaemia. *Arch Ophthalmol* 1975; **93**: 267–74.

3 Moses RA. The Goldmann applanation tonometer. *Am J Ophthalmol* 1958; **46**: 865–9.

4 Ganias F, Mapstone R. Miotics in closed-angle glaucoma. *Br J Ophthalmol* 1975; **59**: 205–6.

5 Airaksinen PJ, Saari KM, Tiainen TJ, Jaanio E-AT. Management of acute closed-angle glaucoma with miotics and timolol. *Br J Ophthalmol* 1979; **63**: 822–5.

6 Edwards RS. A comparative study of Ocusert Pilo 40, intensive pilocarpine and low-dose pilocarpine in the initial treatment of primary acute angle-closure glaucoma. *Curr Med Research & Opinion* 1997; **13**: 501–9.

7 Yoles E, Muler S, Schwartz M, Burke J, WoldeMussie E, Wheeler L. Injury-induced secondary degeneration of rat optic nerve can be attenuated by α2–adrenoceptor-agonists AGN 191103 and brimonidine. *Invest Ophthalmol Vis Sci (ARVO Suppl)* 1996; **37**: S114.

8 Ritch R. Argon laser treatment for medically unresponsive attacks of angle-closure glaucoma. *Am J Ophthalmol* 1982; **94**: 197–204.

9 Anderson DR. Corneal indentation to relieve acute angle-closure glaucoma. *Am J Ophthalmol* 1979; **88**: 1091.

10 Ritch R. Definitive signs and gonioscopic visualization of appositional angle closure are indications for prophylactic laser iridectomy. *Surv Ophthalmol* 1996; **41**: 33–6.

11 Del Priore LV, Robin AL, Pollack IP. Neodymium: YAG and argon laser iridotomy. Long-term follow-up in a prospective, randomised clinical trial. *Ophthalmology* 1988; **95**: 1207–11.

12 Fleck BW. How large must an iridotomy be? *Br J Ophthalmol* 1990; **74**: 583–8.

13 Ho T, Fan R. Sequential argon-YAG laser iridotomies in dark irides. *Br J Ophthalmol* 1992; **76**: 329–31.

14 Schwartz LW, Moster MR, Spaeth GL, Wilson RP, Poryzees EM. Neodymium: YAG laser iridectomy in glaucoma associated with closed or occludable angles. *Am J Ophthalmol* 1986; **102**: 41–4.

15 Quigley HA. Long-term follow-up of laser iridotomy. *Ophthalmology* 1981; **88**: 218–24.

16 Fleck BW, Wright E, Fairley EA. A randomised prospective comparison of operative peripheral iridectomy and Nd:YAG laser iridotomy treatment of acute angle closure glaucoma: 3 year visual acuity and intraocular pressure control outcome. *Br J Ophthalmol* 1997; **81**: 884–88.

17 Yamamoto T, Shirato S, Kitazawa Y. Treatment of primary angle-closure glaucoma by argon laser iridotomy: A long-term follow-up study. *Jpn J Ophthalmol* 1985; **29**: 1–12.

18 Wong JS, Chew PT, Alsagoff Z, Poh K. Clinical course and outcome of primary acute angle-closure glaucoma in Singapore. *Singapore Med J* 1997; **38**: 16–8.

19 Salmon JF. Long-term intraocular pressure control after Nd:YAG laser iridotomy in chronic angle-closure glaucoma. *J Glaucoma* 1993; **2**: 291–6.

20 Gieser DK, Wilensky JT. Laser iridectomy in the management of chronic angle-closure glaucoma. *Am J Ophthalmol* 1984; **98**: 446–50.

21 Yassur Y, Melamed S, Cohen S, Ben-Sira I. Laser iridotomy in closed-angle glaucoma. *Arch Ophthalmol* 1979; **97**: 1920–1.

22 Robin AL, Pollack IP. Argon laser peripheral iridotomies in the treatment of primary angle closure glaucoma. long-term follow-up. *Arch Ophthalmol* 1982; **100**: 919–23.

23 Watson P. Trabeculectomy: long-term follow-up. *Br J Ophthalmol* 1977; **61**: 535–8.

24 Greve EL. Primary angle-closure glaucoma: Extracapsular cataract extraction or filtering procedure? *Int Ophthalmol* 1988; **12**: 157–62.

25 Acton J, Salmon JF, Scholtz R. Extracapsular cataract extraction with posterior chamber lens implantation in primary angle-closure glaucoma. *J Cataract Refract Surg* 1997; **23**: 930–4.

26 Yoles E, Schwartz M. Potential neuroprotective therapy for glaucomatous optic neuropathy. *Surv Ophthalmol* 1998; **42**: 367–72.

27 Wilensky JT, Kaufman PL, Frohlichstein D, et al. Follow-up of angle-closure glaucoma suspects. *Am J Ophthalmol* 1993; **115**: 338–46.

28 Lowe RF. Acute angle-closure glaucoma. The second eye: an analysis of 200 cases. *Br J Ophthalmol* 1962; **46**: 641–50.

29 Snow JT. Value of prophylactic peripheral iridectomy on the second eye in angle-closure glaucoma. *Trans Ophthalmol Soc UK* 1977; **97**: 189–91.

19 The childhood glaucomas: assessment

P T KHAW, S G FRASER, M PAPADOPOULOS, A WELLS, P SHAH

The glaucomas occurring in children are actually a varied group of disorders. There are some similarities with adult glaucoma, but the approach to many of the disorders is not the same; examination, diagnosis and treatment require many different skills in children with glaucoma.

Over the last 50 years there has been a dramatic improvement in the prognosis of the paediatric glaucomas due to changes in the techniques available for treatment and modifications of these treatments. It is not an over-exaggeration to state that for these children, their lifetime of vision and quality of their future lives, depends on prompt and accurate diagnosis and appropriate treatment of their disease.

Incidence

There are many types of childhood glaucoma. They are very rare conditions and a consultant ophthalmologist in a non-specialist centre would expect to see only one case every few years. The most common form, primary congenital glaucoma (PCG) has an incidence of about 1 in 10 000–20 000 live births.[1] This figure is higher in areas where consanguineous marriages are more common. The paediatric glaucomas account for 2–15% of individuals in blind institutions for children around the world and a large percentage of childhood blindness in both developed and developing countries.[2] Untreated or suboptimally treated, the prognosis is poor. The World Health Organization (WHO)/World Bank survey esti-

mated that there were 300 000 cases of the childhood glaucomas worldwide, of whom 200 000 were blind.[3] In a significant proportion of these cases early diagnosis and appropriate treatment could prevent blindness.

Classification of the childhood glaucomas

There are many different classifications of childhood glaucoma, mainly because there is still an incomplete understanding of the pathophysiology of many of the variants. It is important to classify the childhood glaucomas as it gives us some idea of prognosis and treatment, and may guide genetic counselling. The principal types of childhood glaucoma are summarised in Table 19.1.[4–6] The childhood glaucomas can be primary, in which there is a developmental abnormality of the anterior chamber angle, or secondary. In the case of secondary glaucomas, developmental anomalies of the eye or a variety of other pathological processes may cause reduction of aqueous outflow. As we learn more about the genetics of each of these conditions, it is likely that the classifications will change. Some of the major causes of paediatric glaucoma are discussed below.

Primary congenital glaucoma (PCG)

One of the commonest forms of childhood glaucoma is primary congenital. Although the true cause of PCG is unknown, it appears to be

Table 19.1   Classification of the childhood glaucomas

1. Primary childhood glaucoma (primary congenital glaucoma)

2. Secondary childhood glaucoma:
    associated with anterior segment dysgenesis
        Axenfeld/Riegers type anomalies
        Peter's type anomaly
        aniridia
        microphthalmos
        congenital ectropion uveae
        iris hypoplasia
    associated with ocular disease/treatment
        following congenital cataract surgery (especially
            after full lensectomy)
        persistent hyperplastic vitreous
        retinopathy of prematurity
        trauma hyphaema
        angle recession
    associated with phakomatoses
        neurofibromatosis
        Sturge–Weber syndrome
        portwine stains
        cutis marmorata telangiectasia congenita
        Klippel–Trenaunay–Weber syndrome
        oculodermal melanocytosis
        von Hippel–Lindau syndrome
    associated with metabolic disease
        Lowe's syndrome
        homocystinuria
        mucopolysaccharidoses, e.g. Hurler's syndrome
    associated with inflammatory /infective disease
        aeronegative arthropathies
        congenital rubella, cytomegalovirus and other
            infective causes
        juvenile xanthogranuloma
    associated with ocular tumours
        benign, e.g. iris cysts, juvenile xanthogranuloma
        malignant, e.g. retinoblastoma, leukaemia
    associated with chromosomal/systemic disorders
        Down's syndrome (trisomy 21)
        Patau's syndrome (trisomy D 13–15)
        Turner's syndrome (XO)
        Rubinstein–Taybi syndrome
        Pierre Robin syndrome
    associated with connective tissue abnormality
        Marfan's syndrome
        Weill–Marchesani syndrome
        homocystinuria
        Ehlers–Danlos syndrome
        sulphite oxidase deficiency

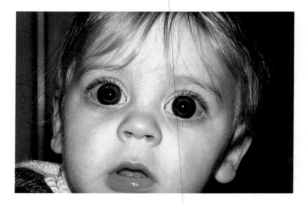

Figure 19.1   Child with buphthalmos
Symmetrical enlargement may delay diagnosis

and splits in Descemet's membrane. The condition is usually bilateral, although IOP may only be raised in one eye in up to 25% of cases (Fig 19.1). However, many of these eyes have abnormal angles or corneal diameters and may represent late opening drainage angles. These eyes have an increased incidence of late onset glaucoma. Caucasian patients respond very well to angle procedures such as goniotomy or trabeculectomy, unless the condition is present at birth or if they have very large eyes (> 14 mm diameter).

The inheritance of PCG has classically been described as either autosomal recessive (hence its high prevalence in consanguineous marriages) or sporadic, although we will only be certain of the latter when we know more of the genetics. In Caucasian patients the risk of another affected sibling in the absence of a family history is < 2%. The first locus for PCG has been found on chromosome 2 and mutations have been found in the CYP1B1 gene in a number of affected families[8] (see Chapter 21). The gene product is responsible for the metabolism of a molecule (cytochrome P450) presumably important for the normal development of the anterior segment.

Juvenile onset open angle glaucoma (JOAG)

Juvenile glaucoma is a non-specific term that traditionally has been used to describe a group

due to an abnormality of the trabecular meshwork – hence the alternative name trabeculodysgenesis. It may be due to abnormal differentiation of intertrabecular spaces rather than a Barkan membrane obstructing flow.[7] There are no other ocular or systemic abnormalities apart from changes induced by raised intraocular pressure (IOP) such as buphthalmos

of patients presenting after the first few years of life and before the age of 35 years. Some of these patients may be misclassified and have late onset PCG or mild variants of the other secondary paediatric glaucomas. There is a sub group of patients who have juvenile onset glaucoma associated with a distinctive hypoplastic iris stroma, which is probably part of the anterior segment dysgeneses covered in the next section. However, there is also a distinct group of patients who have no anterior segment abnormalities and present in their later childhood years (10+ years, average age 18 years) with glaucoma. They often have a family history of glaucoma. Several of these families have mutations at the GLC1A locus on 1q23–q25. There is a suggestion that these patients have high pressures (range 40–50 mm Hg) and do not respond well in the long term to medical or laser treatment and require filtration surgery.

Anterior segment dysgenesis

This has replaced the term "anterior segment cleavage syndrome" simply because no cleavage plane develops during anterior segment differentiation[9] and more likely they are a result of aberrant migration/induction of neural crest cells.[10] Although it is likely that these are a spectrum of disease when certain features are present, eponymous names are given. Thus when there is a posterior embryotoxon (anteriorly displaced, prominent Schwalbe's line) with attached iris strands, this is classically called "Axenfeld's anomaly". The addition of iris abnormalities such as atrophy or corectopia would then be called "Rieger's anomaly" and the addition of systemic abnormalities such as abnormal teeth and facial abnormalities particularly hypertelorism, would change the suffix to "Rieger's syndrome". The clinical overlap between Axenfeld and Rieger anomalies is such that they are often combined as the Axenfeld/Rieger anomaly. The risk of glaucoma with this anomaly is approximately 50%[11] and patients have to be followed up for life. This group normally present with glaucoma in childhood or early adulthood. If they do present in the first few years of life they may have all the secondary features of raised pressure in children, including buphthalmos and Haab's striae. Goniotomy is technically difficult due to the angle changes, and trabeculotomy has a lower success rate in Axenfeld/Rieger anomaly compared with PCG. Filtration surgery with antimetabolites is usually the treatment of choice in these conditions.

Our understanding of this range of conditions will only be improved with the use of molecular and cellular genetics. Families with Axenfeld/Rieger anomaly show an autosomal dominant pattern of inheritance. To date two loci have been identified – REIG 1 at 4q25, and REIG 2 at 13q14[12] (see Chapter 4). "Iris hypoplasia", which is anterior segment dysgenesis with early onset glaucoma and characteristic maldevelopment of the anterior stromal layer of the iris, has been mapped to the same locus as REIG 1, (Heon et al. 1997) and can have the same systemic features as Axenfeld/Rieger syndrome.

"Peter's anomaly" is characterised by a congenital central corneal opacity and underlying defects in stroma, Descemet's and endothelium with iris strands, and sometimes the lens attached to the periphery of this opacity. It is usually bilateral (80%) and sporadic. Approximately 50–70% of patients go on to develop glaucoma. It has been suggested that Peter's anomaly may result from an abnormality in the PAX 6 gene.[13] PAX genes (from "paired box") are thought to be controllers of other genes and thus very important in development with the PAX 6 being involved in ocular development.[9] Goniotomy is not possible in this condition. Lowering of the pressure to the low teens may significantly improve the corneal opacification, and this may only be possible with antimetabolite assisted filtration surgery. Optical iridectomy may also be useful, as penetrating keratoplasty has very variable results.

"Aniridia" (Fig 19.2) has also been associated

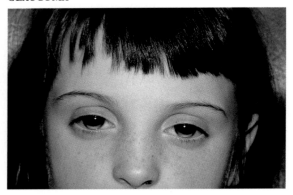

Figure 19.2   Child with aniridia and subluxed lenses

with PAX 6 gene mutations.[14] Clinically, aniridia is characterised by variable loss of iris with a high incidence of glaucoma, cataract, foveola hypoplasia, and corneal surface abnormalities including pannus, presumed due to early corneal epithelial stem cell failure. Inheritance is usually autosomal dominant (although recessive transmission has been recorded) or sporadic. The affected chromosome is the short arm of 11. Wilms' tumour is associated with a deletion on the chromosome 11p13 locus. All patients with apparent sporadic aniridia need screening for Wilms' tumour, including urinalysis for blood and renal ultrasounds. Angle procedures have been recorded to work. Filtration surgery may be especially difficult due to the danger of lens-corneal touch.

Aphakic glaucoma

Glaucoma after childhood cataract surgery has an incidence ranging from 6–65%[15] and increases with length of follow-up. Given this incidence of glaucoma, all patients who have had childhood cataracts removed should be followed up to exclude the development of glaucoma. It occurs in three situations:

- Pupillary-block: if pupil-block occurs there is a very high chance of developing glaucoma even after pupil-block has been relieved by iridectomy
- Late onset chronic angle closure
- Late onset chronic open angle: this type of

glaucoma is the commonest type and can occur many years after surgery. Factors implicated in its development may include postoperative inflammation, retained cortex, coexisting angle anomalies (e.g. Peter's or aniridia), surgery performed on children under 1 year, poor pupil dilation, microphthalmia or microcornea. It is our impression that aphakic glaucoma is relatively rare (<5%) if the capsule is preserved, and removal of the capsule and dispersion of vitreous proteins may also be an important factor.

Aphakic glaucoma can be treated medically. Angle procedures do not work. Cyclodestruction with the diode laser lowers pressure in the majority of patients although repeat treatments are required and the medical therapy cannot be discontinued. Filtration surgery with no or weaker antimetabolites (5-fluorouracil [5FU] or radiation) has a poor success rate. Filtration with mitomycin C (MMC) may have a higher success rate but it is still lower than the success rate in phakic eyes. Furthermore, a MMC trabeculectomy probably excludes post operative contact lens use due to the cystic bleb and the risk of endophthalmitis. Tube implants probably have the highest chance of long-term success particularly if combined with MMC but carry the highest short-term risks of complications.[16]

Sturge–Weber syndrome (encephalotrigeminal encephalosis)

The main feature of this condition is a facial cutaneous angioma (portwine stain, naevus flammeus) which is present at birth and affects the regions innervated by the first and second divisions of the trigeminal nerve. This is associated with a meningeal haemangioma. Iris hyperchromia appears in about 8% of cases. Glaucoma in these patients may arise as result of changes in uveoscleral pressure but there may also be changes in the angle at the macro and microscopic level. Glaucoma can occur at any time from birth to adulthood[17] and develops in around one third of all Sturge–Weber patients, although if the eyelid skin has a haemangioma the glaucoma risk is higher, approximately 50%.

The long-term response rate to goniotomy is inferior to that seen in PCG. Associated choroidal haemangiomas are present in up to 80% if glaucoma is present, and a rapid decompression of the globe may give rise to expulsive choroidal haemorrhage or effusion. Filtration surgery in these patients must be coupled with measures to minimise any period of hypotony such as an anterior segment infusion, pre-placed sutures and viscoelastic. Filtration surgery has to be combined with antimetabolites to provide long-term lowering of IOP without medications in these patients.

The other phakomatoses can be associated with glaucoma although with a lower incidence than Sturge–Weber. Neurofibromatosis is associated with glaucoma, and may present first with iris abnormalities like ectropion uveae, and glaucoma before the systemic disease is apparent. Management depends on the individual patient characteristics, although angle procedures such as goniotomy or trabeculotomy are not usually effective.

Inflammatory glaucoma

Glaucoma may arise following intraocular inflammation from any cause. Inflammation as a cause of glaucoma in the first few years of life is very rare. In later years the juvenile chronic arthropathies can give rise to glaucoma by a variety of mechanisms including chronic trabecular obstruction, pupil-block secondary to cataract removal, and following chronic topical steroid usage. If chronic steroid usage is an essential part of the disease management, then it is best to manage the IOP as if the steroids were an integral part of the disease, rather than constant changing of the steroid regimen to reduce IOP. Patients with juvenile glaucoma must be monitored for the development of ocular hypertension and glaucoma. Unassisted trabeculectomy does not work well in the

inflammatory glaucomas, and MMC trabeculectomy or tube surgery may be indicated.

Miscellaneous conditions

A wide variety of other conditions are associated with childhood glaucoma. Many syndromes and congenital malformations are associated with glaucoma (Table 19.1). Many of these are rare and there is very little precedent in the literature of the right treatment for these glaucomas. The best treatment plan is arrived at by a thorough history and examination and devising a plan based on a rational assessment of all the factors.

For instance, a variety of diseases such as Marfan's syndrome, Weill–Marchesani syndrome, homocystinuria and high myopia, may give rise to childhood glaucoma which may be due to abnormalities in the trabecular meshwork or a subluxed lens, although as a rule glaucoma in childhood is unusual. Early onset glaucoma in these conditions is usually associated with lens displacement. A prophylactic iridectomy may sometimes be required to prevent pupil block glaucoma.

It is important to mention the childhood tumours, such as leukaemia or retinoblastoma, which may give rise to glaucoma by way of obstruction of the outflow tracts from tumour cells or secondary haemorrhage. These rare conditions are important in that the primary disorder must be diagnosed because inadvertent surgery, and release of cells outside the eye may worsen the prognosis for life, e.g. in retinoblastoma. The treatment is generally conservative and involves treating the primary disorder and medical treatment.

Assessment in clinic

The consultation and initial assessment in clinic is an absolutely vital part of the management of the childhood glaucomas. An accurate history and examination in the clinic usually provides the correct diagnosis in the majority of cases. Furthermore, it is the beginning of what may be a lifetime relationship between the ophthalmologist and the patient and his/her parents. The symptoms, signs and differential diagnosis are outlined in Table 19.2.

It is important at this stage to inquire about age of onset as patients with PCG aged less than 3 months or older than 2 years have a worse surgical prognosis with goniotomy. Other questions should include any family history of childhood onset glaucoma, any associated congenital defects or general problems, and any history of maternal problems during pregnancy including the birth history. If the glaucoma starts after the age of 2 years, symptoms may be less marked or even absent. Children with this later onset presentation may have progressive myopia,

strabismus, or may only be detected when they fail routine school vision testing.

A complete general examination may also be important to detect any systemic abnormalities that may be associated with the glaucoma. It is important to work closely with a paediatrician and geneticist who are highly experienced in the assessment, care and counselling of patients with various systemic disorders associated with childhood glaucoma. It is important to develop a teamwork approach to the management of the paediatric glaucomas. These children require a range of skills to be optimally managed from specialised surgical procedures and anaesthetics to support for their play activities and home environment and schooling (Table 19.3).

Examination in the clinic very much depends

Table 19.2   Differential diagnosis of the childhood glaucomas[4-6]

Enlarged cornea (No splits or corneal oedema in these conditions)
  axial myopia
  megalocornea/megalophthalmos
  osteogenenis imperfecta
  connective tissue disorder, e.g. fibrillin mutation

Corneal splits (no corneal enlargement in this condition)
  birth trauma (history)
  hydrops (obvious)

Corneal oedema or opacity (usually no corneal enlargement unless associated with glaucoma which is not common in these
      conditions)
  birth trauma
  congenital hereditary endothelial dystrophy
  metabolic, e.g. mucopolysaccharidoses/cystinosis
  sclerocornea
  rubella/herpes simplex keratitis

Watering and "red eye" (no splits, oedema or corneal enlargement in these conditions)
  conjunctivitis
  nasolacrimal duct obstruction
  corneal epithelial defect, abrasion, very occasionally dystrophy
  occular inflammation

Secondary glaucomas need to be excluded (Table 19.1).

If there is corneal enlargement with corneal oedema and splits then there has been raised IOP at some stage in infancy.

Table 19.3   The paediatric glaucoma service team

• paediatric anaesthetist
• paediatrician (with a special interest in syndromes associated with glaucoma)
• geneticist (with a special interest in ocular genetic disease)
• paediatric nurse co-ordinator (co-ordinates child and family care)
• orthoptist (sees patients pre- and post-examination/refraction and supervises occlusion therapy)
• optometrist (special skills in assessing vision and refraction in children with glaucoma)
• care co-ordinator for children with visual problems (social support, education)
• play leader

on the age and behaviour of the child. It is difficult to underestimate the impact of previous medical experiences of the child and its parents in co-operation with the examination. The first step should always be "hands off". Just by observing the child it may be possible to assess the relative and actual sizes of the eyes, the presence or absence of corneal oedema and the presence of lacrimation, photophobia, and blepharospasm. Reducing the level of ambient illumination can often have a profound effect on the child, who may then open the eyes and allow a more complete examination.

If a neonate has been fed recently it may be possible to carry out quite a thorough examination including applanation tonometry, particularly if a Tono-pen is used. In an older child, examination and applanation tonometry on the slit lamp microscope may be possible from the age of 3 in exceptional cases (Figure 19.3), but in the majority examination under anaesthesia is necessary until about the age of 5. Although it is important to get the child used to the concept of the slit lamp, the surgeon must gain the

confidence of the child and parents. Children with glaucoma will need to have frequent, repeated ophthalmic assessments throughout their childhood and it is essential that they do not develop phobias to any component of the examinations. If there is any doubt and there is possible glaucoma, then the child should be examined under general anaesthesia.

The presence of subtle signs of anterior segment dysgenesis in the parents, such as an abnormal iris and posterior embryotoxon (Figure 19.4), may change the genetic advice that the parents receive and may alter the management of subsequent siblings. Therefore, it is also important to examine the patient's parents if possible.

Following the consultation it is important to explain at the beginning to parents the nature of the condition, and that their child may require lifelong follow-up. When explaining the need for an examination under anaesthetic, it should be explained to the parents that surgical intervention such as goniotomy might be required at the same time. At each follow-up anaesthetic a further procedure may be required, as a subsequent rise in IOP may not be readily detected clinically without an examination under anaesthetic. It is also useful to ask the parents if they are worried about specific issues as misconceptions often can be dealt with. An illustrated booklet explaining the nature of the condition

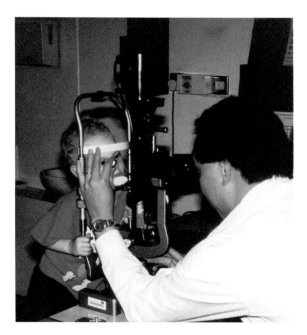

Figure 19.3 Child aged 1 year 10 months being examined at the slit lamp

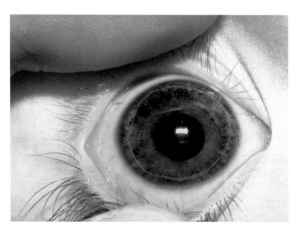

Figure 19.4 Posterior embryotoxon

and the various treatments in lay terms has proved to be extremely helpful.[18] Other investigations such as ultrasound can be carried out before examination under anaesthesia if indicated, to exclude posterior segment pathology, document any changes in axial length, and occasionally detect optic disc cupping.

The differential diagnosis of the child with childhood glaucoma is large and should always be borne in mind (Table 19.2). With experience the initial assessment is usually correct. However, the vast majority of young children are then examined in the operating theatre if there is any question of glaucoma.

Assessment under anaesthesia

Type of anaesthetic

An appropriate anaesthetic is vital for assessment of patients with childhood glaucoma. In preparing the child for anaesthetic we encourage a parent to accompany the child to the anaesthetic room (Figure 19.5). In general, *all* anaesthetics alter the IOP[19] and in particular some such as halothane, and even newer agents such as sevofluorane, lower the IOP substan-

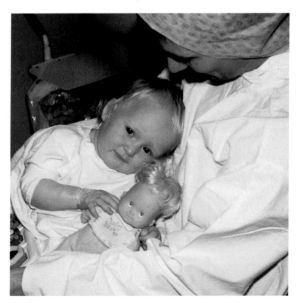

Figure 19.5 Child with father in theatre before examination under anaesthetic

tially.[20] Patients with IOPs of 30–40 mm Hg may measure 10–20 mm Hg under anaesthesia. Whatever agent is used, it is important to have a consistent approach so that the normal range for the chosen anaesthetic regimen can be established.

One approach is to premedicate with oral midazolam and atropine (to reduce bronchial secretions). Ketamine hydrochloride (Ketalar, Parke Davis, Eastleigh, UK) is then given intramuscularly at 5–10 (usually 7) mg/kg. If the child is large, local anaesthetic patches and intravenous ketamine are used. Ketamine can cause a transient rise in IOP, which may last 3–4 minutes, and this can be potentiated if the child is crying when the injection is given. The timing of IOP measurement is thus critical. The duration of ketamine is short, usually lasting 10–15 minutes, although the patient may then sleep on for several hours if left undisturbed.

If intraocular surgery is required it is necessary to convert to full anaesthesia with assisted ventilation, as ketamine alone is inadequate for maintaining sufficient anaesthesia and analgesia during these procedures. Once under ketamine anaesthesia a sequence of procedures needs to be carried out (Table 19.4).

Systemic examination

While the patient is under anaesthesia any general examination that is not possible while the patient is awake, and any venesection for laboratory investigation including screens for

Table 19.4 Examination of the child with suspected glaucoma under anaesthetic

- cornea
- corneal diameter
- anterior chamber
- iris
- lens
- intraocular pressure
- gonioscopy
- disc
- fundus
- refraction
- other indicated examinations, e.g. lids, keratometry, ultrasound, venesection

infective agents and chromosome studies, is performed. If necessary other investigations such as keratometry, pachymetry, elecrodiagnostics, and ultrasonography can be carried out.

Intraocular pressure

Local anaesthetic drops are *always* used before applanation even though the patient is partially anaesthetised, as they may still be sensitive to corneal touch. The majority of normal eyes have pressures < 22 mm Hg with this regimen. However, judgements are never made on IOP alone and are taken in context with all the other clinical findings. The gold standard for tonometry is the Perkins hand held tonometer with a blue filter after fluorescein has been instilled in the eye. However, if there is any chance that the patient will require a goniotomy, a Schiotz tonometer or the Perkins tonometer with blue filter removed (without fluorescein) is used. This is to avoid the impairment of the gonioscope view of the angle induced by fluorescein in the corneal stroma. The Tono-pen is more expensive but has the advantage of being relatively convenient and requiring only a small area of contact, and therefore may be useful if the cornea has a large central opacity, e.g. Peter's anomaly. Whichever method is used accurate measurement of IOP can be difficult and one should always measure the IOP several times in both eyes.

Cornea

The cornea is examined for the presence of oedema, opacities and splits in Descemet's membrane that are virtually pathognomonic of glaucoma (Figure 19.6). It is useful to have some form of oblique illumination such as a Kowa SL-15 portable slit lamp, even if an operating microscope is used, as this helps to show up abnormalities. It is important to examine the cornea carefully as corneal pathology may give rise to symptoms such as lacrimation, photophobia, and blepharospasm. The diagnosis will be missed in more subtle cases unless the cornea is properly examined with magnification.

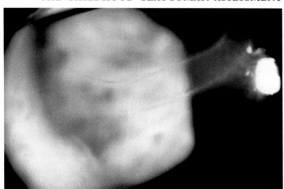

Figure 19.6 Haab's striae
Almost pathognomonic of congenital glaucoma

The corneal diameter is measured along the horizontal meridian with callipers (checked with a graduated ruler) from limbus to limbus (Figure 19.7). Consistency in deciding where to measure from is vital, as eyes with childhood glaucoma often have very abnormal limbal anatomy. The normal horizontal neonatal corneal diameter is 10.5 mm increasing about 1 mm in the first year of life,[20] and a diameter > 12.5 mm in children under the age of 1 year is very suggestive of raised IOP.[21] A measurement > 13 mm in a child of any age is abnormal.

Measurement of corneal diameter is important in management as well as diagnosis. If the corneal diameter is increasing this is an

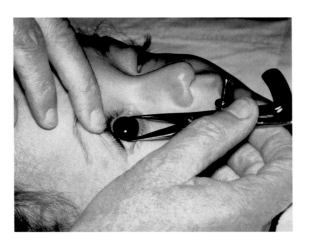

Figure 19.7 Corneal measurement
Important for diagnosis, prognosis and assessment of progression

indication that IOP is not adequately controlled. Similarly, corneal oedema is a sign that the glaucoma may not be controlled, although in some eyes corneal oedema may persist for some weeks after lowering of the IOP. The oedema clears from the peripheral cornea first and then towards the central area. In some patients endothelial function may be reduced, and the cornea may not clear until there is a consistent IOP reduction to the low teens.

Iris and drainage angle

Abnormalities of the iris such as an abnormal stroma and pupil, e.g. corectopia, may suggest anterior segment dysgenesis rather than simple PCG. This is important for management (anterior segment dysgenesis responds better to trabeculotomy than goniotomy) and for genetic counselling. The presence of abnormal masses may suggest secondary glaucoma due to malignant or inflammatory conditions. Examination of the internal sclerostomy to exclude iris incarceration is also vital if the IOP is high following filtration surgery.

Lens

In a number of paediatric glaucomas there may be co-existing lens opacities which may require treatment. When cataract extraction in patients with glaucoma is required, it is vital to try and preserve the posterior capsule to make IOP easier to control in the future. Furthermore if cataract surgery is imminent it may be necessary to place a tube implant, as this is more likely to survive cataract surgery than filtration surgery, even with mitomycin.

The presence of lens subluxation increases the likelihood of vitreous prolapse into the anterior chamber and should be carefully looked for. It is seen in severe cases of childhood glaucoma in association with ocular enlargement, aniridia, microspherophakia, and Marfan's syndrome. A laser or surgical peripheral iridectomy may be required if there is a danger of pupil block. The presence of significant lens subluxa-

tion considerably worsens the surgical prognosis of glaucoma surgery, sometimes requiring extensive surgical intervention such as vitreolensectomy and tube drainage surgery rather than trabeculectomy.

Optic disc

The optic disc assessment is vitally important in the diagnosis and monitoring of the childhood glaucomas. Although the same could be said of adult glaucomas, change in cup:disc ratio (CDR) can occur much more rapidly in children (Figure 19.8).

In regard to diagnosis, the CDR is a useful indicator of disease, even more so than adult glaucoma. Richardson[22] noted a CDR of > 0.3 in only 2.6% of newborn infant eyes, while Shaffer and Hetherington[23] found a CDR > 0.3 in 68% of eyes with congenital glaucoma.

In regard to progression, CDR is probably

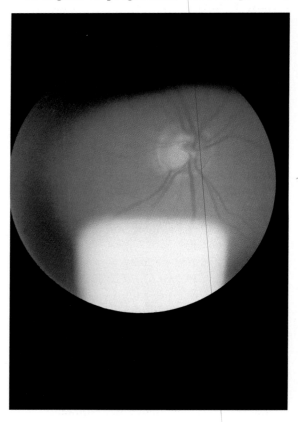

Figure 19.8   Cupped disc in congenital glaucoma

the most important parameter available to monitor visual damage caused by the raised IOP. Often it is not possible to view the disc initially if the IOP is raised and the cornea is oedematous. Viewing through a Keoppe lens to reduce the epithelial irregularities may help. Direct ophthalmoscopy can be used with the undilated pupil and an indirect ophthalmoscope (particularly one with a small pupil facility) can be very helpful in obtaining a binocular view of the disc. The pupil is not dilated preoperatively as this may alter and mask the angle appearance, spuriously increase the IOP, and increase the risk of lens damage if surgery is required.

The status of the optic disc is carefully recorded with drawings or with photographs if possible, and the horizontal and vertical CDR recorded. An increase in the size of the cup indicates that the glaucoma is not controlled and that further treatment is necessary. Conversely, a stable CDR with borderline IOPs and stable corneal diameters, suggests that a more conservative approach may be appropriate. If the disc cannot be visualised b-scan ultrasonography may be useful to detect the presence and degree of cupping.

Retina and vitreous

It is important not to limit inspection of the posterior pole to the optic nerve and the remainder of the fundus should be examined for any associated abnormalities such as foveal hypoplasia associated with aniridia, pigmentary retinopathy associated with systemic disorders such as rubella, and choroidal haemangiomas in Sturge–Weber syndrome.

Refraction

If one cannot obtain a good cycloplegic refraction in the outpatient setting, retinoscopy will need to be performed during the examination under anaesthetic (Figure 19.9). The pupil should not be dilated preoperatively (for the reasons given above) after full examination should the pupils be dilated with cyclopentolate 0.5% and retinoscopy performed. Advantage

can be taken of the dilated pupil and indirect fundoscopy carried out at the same time. Buphthalmic eyes are usually myopic, but usually less than the axial length would suggest due to simultaneous changes reducing the curvature of the cornea. Rapidly progressive myopia may also suggest that the IOP is not fully controlled. The state of refraction is useful as a prognostic sign with respect to the risk of amblyopia and will indicate the need for occlusion therapy. Anisometropia greater than six dioptres is invariably associated with significant amblyopia in the eye, whatever the occlusion regimen.[24,25]

Follow-up

If glaucoma is confirmed then a treatment regimen is usually commenced. If there is a high risk of glaucoma then clearly further follow-up examinations will be required under anaesthetic until the child can be examined in clinic. The frequency of follow-up will depend on individual circumstances.

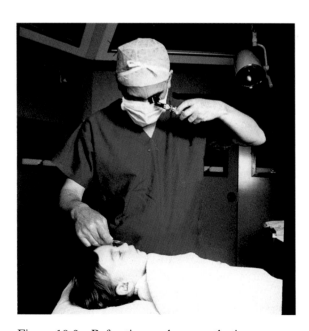

Figure 19.9   Refraction under anaesthetic
It is essential to detect and correct any refractive error

References

1 Miller SJH. Genetic aspects of glaucoma. *Trans Am Ophthalmol Soc UK* 1962; **81**: 425–34.

2 Gilbert CE, Canovas R, Hagan M, Rao S, Foster A. Causes of Childhood Blindness: Results from West Africa, South India and Chile. *Eye* 1993; 7: 184–8.

3 Thylefors B, Negrel A-D. The global impact of glaucoma. *Bulletin* WHO 1994; **72**: 323–6.

4 Shaffer RN, Weiss DI. The congenital and pediatric glaucomas. St Louis: CV Mosby 1970.

5 Hoskins H, Hetherington J, Shaffer R, Welling A. Developmental glaucomas: diagnosis and classification. In: Anonymous Symposium on glaucoma. *Trans New Orleans Ac Ophthalmol* St Louis: CV Mosby 1975; 194–7.

6 De Luise VP, Anderson DR. Primary Infantile Glaucoma (Congenital Glaucoma). *Surv Ophthalmol* 1983; **28**: 1–19.

7 Knepper PA, Goossens W, McLone DG. Ultrastructural studies of primary congenital glaucoma in rabbits. *J Ped Ophthalmol Strabismus* 1997; **34**: 365–71.

8 Sarfarazi M, Akarsu AN, Hossain A, *et al*. Assignment of a locus (GLC3A) for primary congenital glaucoma (buphthalmos) to 2p21 and evidence for genetic heterogeneity. *Genomics* 1995; **30**: 171–7.

9 Churchill A, Booth A. Genetics of aniridia and anterior segment dysgenesis. *Br J Ophthalmol* 1996; **80**: 669–73.

10 Kupfer C, Kaiser-Kupfer. Observations on the development of the anterior chamber angle with reference to the pathogenesis of congenital glaucoma. *Am J Ophthalmol* 1979; **88**: 424.

11 Walter MA, Mirzayans F, Mears AJ, Hickey K, Pearce WG. Autosomal-dominant iridogonidysgenesis and Axenfeld/Reiger syndrome are genetically distinct. *Ophthalmology* 1995; **103**: 1907–15.

12 Sarfarazi M. Recent advances in molecular genetics of glaucomas. *Human Molec Genet* 1997; **6**: 1667–77.

13 Hanson IM, Fletcher J, Jordan T, Brown A, Taylor D, Adams R. Mutations in the PAX6 locus are found in the heterogenous anterior segment malformations including Peter's anomaly. *Nature Genetics* 1994; **6**: 168–73.

14 Axton R, Hanson I, Danes S, Sellar G, van Heyningen V, Prosser J. The incidence of PAX 6 mutation in patients with simple aniridia: an evaluation of mutation detection in 12 cases. *J Med Genetics* 1997; **34**: 279–86.

15 Asrani SG, Wilensky JT. Glaucoma after congenital cataract surgery. *Ophthalmology* 1995; **102**: 863–7.

16 Wallace DK, Plager DA, Snyder SK, Raiesdana A, Helveston EM, Ellis FD. Surgical results of secondary glaucomas in childhood. *Ophthalmology* 1997; **105**: 101–11.

17 Phelps CD. The pathogenesis of glaucoma in Sturge–Weber syndrome. *Ophthalmology* 1978; **85**: 276–86.

18 Khaw PT. Childhood Glaucoma: A guide for parents. Moorfields Eye Hospital. London, UK 1999; **6**. Available on www.moorfields.org.uk.

19 Quigley HA. Childhood Glaucoma: Results with trabeculectomy and study of reversible cupping. *Ophthalmology* 1982; **89**: 219–25.

20 Kwitko ML. The paediatric glaucomas. In: McAllister JA, Wilson RP, (eds). *Glaucoma* London: Butterworths, 1986; 111–37.

21 Becker B, Shaffer RN. Diagnosis and Therapy of the Glaucomas. St Louis: Mosby Febiger, 1965.

22 Richardson KT, Shaffer TN. Optic nerve cupping in congenital glaucoma. *Am J Ophthalmol* 1966; **62**: 507–9.

23 Shaffer RN, Hetherington J. Glaucomatous disc in infants. A Suggested hypothesis for disc cupping. *Trans Am Acad Ophthalmol Otolaryngol* 1969; **73**: 929–35.

24 Rice NSCR. Management of infantile glaucoma. *Br J Ophthalmol* 1972; **56**: 294–8.

25 Clothier CM, Rice NS, Dobinson P, Wakefield R. Amblyopia in congenital glaucoma. *Trans Ophthalmol Soc UK* 1979; **99**: 427–31.

20 The childhood glaucomas: management

P T KHAW, S G FRASER, M PAPADOPOULOS, A WELLS, P SHAH

The decision to commence treatment for glaucoma is never one to be taken lightly, particularly in children. Nonetheless, if uncontrolled glaucoma is present the prognosis is very poor without treatment.[1] This decision to treat, while based in the context of the overall clinical situation, relies on many parameters, including visual potential, intraocular pressure (IOP), corneal enlargement, corneal oedema at low pressures, cupping of the optic disc, axial length, and IOP. The finding of an enlarged corneal diameter, corneal oedema with splits, raised IOP and a cupped optic disc, usually leaves no doubt that immediate treatment is necessary. If the corneal diameter and cup:disc ratio is increasing, treatment should be considered even if the IOP is borderline or normal. On the other hand, if the IOP is slightly raised or borderline but there is no change in disc or corneal diameter, further measures need not be introduced immediately. As with all clinical situations, the risks of treatment have to be balanced against the risk of disease progression.

Medical treatment

The main treatment of the childhood glaucomas, particularly primary congenital glaucoma (PCG), is usually surgical. However, the older the child the more likely it is that medical therapy becomes the initial treatment. Medical treatment is necessary if surgical treatment is not possible or too high risk, before surgical treatment can be undertaken, or as adjuncts to maximise IOP lowering after surgery (see also Chapter 9).

Children run a higher risk of systemic side effects as high blood levels may be achieved following topical administration of drops that occasionally approach or even exceed therapeutic levels after oral administration.[2] Young children have smaller blood volumes and immature metabolic systems and this can result in a drug halflife two to six times longer than in the adult[3] and great care has to be exercised when prescribing. To reduce the chance of systemic toxicity parents can be instructed to use punctal occlusion for 3–5 minutes[4] after instilling drops. In younger children it may be useful to commence treatment while the child is in a hospital setting to monitor for initial adverse effects.

β-blockers

Topical β-blockers have also been used with some success for patients with childhood glaucoma, but this is usually in patients who have already undergone previous surgery. We only occasionally use topical β-blockers in neonates because of the risk of systemic side effects. If these drugs are used, we prefer a drug such as betaxolol, which may have a larger safety margin, and we advise punctal occlusion. In older children it is important to inquire about symptoms of asthma, which at this age may present as persistent nocturnal coughing rather than wheezing. Parents should be told to report symptoms of respiratory problems, to stop the drops if these became a problem, and return for reassessment.

Parasympathomimetics

One drop of pilocarpine 1% every 6–8 hours may be given as temporary treatment before surgical intervention in infants with PCG. An improvement in symptoms with treatment is a sign that the eye will respond to angle surgery. This may be continued for a few weeks after goniotomy to enhance outflow. At this dose, systemic toxicity has not been a problem, although it still remains a possibility. With stronger anticholinergic drugs such as phospholine iodide,[5] diarrhoea has been reported, and there is a risk of prolonged muscle paralysis if agents such as succinyl choline are used during general anaesthesia. In view of this, the only anticholinergic agent we use is pilocarpine. The drops are usually stopped the night before surgery to allow the IOP to return to actual levels for assessment. For longer-term use, it is important to bear in mind that the use of topical pilocarpine may increase the long-term risk of surgical failure.

Sympathomimetics

Both adrenaline and dipivefrin may greatly increase the risk of failure of subsequent filtration surgery. The role of topical α_2-agonists such as apraclonidine and brimonidine and is not yet clear. Additionally, approximately 5–10% of the children on α-agonists get side effects which necessitate termination of treatment, of which lassitude is most prominent.

Prostaglandin agonists

The role of the newer prostaglandin analogues such as latanoprost is not clear. The unknown long-term side effects and the moderate additive effect in the majority of cases limit their use. Parents should be advised about the effects of latanoprost on iris colour and the permanent nature of this change. The effects on eyelashes and eyelid pigmentation also need to be mentioned. If patients are on multiple therapy the addition of latanoprost significantly lowers pressure in about one third of patients.

Carbonic anhydrase inhibitors

Topical carbonic anhydrase inhibitors appear to have minimal systemic side effects, although caution must be used in a compromised cornea with poor endothelial function as corneal oedema may be worsened. Oral acetazolamide has been used as crushed tablets or elixir,[6,7] although we very rarely use it in young children. Children on oral carbonic anhydrase inhibitors may have unusual side effects such as bed-wetting and disturbed hyperactive behaviour, and may present with failure to thrive. Carbonated drinks also taste bad.

Surgical treatment

There are several surgical procedures used in the childhood glaucomas. All these procedures have advantages and disadvantages and varying indications. The best treatment of choice for the different types of glaucoma depends on the type of glaucoma, associated ocular disease and the experience of the surgeon.[8] An example of a surgical treatment flow chart for Axenfeld–Rieger anomaly is shown in Figure 20.1. The surgical treatment of choice will vary from unit to unit (see also Chapter 11).

The cornea in many of these children may be oedematous. Removal of the surface epithelium with alcohol (Figure 20.2) may improve the clarity of the cornea sufficient to perform surgical procedures such as goniotomy. However, residual stromal opacification can prevent a sufficiently clear view of the angle structures, necessitating an alternative approach.

Goniotomy

Goniotomy was first described in its current form by Otto Barkan[9] and is the operation of

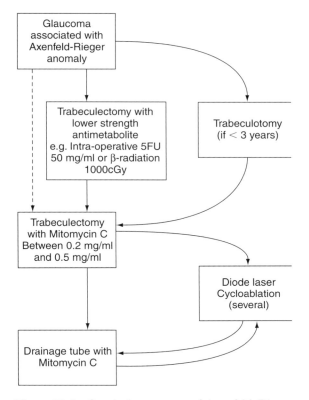

Figure 20.1 Surgical treatment of Axenfeld–Rieger anomaly.

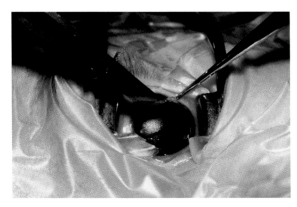

Figure 20.2 Removal of epithelium with alcohol allowing a clear view for goniotomy.

choice where there is primary trabecular meshwork dysgenesis (primary congenital glaucoma) without other significant anterior segment dysgenesis.[10] It is not usually indicated after the age of 3–4 years, and if the patient presents before the age of 3 months the surgical prog-

nosis after goniotomy is poorer. It is an extremely effective operation with reports of 70–90% of patients having controlled IOPs (usually IOP < 21 mm Hg) after 5 years.[11–16]

Goniotomy is less invasive than trabeculotomy and avoids damage to the conjunctiva, thereby increasing the chance of subsequent success if trabeculectomy is required.[17] It is however a difficult procedure to perform, requiring surgical techniques not commonly used. Although safe in experienced hands, potential complications include lens and corneal damage, inadvertent cyclodialysis and scleral perforation. It cannot be performed safely without an operating microscope and special instruments (Figure 20.3). The advantages and disadvantages of goniotomy are summarised in Table 20.1. Preoperative pilocarpine is useful to constrict the pupil. The technique of goniotomy is described in detail elsewhere.[18] In Caucasian patients with PCG, the majority of corneas can be cleared with alcohol to allow good visualisation for goniotomy. Goniotomy can be repeated in a non-operated part of the angle if there has been a reasonable lowering after the first goniotomy.

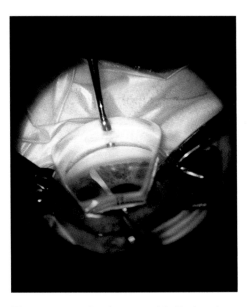

Figure 20.3 Goniotomy with Barkan lens and knife
The iris falls back as the knife moves across the angle.

Table 20.1 Advantages and disadvantages of goniotomy

Advantages

- Conjunctiva left for future surgery
- Probably no adverse effect on future filtration surgery
- More "physiological" approach opening channels that have not opened
- Minimal risk of significant hypotony
- Rapid
- No long term risk of bleb endophthalmitis
- 80–90% success in primary congenital glaucoma over 3–5 years in best series

Disadvantages

- Technically very demanding, particularly if only rarely performed by surgeon. Very difficult in smaller eyes
- Uncomfortable for first few days if epithelium has to be stripped
- Works mainly for primary congenital glaucoma. Difficult if significant anterior segment dysgenesis present
- Requires special instruments
- Complications include endothelial, angle and lens damage
- Not possible if cornea cannot be cleared with alcohol (but possible in 90% of cases of PCG in Caucasians)
- Requires debridement of epithelium in the majority of cases to get an excellent view
- < 50% success in one series when performed by general ophthalmologists

The Q-switched Nd:YAG laser is not a useful tool for goniotomy and does not work in the long term.

Trabeculotomy

Trabeculotomy is described in its modern form by both Redmond Smith[19] and Burian.[20] In theory, trabeculotomy can be used for any condition where a goniotomy is required. It is particularly useful where a goniotomy cannot be performed due to corneal opacification,[21] very early onset PCG (< 3 months), and in patients with anterior segment dysgeneses such as Axenfeld-Rieger anomaly, Peter's anomaly, or aniridia.[22] Like goniotomy, primary angle opening procedures are much less likely to work if the patients are older than 3 years. Many surgeons use trabeculotomy as the primary procedure in all patients with PCG. However, there is an increase in surgical trauma associated with the procedure compared with goniotomy, and the conjunctival incision has a long-term prejudicial effect on future glaucoma filtration surgery.[23]

Trabeculotomy has the advantage of being technically possible even if the cornea is opaque. It also involves some surgical techniques and approaches, e.g. conjunctival flap, scleral flap, which are more familiar to ophthalmic surgeons, than goniotomy. Despite having these techniques in common with trabeculectomy, the trabeculotomy technique remains difficult, particularly for the surgeon who only sees the occasional case of congenital glaucoma. The conjunctiva is damaged which prejudices future glaucoma filtration surgery near the area, and it is essentially more traumatic than a goniotomy. The advantages and disadvantages of trabeculotomy are summarised in Table 20.2. An inferior trabeculotomy spares the superior conjunctiva. An operating microscope and special trabeculotome are essential. Complications include tears of Descemet's membrane, hyphaema and cyclodialysis with persistent hypotony. The technique is reviewed in detail elsewhere.[18] Beck and Lynch[24] have described a variation on the standard trabeculotomy technique in which a 6/0 suture is used rather than a trabeculotome. This has the advantage of a 360° trabeculotomy in one procedure.

Trabeculotomy/trabeculectomy

Some authors have suggested that trabeculotomy combined with trabeculectomy may be superior to trabeculotomy or trabeculectomy alone.[25,26] This may have the advantages of

Table 20.2 Advantages and disadvantages of trabeculotomy (with trabeculectomy).

Advantages

- Many components of technique similar to trabeculectomy
- Can be performed even if cornea is opaque
- More "physiological" approach opening channels that have not opened
- Minimal risk of significant hypotony
- Success rates at best about 80–90% at 3 years in primary congenital glaucoma
- Unlike goniotomy, can often be used for anterior segment dysgenesis such as Axenfeld– Riegers
- (When combined with trabeculectomy some reports of higher success rate – may reduce number of anaesthetics as reduced need for angle surgery followed later by trabeculectomy)

Disadvantages

- Damages conjunctiva and significantly increases risk of subsequent trabeculectomy failure
- Not under direct visualisation which may lead to significant complications, e.g. iris disinsertion
- Schlemm's canal may not be found in 10–20% of cases
- Converting a trabeculotomy entry site to trabeculectomy places the sclerostomy very close to the iris root predisposing to iris incarceration
- Requires special trabeculotomy probes
- (When combined with trabeculectomy may be technically more difficult.)
- (Entry site to eye has to be closer to base of iris to cannulate Schlemm's canal, increases risk of iris and ciliary body incarceration)
- (May be more difficult to secure scleral flap because of posterior position resulting in hypotony – particularly a problem if antimetabolites are used)

trabeculotomy in eyes with opaque corneas possibly with increased efficacy. However, it is a more complex operation and requires experience. Combined surgery requires the placement of a scleral flap closer to the iris root. In inexperienced hands this may predispose to iris/ciliary process prolapse, incarceration, vitreous loss, and hypotony if strong antimetabolites are used.

Filtration surgery (trabeculectomy) usually with antimetabolite

Indications for glaucoma filtration surgery (GFS) in childhood include previous failed angle procedures, e.g. goniotomy or trabeculotomy. Other indications include when a low IOP (10–15 mm Hg) is needed in order to enable clearing of corneal oedema or opacification. An antimetabolite is usually required to consistently achieve this degree of pressure lowering.

Filtration surgery has the advantage that most surgeons have experience performing this procedure in adults with glaucoma, and are performing this surgery much more regularly. If the operating surgeon has no or minimal experience of goniotomy or trabeculotomy and it is

not possible to refer the patient to a specialised centre, it would be safer to carry out a trabeculectomy. The disadvantage of GFS is that it is a more invasive procedure compared to goniotomy and trabeculotomy and probably has the highest complication rate of the three procedures, even in the hands of surgeons experienced in carrying out all three procedures (Figure 20.4). It is technically a more difficult procedure in childhood glaucoma compared with adult glaucoma because of abnormal

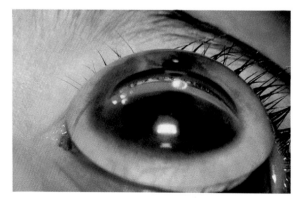

Figure 20.4   Patient referred because of flat anterior chamber post trabeculectomy due to lens incarceration.

limbal anatomy, thin sclera, difficult access, and a greater risk of intra- and postoperative hypotony. The advantages and disadvantages of trabeculectomy are summarised in Table 20.3.

The failure rate of primary filtration surgery is variable, being higher than primary trabeculotomy and goniotomy in some studies (Figure 20.5)[27,28] but not in others.[26,29] The technique of trabeculectomy in children may have to be modified to address the unique problems encountered in these eyes. These modifications are described in Table 20.4.

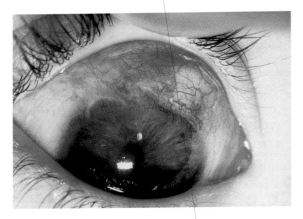

Figure 20.5   Failed surgery due to inflammation and fibrosis at surgical site.

Antifibrosis treatment

It has been shown that the long-term success rate of children with PCG after glaucoma filtration surgery is reduced, particularly if previous conjunctival surgery has been performed, such as trabeculotomy.[30] The use of postoperative injections of 5-fluorouracil has considerably increased the success rate of adult patients who have a high risk of failing glaucoma filtration surgery,[31] but regular injections are not a practical proposition in children with glaucoma. Therefore single intraoperative application regimens for the prevention of postoperative fibrosis are of particular use in children undergoing filtration surgery. There are a number of options available:

Intraoperative β-radiation

The use of intra-operative β-radiation has considerably increased the success rate of glaucoma filtration surgery in PCG (Figure 20.6).[30] This is with few associated complications, even in the long term. A single application of 750 cGy can inhibit the proliferation of Tenon's capsule fibroblasts *in vitro* for several weeks without resulting in significant fibroblast cell death.[32] A semicircular Strontium-90 probe

Table 20.3 Advantages and disadvantages of trabeculectomy (with antimetabolites)

Advantages

- Familiarity – most surgeons perform trabeculectomy on a regular basis and have experience and can deal with complications
- Reasonable results in low risk category of primary congenital glaucoma
- (80–90% 3 year success rate achievable in both lower and higher risk individuals using appropriate antimetabolites)
- (Lower pressures achievable with antimetabolites)
- (In patients with cloudy corneas lower pressures with trabeculectomy and antimetabolites may clear cornea significantly)
- (Postoperative pressures "titratable" compared with angle surgery by using techniques such as releasable sutures and post operative antimetabolites)

Disadvantages

- Damages conjunctiva and significantly increases risk of subsequent trabeculectomy failure
- Not under direct visualisation which may lead to significant complications, e.g. iris disinsertion
- Poor results due to scarring in high risk eyes particularly early onset cases and those with previous surgery
- Damages conjunctiva compared to goniotomy and makes secondary surgery more difficult
- (Greater risk of endophthalmitis than angle surgery particularly with mitomycin C and limbus based flaps)
- (Greater risk of hypotony with choroidal effusion and haemorrhage than angle surgery, particularly with mitomycin C)
- (Poor results in aphakic glaucoma even with antimetabolites)
  (Risk of intraocular damage if antimetabolites enter eye)

Table 20.4 Important surgical points in paediatric trabeculectomy

POINT	ACTION	RATIONALE
Exposure	Corneal traction suture (7–0 silk) Fornix based Conjunctival flap	Allows maximum inferoduction of globe Allows good visualisation of limbal anatomy Easier placement of sutures in scleral flap Superior limbal flap may not be possible in neonate
Haemostasis	Corneal traction suture Wetfield cautery	Avoids haemorrhage from superior rectus Avoids scleral shrinkage (very important in thin sclera)
Prevention of scarring	Antimetabolites	See text
Scleral flap	Anterior placement Larger (4 × 3–4 mm) Anterior pocket valve	To avoid the ciliary body and vitreous incarceration Easier to suture without cheese wiring in thin sclera Greater resistance to aqueous outflow (vital in large buphthalmic eyes, particularly if antimetabolites are used) Valve effect to prevent hypotony and direct aqueous posteriorly to prevent cystic blebs
Paracentesis	Oblique tunnel Long tunnel (2+ mm)	A paracentesis allows an assessment of the opening pressure of the scleral flap and reformation of the AC post-op. Oblique long tunnel paracentesis removes the risk of inadvertent lens damage during the manoeuvre and is less likely to leak
Maintenance of IOP during Procedure	Anterior chamber maintainer	Prevents eye from becoming hypotonous during procedure with choroidals (e.g. Sturge–Weber) Can be used to gauge flow through the sclerostomy To ensure adequate closure
Sclerostomy	Small (1–2 punch bites) Anterior as possible	Increased control of aqueous outflow intra- and post-op. Quick therefore less intra-op hypotony To prevent ciliary body/iris/vitreous incarceration
Scleral flap closure	Tight releasable/adjustable (preplaced before sclerostomy) Loop buried (in cornea) Adjustable knots	Allows control of opening pressures Easier to place with intact globe Faster to tie therefore reduced period of intra-operative hypotony Allows releasable sutures to be left safely in place long-term if necessary (particularly important with MMC). Can be removed under anaesthetic without the need for a laser Adjustable allows tight closure but are easily loosened without complete removal
Conjuntival closure (fornix based)	10–0 nylon purse string (corners)	Retains tension longer than dissolvable sutures Minimal associated inflammation Ends of nylon buried under conjunctiva
Post operative prevention of hypotony	Viscoelastic in anterior chamber	May be necessary if flow rate too high despite maximal suturing Can be repeated

(Amersham International, Amersham, UK) is gently placed over the closed conjunctiva of the filtration area at the end of surgery and left there for the time required to deliver a surface dose of 750–1000 cGy. The resulting bleb is usually diffuse and non-cystic.

Intraoperative topical antimetabolites

Intraoperative 5-fluorouracil (5FU) is equivalent in cell culture to the effect of β-radiation. A titratable regimen of 3 minute intraoperative exposures to either 5FU 50 mg/ml or mitomycin C (MMC) 0.2 or 0.4 mg/ml are used in an attempt to achieve maximal benefit with a minimum of side effects. Intraoperative β-radiation may be preferable to 5FU in children because of the long record of safety in children and the more diffuse less cystic blebs.

The use of single application MMC[33] is now widely used in adult glaucoma surgery and

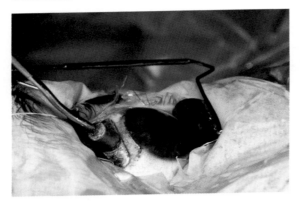

Figure 20.6 Strontium 90 probe delivering β-radiation to surgical site after trabeculectomy.

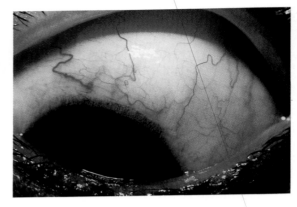

Figure 20.8 β-radiation bleb-diffuse and non-cystic.

increasingly in children.[34–36] (see also Chapter 11). MMC 0.4 mg/ml is used for patients who have failed filtration surgery with previous adjunctive β-radiation or 5FU, or have a combination of high-risk characteristics (Figures 20.7, 20.8), (Table 20.5). If the subconjunctival tissues are thin, or there is a particular worry about hypotony or endophthalmitis, MMC 0.2 mg/ml should be used.

The result of IOP reduction on corneal clarity can be dramatic (Figures 20.9, 20.10).

MMC has the potential to produce thin, cystic, avascular blebs that are prone to develop delayed leaks and may result in hypotony and endophthalmitis. Our modifications to the intraoperative application of MMC involve treating much larger areas of conjunctiva and

Table 20.5 Risk factors for trabeculectomy failure in childhood glaucoma (even with antimetabolites)

- Corneal diameter > 14 mm
- Very disordered anterior segment (e.g. Riegers with marked iris/angle abnormalities)
- Previous conjunctival surgery (including squint/retinal detachment surgery and trabeculotomy)
- Indian subcontinent origin
- Red eye/persistent ocular inflammation
- Aphakia
- Neovascularisation
- Previous failed trabeculectomy with β-radiation or 5FU
- Very early onset disease (at birth or "before")
- ? Recent previous surgery including laser

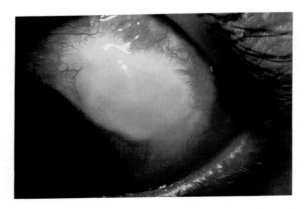

Figure 20.7 Mitomycin bleb after limbus-based conjunctival flap and small surface area of treatment.

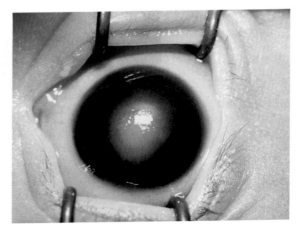

Figure 20.9 Eye with central corneal opacification before IOP reduction.

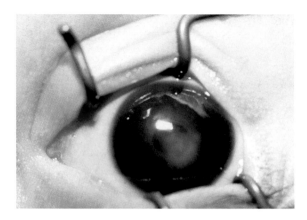

Figure 20.10 Eye in Figure 20.9 with central corneal opacification after IOP control.

Tenon's capsule,[37] seem to result in better post-operative bleb morphology. MMC blebs using this technique appear more likely to be diffuse, non-cystic, posterior draining, and have normal conjunctival vasculature and architecture without encapsulation.

Postoperative antimetabolites and treatments

Subconjunctival injections of 5FU can be given while the child is under anaesthesia if necessary (Figure 20.11). When intraoperative anti-scarring treatment has been used, this prolongs the period in which the postoperative subconjunctival injections of 5FU may be useful for up to several months. Care should be taken to

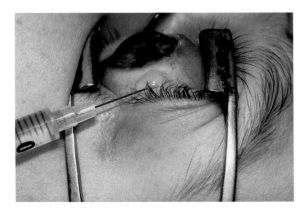

Figure 20.11 Subconjunctival injection of 5 FU adjacent to but not into the bleb.

avoid intraocular entry of 5FU as it has a pH of 9.0. Although not an antimetabolite, it is useful to remember that subconjunctival steroids, e.g. Betamethasone (Betnesol), can be used for its anti-inflammatory properties when it is felt inappropriate to use 5FU.

Tube drainage devices

Drainage tubes of various types have been used with some success for patients with childhood glaucoma.[38] Similar complications develop as for adult eyes (see Chapter 11). Because children tend to have large eyes and reduced scleral rigidity there is more likely to be leakage around the tube, and hypotony results in much more scleral collapse. This increases the risk of suprachoroidal haemorrhages (aphakic eyes are at highest risk). If a tube is to be used *without* anti-scarring agents, a large surface area plate is required, e.g. a two plate rather than single plate Molteno implant, and measures should be taken to avoid prolonged hypotony such as an intratube occlusive suture. The advent of single application antifibrosis treatments and the ease of use of the diode laser has reduced the indication for glaucoma tube surgery. The advantages and disadvantages of tube drainage surgery are summarised in Table 20.6.

In certain groups of patients tubes remain an important part the therapeutic repertoire. These groups include aphakic eyes that have developed glaucoma following congenital cataract surgery[39] and eyes that have failed MMC trabeculectomy.[40] Aphakic eyes also respond less well to MMC trabeculectomy than phakic eyes. Drainage tubes are also useful if further intraocular surgery such as cataract extraction or vitrectomy will be required later, as a tube seems to be more likely to maintain IOP control after these procedures.

Modification of tube surgery can reduce complications and improve success.[41] Placement of a tube in an aphakic eye should be combined with a complete anterior and partial core vitrectomy to prevent tube blockage. At the

Table 20.6 Advantages and disadvantages of tube surgery (with antimetabolites)

Advantages

- Very effective in reducing intraocular pressure
- Most effective long-term treatment even if previously failed trabeculectomy with antimetabolites
- Most likely to survive further surgery, e.g. graft, lensectomy, vitrectomy therefore best drainage option if further surgery likely
- Modifiable later, e.g. tube needling, antimetabolite treatment of capsule
- (With mitomycin C > 70% off all treatment with diffuse non-cystic blebs)
- (Even combined with antimetabolites gives diffuse posterior bleb with minimal risk of endophthalmitis)
- (In aphakic glaucoma makes contact lens wear possible)

Disadvantages

- Highest complication rate short term, particularly hypotony related complications including sight threatening complications
- Longest rehabilitation period
- Long term complications include tube extrusion, tube blockage, endothelial damage and plate encapsulation
- ? Higher rate of graft rejection
- Longest surgical time
- Foreign tissue if patch graft (sclera, pericardium, dura mater) used

end of the operation C3F8 20% is injected into the anterior chamber[42] (after clearing anaesthetic nitrous oxide from the systemic circulation) to prevent postoperative hypotony. The use of intraoperative MMC gives > 80% with an IOP < 21 mm Hg of all treatment at one year with single plate Molteno tubes without any focal high encapsulation (Figure 20.12). When using intraoperative MMC in tube surgery, obsessive measures have to be taken to protect the eye from early *hypotony*. This includes very tight entry holes (long tunnel with a 25 gauge needle), intraluminal 3/0 supramid nylon sutures, external 6/0 vicryl occlusion, a Tenon's

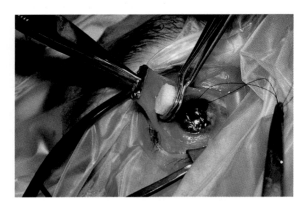

Figure 20.12   Mitomycin pre-treatment of the conjunctiva and Tenon's capsule, before tube placement The sclera is protected from the mitomycin.

capsule patch and high viscosity viscoelastics in the anterior chamber if required.

Cyclodestruction

Ciliary body destruction has been used in the management of childhood glaucoma, most usually with the cryoprobe. However, cyclocryotherapy is associated with complications such as postoperative discomfort, inflammation and phthisis.[43] Cyclodestructive procedures are reserved for eyes with a poor visual prognosis, or where drainage surgery is technically not possible.

Contact diode cyclodestruction has replaced the use of cyclocryotherapy and Nd:YAG cyclodestruction. It is important to transilluminate the eye to ensure accurate placement of the laser burns on the ciliary body, as the normal anatomical landmarks are often distorted. The probe is then placed over the eye in the appropriate position. 40 burns are placed (sparing the area of the long ciliary vessels and nerves at 3 and 9 o'clock) at 1,500–2,000 mW over 1500–2000 ms (Figure 20.13).[44] Avoid overtreatment and pigmented areas as there has been one report of a perforation in a buphthalmic eye during diode laser treatment. The advantage of diode laser ciliary ablation is ease of use, good pressure lowering and an appar-

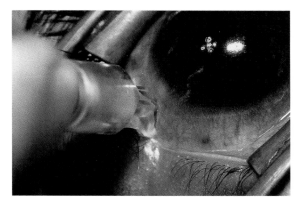

Figure 20.13 Diode laser cycloablation
In the buphthalmic eye the probe is placed further back from the limbus.

ently low risk of phthisis. The disadvantages are that medical treatment is usually required after the laser, and that the pressure lowering effect is usually temporary and may need to be repeated. In addition the eye may be more prone to hypotony if future filtration or tube surgery is required, and destruction of the blood aqueous barrier may predispose to long-term filtration failure and inflammation. The advantages and disadvantages of diode laser cyclodestruction are summarised in Table 20.7.

Postoperative follow-up

Following a surgical procedure the child is examined again under anaesthesia (if necessary) about two to three weeks later, and then at increasing intervals after that if progress is satisfactory. This intensive follow up is important to allow detection of "early failure" with post-operative incipient pressure rise. Should this develop the process can be bypassed with releasable sutures that can be pulled or cut, and needlings of the bleb. Alternatively it can be overcome with subconjunctival 5FU.

Parents are told to return with the child if they notice worsening symptoms such as photophobia or blepharospasm, or signs such as in increase in corneal cloudiness or size, all of which may indicate loss of IOP control. As the children get older, they should be introduced to the concept of slit lamp examination and tonometry without unduly stressing or frightening them for further visits. Usually the majority of children can be examined at the slit lamp by the time they are 5 years old, although some may require examination under anaesthesia for a longer period. Conversely, some children may allow a complete examination from as early as 3 years of age. It may be helpful to get the parents to use torches brought close to the eye while the child is sitting backwards on a chair with their chin resting on the back – simulating the tonometer.

All forms of childhood glaucoma need lifelong follow-up as they continue to relapse for many decades after the primary treatment,[11] and this must be stressed to the parents. If children are likely to have significantly impaired

Table 20.7 Advntages and disadvantages of diode laser cyclodestruction

Advantages

- Short surgical time
- Low complication rate and rapid rehabilitation
- Good short term response rate
- Very useful where surgery has high risks particularly in only eyes
- Technically less demanding than other procedures in difficult eyes

Disadvantages

- Has to be repeated several times in more than 50% of cases due to recovery of ciliary body in paediatric patients
- Most patients remain on medical therapy
- Pressure control is worse than drainage surgery; pressures in the low teens not usually achievable
- Danger of long term phthisis due to recurrent damage to ciliary body
- ? May affect future drainage surgery; hypotony due to hyposecretion, and fibrotic failure due to destruction of blood aqueous barrier releasing stimulatory cytokines into aqueous and drainage site

acuity or the treatment requires periods of absence from education, it is important that arrangements are made for the early assessment of any special schooling requirements. It is easy to overlook the effect that the disease and its treatment can have on the parents' relationship with their child, with each other and with their other children.

Occlusion therapy and refractive correction

The development of amblyopia is a significant complication of childhood glaucoma and is important as a cause of poor vision in these patients.[45-47] Vision may be significantly improved for patients with childhood glaucoma if a regimen of occlusion in the better eye is commenced (Figure 20.14). Findings which suggest the need for occlusion therapy include unequal visual acuity, strabismus (vision is almost always worse in the squinting eye), and anisometropia on refraction of more than one dioptre (the amblyopic eye is usually the most ametropic) (Figure 20.15).

The orthoptist plays a critical role managing these patients and is involved in assessing patients, detecting signs suggesting amblyopia and supervising the occlusion treatment. The importance of the occlusion treatment should be explained to the parents as the child is likely to be resistant – generally several hours of

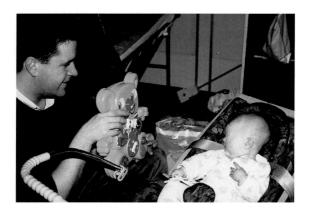

Figure 20.14 Occlusion therapy in a child.

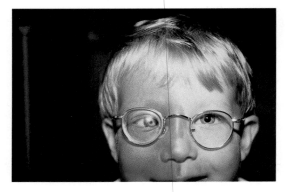

Figure 20.15 Sturge–Weber with secondary glaucoma.
The affected eye is myopic and requires optical correction.

occlusion therapy, although this is very much dependent on the child, their age and visual acuity.

Genetic counselling

Primary congenital glaucoma is inherited as an autosomal recessive gene from both parents. It is most commonly seem in cousin-cousin marriages, and therefore prevalent in some ethnic and religious groups. Counselling should be offered to the parents of such children, telling them of the risk of subsequent children being affected (see Chapter 4).

References

1 Anderson JR. Hydrophthalmia or congenital glaucoma. London: Cambridge University Press, 1939; 14–6.
2 Passo MS, Palmer EA, Van Buskivk EM. Plasma timolol in glaucoma patients. *Ophthalmology* 1984; **91**: 1361–3.
3 Harte VJ, Timoney RF. Aspects of the prescribing of drugs for children. *Pharm Int* 1981; **2**(6): 132–5.
4 Zimmerman TJ, Kooner KS, Kandarakis AS, Ziegler LP. Improving the therapeutic index of topically applied ocular drugs. *Arch Ophthalmol* 1984; **102**: 551–3.
5 Becker B, Shaffer RN. Diagnosis and Therapy of the Glaucomas. St Louis: CV Mosby Febiger 1965.
6 Boger WP, Walton DS. Timolol in uncontrolled childhood glaucoma surgery. *Ophthalmology* 1981; **88**: 253–8.
7 McMahon CD, Hetherington J, Hoskins HD, Shaffer RN. Timolol and pediatric glaucoma. *Ophthalmology* 1981; **88**: 249–52.
8 Khaw PT. What is the best primary surgical treatment for the infantile glaucomas? *Br J Ophthalmol* 1996; **80**: 495–6.
9 Barkan O. Techniques of goniotomy. *Arch Ophthalmol* 1938; **19**: 217–221.

10 Gramer E, Krieglstein. Infantile glaucoma in unilateral uveal ectropion. *Graefe's Arch Ophthalmol* 1979; **211**: 215.

11 Russell Eggitt IM, Rice NS, Jay B, Wyse RK. Relapse following goniotomy for congenital glaucoma due to trabecular dysgenesis. *Eye* 1992; **6**: 197–200.

12 Moller PM. Goniotomy and congenital glaucoma. *Acta Ophthalmol* 1977; **55**: 436–42.

13 Bietti GB. Contribution a la connaissance des resultats de la goniotomie dans le glaucoma congenitale. *Ann Ocul (Paris)* 1966; **199**: 481–5.

14 Haas J. End results of treatment. *Trans Am Acad Ophthalmol Otolaryngol* 1955; **59**: 333–40.

15 Morin JD. Congenital glaucoma. *Trans Am Acad Ophthalmol Otolaryngol.* 1980; **78**: 123.

16 Anderson DR. Discussion of Quigley HA: Childhood glaucoma. *Ophthalmology* 1982; **90**: 225–6.

17 Murthy U, Basu M, Sen-Majumdar A, Das M. Perinuclear location and recycling of epidermal growth factor receptor kinase: Immunofluorescent visualization using antibodies directed to kinase and extracellular domains. *J Cell Biol* 1986; **103**: 333–42.

18 Khaw PT, Rice NSC, Baez KA. The congenital glaucomas. In: El Sayyad F (ed). *The refractory glaucomas* Igaku-Shoin 1995; 1–21.

19 Smith R. A new technique for opening the canal of Schlemm. Preliminary report. *Br J Ophthalmol* 1960; **44**: 370.

20 Allen L, Burian HM. Trabeculotomy *ab externo.*. A new glaucoma operation. Technique and results of experimental surgery. *Am J Ophthalmol* 1962; **53**: 19–26.

21 DeLuise VP, Anderson DR. Primary infantile glaucoma (congenital glaucoma). *Surv Ophthalmol* 1983; **28**: 1.

22 Adachi M, Dickens CJ, Hetherington J, *et al.*. Clinical experience of trabeculotomy for the surgical treatment of aniridic glaucoma. *Ophthalmology* 1997; **104**: 2121–5.

23 Miller MH, Rice NSC. Trabeculectomy combined with β-irradiation for congenital glaucoma. *Br J Ophthalmol* 1991; **75**: 584–590.

24 Beck AD, Lynch MG. 360 trabeculotomy for primary congenital glaucoma. *Arch Ophthalmol* 1995; **113**: 1200–2.

25 Mandal AK, Naduvilath TJ, Jayagandan A. Surgical results of combined trabeculotomy-trabeculectomy for developmental glaucoma. *Ophthalmology* 1998; **105**: 974–82.

26 Elder MJ. Combined trabeculotomy-trabeculectomy compared with primary trabeculectomy for congenital glaucoma. *Br J Ophthalmol* 1994; **78**: 745–8.

27 Beauchamp GR, Parks MM. Filtering surgery in children: barriers to success. *Ophthalmology* 1979; **86**: 170–80.

28 Debnath SC, Teichmann KD, Salamah K. Trabeculectomy versus trabeculotomy in congenital glaucoma. *Br J Ophthalmol* 1989; **73**: 608–11.

29 Fulcher T, Chan J, Lanigan B, Bowell R, O'Keefe M. Long-term follow-up of primary trabeculectomy for infantile glaucoma. *Br J Ophthalmol* 1996; **80**: 499–502.

30 Miller M, Rice N. Trabeculectomy combined with β-radiation for congenital glaucoma. *Br J Ophthalmol* 1991; **75**: 584–90.

31 The Fluorouracil Filtering Surgery Study Group. Fluorouracil filtering surgery study one-year follow-up. *Am J Ophthalmol* 1989; **108**: 625–35.

32 Khaw PT, Ward S, Grierson I, Rice NSC. The effects of β-radiation on proliferating human Tenon's capsule fibroblasts. *Br J Ophthalmol* 1991; **75**: 580–3.

33 Chen C-W, Huang H-T, Bair JS, Lee C-C. Trabeculectomy with simultaneous topical application of mitomycin-c in refractory glaucoma. *J Ocul Pharmacol* 1990; **6**: 175–82.

34 Susanna R Jr, Nicolela MT, Takahashi WY. Mitomycin-C as adjunctive therapy with glaucoma implant surgery. *Ophthalmic Surg* 1994; **25**: 458–62.

35 Mandal AK, Walton DS, John T, Jayagandan A. Mitomycin-C-augmented trabeculectomy in refractory congenital glaucoma. *Ophthalmology* 1997; **104**: 996–1003.

36 Khaw PT, Doyle JW, Sherwood MB, Grierson I, Schultz GS, McGorray S. Prolonged Localized Tissue Effects From 5–Minute Exposures to Fluorouracil and Mitomycin-C. *Arch Ophthalmol* 1993; **111**: 263–7.

37 Cordeiro MF, Constable PH, Alexander RA, Bhattacharya SS, Khaw PT. The effect of varying mitomycin-C treatment area in glaucoma filtration surgery in the rabbit . *Invest Ophthalmol Vis Sci* 1997; **38**: 1639–46.

38 Netland PA, Walton DS. Glaucoma Drainage implants in paediatric patients. *Ophthalmic Surg* 1993; **24**: 723–9.

39 Asrani SG, Wilensky JT. Glaucoma after congenital cataract surgery. *Ophthalmology* 1995; **102**: 863–7.

40 Eid TE, Katz LJ, Spaeth GL, Augsburger JJ. Long-term effects of tube-shunt procedures on management of refractory childhood glaucoma. *Ophthalmology* 1997; **104**: 1011–6.

41 Lim KS, Allan BDS, Lloyd AW, Muir A, Khaw PT. Glaucoma drainage devices; past, present and future. *Br J Ophthalmol* 1998; **92**: 1083–9.

42 Franks WA, Hitchings RA. Injection of perfluoropropane gas to prevent hypotony in eyes undergoing tube implant surgery. *Ophthalmology* 1990; **97**: 899–903.

43 Eid TE, Katx JJ, Spaeth GL, Augsburger JJ. Tube-shunt surgery versus neodymium: YAG cyclophotocoagulation in the management of neovascular glaucoma. *Ophthalmology* 1997; **104**: 1692–700.

44 Bloom PA, Tsai JC, Sharma K, *et al.*. "Cyclodiode" Trans-scleral diode laser cyclophotocoagulation in the treatment of advanced refractory glaucoma. *Ophthalmology* 1997; **104**: 1508–20.

45 Clothier CM, Rice NS, Dobinson P, Wakefield R. Amblyopia in congenital glaucoma. *Trans Ophthalmol Soc UK* 1979; **99**: 427–31.

46 Richardson KT, Ferguson WJ Jr, Shaffer RN. Long-term functional results in infantile glaucoma. *Trans Am Acad Ophthalmol* 1967; **71**: 833–6.

47 Rice NSC. Management of infantile glaucoma. *Br J Ophthalmol* 1972; **56**: 294–8.

21 Secondary glaucomas: classification and management

K BARTON

This chapter classifies and outlines general principles of management of secondary glaucomas before examining issues specific to individual types.

Classification

Most secondary glaucomas are diagnosed when intraocular pressure (IOP) elevation occurs in the presence of a potential cause such as ocular disease, orbital disease or corticosteroid usage, which should have predated the IOP rise. The optic disc need not be cupped, nor the visual field constricted, but to be clinically significant there should be an element of chronicity.

A diverse group of conditions may elevate the IOP, mostly by reducing conventional aqueous outflow. In some circumstances movement of fluid into the eye from the intravascular space may contribute to the IOP rise, e.g. reduced plasma osmolality after haemodialysis,[1,2] or increased aqueous protein content in neovascular glaucoma, but this is not believed to have a significant effect in the presence of normal outflow. Aqueous outflow may be obstructed at three points in the outflow pathway, i.e. proximal to the trabecular meshwork (TM), within the meshwork itself, and distal to the meshwork. The secondary glaucomas relevant to these locations have been classified as pretrabecular, trabecular, and post-trabecular respectively (Table 21.1).[3]

Pre-trabecular

Aqueous is prevented from reaching the meshwork by tissue obstructing the angle, or substances surgically introduced into the anterior chamber. This category encompasses clinical secondary angle closure glaucoma and several conditions in which the angle may appear open on gonioscopy when it is closed histologically by overgrowth of, e.g. endothelium in iridocorneal endothelial syndrome (ICE) or epithelium in epithelial downgrowth, sometimes without visible peripheral anterior synechiae (PAS) formation. Increased aqueous viscosity in uveitis and neovascularisation may produce an additional relative reduction in outflow but is usually associated with other physical barriers to outflow such as PAS. Silicone oil emulsion in the anterior chamber may reduce outflow physically but additionally may cause pupil-block or closed angle without pupil-block. Furthermore, histological changes to the TM may result in severe glaucoma in the presence of minimal residual silicone oil emulsion (Figure 21.1). IOP elevation secondary to retained viscoelastic is usually short-lived but may be prolonged in patients with very low outflow facility.

When the angle is visibly closed on gonioscopy, it is important to differentiate between pupil-block and other causes of secondary angle closure such as PAS or anterior movement of iris-lens diaphragm secondary to posterior segment space-occupying lesion, e.g. melanoma or tight encircling band. Indentation gonioscopy will assist in differentiating synechial from appositional closure, but adequate fundus examination either by direct visualisation or ultrasonography is also required to exclude posterior segment disease.

Trabecular (open angle)

The TM may itself become *clogged* with pigment, erythrocytes or macrophages, or permanently altered. Permanent alteration may be the result of degeneration of the meshwork, e.g. in pigmentary glaucoma with migration of trabecular endothelial cells and collapse of trabecular beams, compression of the angle, e.g. in aphakic and post-keratoplasty glaucoma, or acute direct trauma as in angle recession. Less commonly, the TM may suffer from direct inflammation or trabeculitis, e.g. herpes simplex keratouveitis, scleritis, or the chronic foreign body reaction induced by the presence of silicone oil droplets (Figure 21.1).

Post-trabecular (open angle)

In the post-trabecular category, the outwardly-directed pressure gradient from the anterior chamber to the episcleral venous system is reversed because of extraocular venous congestion. Unlike Schlemm's canal, the endothelial-lined spaces of the collector channels and venous plexuses do not have vacuoles and the absence of a valve permits retrograde movement of blood into Schlemm's canal if the pressure in the venous outflow bed exceeds that in the canal. This may occur with: 1) congenital vascular abnormalities, e.g. Sturge–Weber syndrome, 2) arterio-venous shunts which allow blood at arterial pressure to enter the venous system, e.g. caroticocavernous fistulas and dural arterio-venous shunts, 3) systemic venous obstruction, e.g. superior vena caval syndrome, or 4) localised venous obstruction within the orbit, e.g. dysthyroid ophthalmopathy. Again the angle is open, but blood may be visualised in Schlemm's canal.

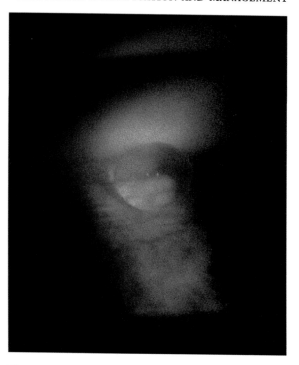

Figure 21.1(a) Silicone oil droplet in the angle of gonioscopy

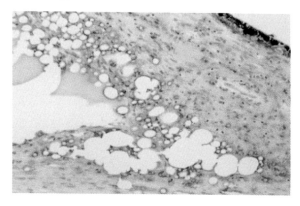

Figure 21.1(b) Gross histological damage to the trabecular meshwork from silicone oil emulsion in the iridocorneal angle

Management: general principles

Initial management is to treat the causative condition appropriately where possible and to protect the eye from the effects of high IOP. In many cases the aim of lowering the IOP will be to protect the optic nerve from glaucomatous damage, but alternatively may be to protect a

Table 21.1   Anatomical classification of mechanisms of secondary glaucoma

Mechanism	Category	Example
Pre-trabecular		
Closed angle: Pupil-block	Secluded pupil: posterior synechiae	Uveitis
	Secondary pupil-block glaucoma	Vitreous or silicone oil pupil-block in the aphakic patient. Anterior chamber IOL in pseudophakic patient
Closed angle: No pupil-block	Peripheral anterior synechiae	Chronic anterior segment inflammation, chronic appositional angle closure
	Posterior segment space-occupying lesion	Melanoma, surgical explant, pan-retinal photocoagulation, posterior scleritis
	Aqueous misdirection	Malignant glaucoma
	Fibrovascular	Neovascular glaucoma, chronic inflammation
	Endothelial	Iridocorneal endothelial syndrome, neovascular glaucoma
	Epithelial	Epithelial downgrowth
Open angle	Extraneous substances	Silicone oil, viscoelastic
	Altered aqueous (chronic blood-aqueous barrier incompetence)	Chronic uveitis, Fuchs' heterochromic cyclitis
Trabecular		
Clogged meshwork	Pigment	Pigmentary glaucoma, pseudoexfoliative glaucoma
	Proteinaceous material	Pseudoexfoliative glaucoma, phacolytic glaucoma
	Red blood cells	Hyphaema, vitreous haemorrhage
	Erythroclasts (ghost cells)	Ghost cell glaucoma
	Macrophages	Phacolytic glaucoma
Damaged meshwork	Trabecular collapse	Pigmentary glaucoma
	Trabecular inflammation/fibrosis	Trabeculitis, e.g. herpes simplex keratouveitis, Posner–Schlossman syndrome, silicone oil emulsion
	Trabecular compression	Post-keratoplasty, possibly aphakic glaucoma
	Trabecular trauma	Traumatic angle recession
	Drug-induced	Corticosteroid-induced glaucoma
Post-trabecular		
Elevated episcleral venous pressure	Arterio-venous shunts	Sturge–Weber syndrome, carotico-cavernous fistula, dural shunts
	Venous obstruction	Superior vena caval syndrome, dysthyroid ophthalmopathy

poorly-sighted eye from pain and the development of phthisis or to maintain residual vision in a poorly-sighted eye. The visual potential may therefore dictate the degree of aggression to which IOP lowering is sought.

Medical therapy

In most secondary glaucomas, medical therapy to lower the IOP is the first line. In some cases aggressive medical therapy will be required from the start to achieve a safe IOP level, in which case oral carbonic anhydrase inhibitors such as acetazolamide, methazolamide or dichlorphenamide will be required. A logical adjunct will be a topical non-selective β-blocker and a topical α_2-agonist (apraclonidine or brimonidine). There is no added benefit from the combination of topical and systemic carbonic anhydrase inhibitors. Drugs which facilitate outflow, such as prostaglandin agonists or cholinergics may sometimes be appropriate but should be used with caution in secondary glaucomas, e.g. prostaglandin agonists may exacerbate inflammatory disease, or precipitate cystoid macular oedema in aphakes. Pilocarpine may cause vasodilation, exacerbating blood-aqueous barrier breakdown and predisposing to synechial formation, e.g. in uveitis, pseudoexfoliation and neovascular glaucoma.

Many secondary glaucomas respond poorly to maximum tolerated medical therapy in the long-term. Surgical or laser treatment is then indicated. Nevertheless, medical therapy often provides an essential stopgap while more definitive intervention is planned, both to protect from the effects of high IOP prior to surgery, and to reduce the risk of suprachoroidal haemorrhage at the time of surgery.

Surgery

Numerous procedures have been described for the surgical management of secondary glaucomas, such as cyclocryotherapy, trabeculodialysis,[4] and partial cyclectomy.[5] However, the most commonly performed procedures are cyclophotocoagulation (CPC), trabeculectomy and seton implantation. Where the TM is heavily pigmented, argon laser trabeculoplasty (ALT) may be appropriate, whereas in cases of pupil-block, iridotomy, synechiolysis or lens extraction is usually indicated.

Filtration surgery

The general principles of maximising success and avoiding complications of filtration surgery as applied to the primary glaucomas are even more important for the secondary types as there are usually more risk factors present for failure. The patients are often younger and inflammation is common. It is important to perform filtration surgery under circumstances which are as close as possible to ideal. Secondary glaucoma patients may have undergone one or more previous surgical procedures reducing the long-term prospects of successful trabeculectomy function. If the inflammatory episode or previous surgery is recent, the prospect of successful trabeculectomy is enhanced by delaying surgery.[6] It may be difficult to manage the

IOP medically in the interim, and judicious use of CPC may be helpful.

Trabeculectomy is less successful in some types of secondary glaucoma, irrespective of adjunctive antiproliferative usage. In conditions such as neovascularisation, iridocorneal endothelial (ICE) syndrome, and epithelial downgrowth, further proliferation of abnormal tissue may block the filter. In patients with anterior chamber silicone oil emulsion following vitreoretinal surgery, silicone droplets or macrophages laden with engulfed silicone may obstruct trabecular outflow or a trabeculectomy filter. In addition, a chronic granulomatous or fibrotic reaction to silicone in the anterior chamber may compromise trabeculectomy function (Figure 21.1).[7] Finally, eyes with long-term breakdown of the blood aqueous barrier may always be at risk of fibroblast activation and scar tissue formation.[8]

Cyclophotocoagulation

While the outcome of cyclocryotherapy was somewhat unpredictable with a high rate of progression to phthisis,[9] transscleral laser CPC formerly with Neodymium:YAG laser and more recently with the semiconductor diode laser, allows titration of effect and a more controlled outcome as well as reducing the risk of phthisis.[10,11]

Transscleral diode CPC is effective in reducing the IOP to some degree in most cases. Multiple treatments may be required to maintain the IOP at an acceptable level and repeat treatment at a higher energy level may be effective in a patient with no initial response. Even when long-term acceptable IOP control is not achieved, CPC may be used to "buy time" for patients with secondary glaucomas in whom it would be inappropriate to operate immediately for other reasons, e.g. a recent early filtration failure.

Seton implantation

Seton implantation should not be undertaken lightly because of the potential risks of serious complications from early hypotony and the significant long-term risk of failure of pressure control from plate encapsulation. Nevertheless, drainage devices may still offer the best prospect of long-term IOP control in some intractable types of secondary glaucoma. Secondary glaucomas where setons should be considered include cases where a trabeculectomy may become blocked by vitreous (aphakic glaucoma), abnormal endothelium (ICE),[12] fibrovascular tissue neovascular glaucoma (NVG),[13-15] epithelium (epithelial downgrowth),[16] or in the presence of uveitis[17] where chronic inflammation may continually challenge the drainage site. In these cases setons have been reported by some authors to produce better long-term IOP control.

Specific characteristics and management of individual secondary glaucomas

Pseudoexfoliative (PXF) glaucoma

Pseudoexfoliation syndrome manifests clinically as PXF deposits on anterior lens surface and iris, pigmentary abnormalities of peripupillary iris and TM, breakdown of the blood-aqueous barrier due to PXF protein accumulation in the iris vasculature, zonular instability, and glaucoma.[18] It is worth remembering that histologically almost all cases are bilateral,[19] and that pseudoexfoliation has been recognised in virtually every ethnic group.

Glaucoma develops in approximately 50% of clinically affected eyes (the reported rates are highly variable) and the deposition of PXF material and iris pigment in the TM in combination with active production of exfoliative material by TM cells is believed to obstruct aqueous outflow. The drainage angle is usually open on gonioscopy but the meshwork may be heavily pigmented. The response to medical therapy may be poor but argon laser trabeculoplasty may be beneficial. Incompetence of the blood-aqueous barrier as a result of deposition

of PXF material within the iris vascular endothelial lining and possibly also an effect of chronic miotic therapy, contribute to the development of posterior synechiae. Pilocarpine is therefore best avoided if appropriate alternatives exist.

Cataract commonly coexists with glaucoma in PXF eyes and because of the progressive nature of PXF zonular instability, it is desirable to perform cataract surgery relatively early, if clinically justifiable on visual grounds. Combined phacotrabeculectomy is often appropriate for patients without evidence of zonular instability and moderately uncontrolled IOP. However, under certain circumstances separate filtering and cataract surgery should be considered. These would include a high preoperative IOP, suspect zonules, or if the lens showed advanced nuclear sclerosis. Similar surgical outcomes have been reported after trabeculectomy in PXF glaucoma as in primary open angle glaucoma.[20]

Pigmentary glaucoma

Pigment dispersion is usually bilateral and most often seen in young myopic white people, more commonly male than female (2-3:1). The influence of heredity is confounded by the heritability of myopia and no clear pattern has been consistently demonstrated.[21] Approximately 50% of these patients develop glaucoma.

The mechanism of pigment dispersion is presumed to be abrasion of posterior iris surface by anterior zonule causing pigment shedding from the posterior iris surface[22] and deposition throughout the anterior segment. It is hypothesised that a relative negative pressure in the posterior chamber induced by lens accommodation, causes the iris to bow backwards coming into contact with zonular fibres. Posterior bowing is often visible on gonioscopy.

Pigment deposition on the posterior corneal surface (Krukenberg's spindle), usually arouses suspicion of the diagnosis. Deposition may also be seen on the TM, dusting the anterior iris surface, on the anterior lens surface (Figure 21.2), and even peripheral posterior lens surface. Circulating pigment particles suspended in aqueous may in extreme cases be confused with uveitis ("pigment storms"). Mid-peripheral radial iris pigment defects on transillumination coincide with anterior zonule packets[22] and are considered a *sine qua non* for the diagnosis, although they may disappear with time,[23] as may pigment deposition on intraocular structures when shedding stops.

The early stages of pigment dispersion syndrome (PDS) are characterised by trabeculo-

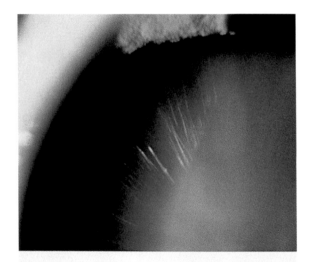

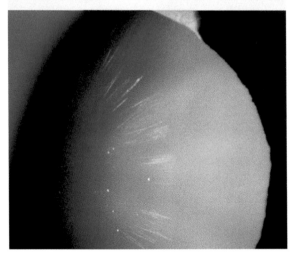

Figure 21.2 Pigment deposition on the anterior lens surface in pigment dispersion syndrome (PDS)

cytes phagocytosing pigment from the TM. Subsequent migration of these trabecular endothelial cells out of the meshwork leads to collapse of trabecular beams. This in turn causes irreversible obstruction of aqueous outflow and ocular hypertension.[21,24] It is worth trying to reduce pigment shedding with miotics. These drugs are not well tolerated by the typical patient with PDS who is younger and more likely to be myopic. However, the visual side effects may often be overcome with pilocarpine gel (Pilogel[TM]) at night or with pilocarpine inserts (Ocuserts[TM]). In all patients with PDS it is necessary to examine the peripheral retina before starting pilocarpine because of the risk of retinal detachment in eyes with pre-existing retinal disease.

Should miotic treatment prove unacceptable, the mainstay of IOP reduction is the topical β-blockers. When maximum tolerated medication is insufficient to control the IOP, ALT may be indicated. Patients with PDS respond well initially to ALT but long-term control may be less than 50%,[25] and because of this the overall usefulness of ALT in pigmentary glaucoma has been questioned.[26] ALT has been reported to be of greatest benefit in younger patients, although one third of patients may still eventually require filtering surgery.[25] Filtering surgery should be approached cautiously in this younger group of patients who are more prone to early postoperative hypotony maculopathy as well as a greater risk of long-term filtration failure. Younger patients also have a lower tolerance of induced astigmatism, and the cataractogenic effect of filtration surgery, especially if visually asymptomatic prior to surgery.

The place of peripheral laser iridotomy in management of PDS is not clear. Posterior bowing can certainly be reversed,[27] but the prevention of pigment shedding has not yet been demonstrated to alter the course of established glaucoma.

Neovascular glaucoma

New vessels in the angle accompany fibrovascular proliferation, the contraction of which causes PAS and ectropion uveae. This fibrovascular membrane becomes covered by an extension of Descemet's membrane and corneal endothelium,[28] further obstructing aqueous outflow. Heavy flare due to protein leakage from incompetent new iris vessels increases aqueous viscosity. This in turn exacerbates the physical outflow obstruction.

The earliest features are subtle, usually at the pupillary margin but occasionally vessels in the angle may be noted prior to any change in the pupillary area. It is important to identify the source of the angiogenic stimulus such as retinal or anterior segment ischaemia. This may not be easy in the presence of corneal oedema. Adequate early management of retinal ischaemia by pan-retinal photocoagulation may cause regression of iris neovascularisation prior to permanent synechial formation with improvement in the glaucoma. Goniophotocoagulation of early vessels has also been suggested as a method of preventing angle closure, but has not gained widespread acceptance.

Once angle closure is established, the IOP elevation can be intractable. Therapy for neovascular glaucoma should initially consist of topical corticosteroids and atropine to improve vascular competence and reduce flare. These are often more effective than ocular hypotensive medications. Neovascular glaucoma is generally resistant to aqueous suppressant therapy and CPC or surgery is often required to achieve IOP control.

Trabeculectomy is usually unsuccessful at controlling the IOP in neovascular glaucoma, and even when adjunctive 5-fluorouracil is used, the five year survival in terms of IOP control may be only 28%.[29] Some authors have reported improved results with mitomycin C. The likelihood of successful filtration may be better in the presence of inactive or regressing neovascularisation than those with active rubeosis.

In contrast, setons do not usually become occluded by neovascular membranes. Additionally setons offer a potential drainage route from the eye for angiogenic factors. While these devices have been used relatively successfully to control the IOP and thereby avoid pain and potentially enucleation,[13,30] in many patients progressive disease results in further visual reduction despite adequate IOP control.[14]

Corticosteroid-induced glaucoma

Normal individuals demonstrate three potential levels of IOP response to treatment with topical corticosteroids. Two thirds have a "low response" (< 5 mm Hg IOP rise), one third has an "intermediate response" (IOP rise 6–15 mm Hg) and 4–5% have a "high response" (> 15 mm Hg IOP rise).[31,32] In open angle glaucoma a high response has been demonstrated in over 50% of patients in one study.[33] Some authors have also reported chronic IOP elevation despite discontinuation of therapy if treatment has been prolonged. Systemic corticosteroids appear to cause IOP elevation less often than topical application. Dermal application and inhaled corticosteroid may also elevate the IOP.[34]

Glucocorticoids appear to reduce facility of outflow by altering the extracellular matrix composition in the angle, and possibly the fluid hydraulic conductivity of TM cells. The clinical significance of corticosteroid-induced glaucoma lies in its detection in patients at risk and its differentiation from glaucoma caused by the condition for which the corticosteroids are being taken, e.g. uveitis. From a practical viewpoint, in most eyes the IOP elevation is present by the end of the second week of treatment. However, in patients on a chronic low dose of corticosteroid, elevation may occur *de novo* after several months of treatment. In a few patients the IOP returns to normal after discontinuing corticosteroid therapy, yet glaucomatous cupping persists potentially leading to the misdiagnosis of normal pressure glaucoma.

Inflammatory glaucoma

Glaucoma secondary to chronic intraocular inflammation can be the most devastating and intractable complication of uveitis. The prevalence varies according to the type of uveitis, but is seen more commonly in patients with chronic than acute inflammatory disease.[35]

Conventional outflow may be reduced in uveitic glaucoma through clogging of TM with debris, direct inflammatory damage to the outflow pathway, PAS, pupil-block, and the effect of corticosteroid therapy. Although outflow may be significantly reduced, the resultant IOP is often a balance between altered outflow and altered inflow. In a cynomolgous monkey model of uveitis, aqueous production has been reported to fall by up to 50% in the acute phase, accompanied by a fourfold increase in uveoscleral outflow and a net fall in IOP.[36] Reduction of aqueous production is presumably a direct result of inflammation of non-pigmented ciliary epithelium, but the contribution of uveoscleral outflow is less important in humans than monkeys, so the resultant IOP is a balance between reduced aqueous production and reduced conventional outflow.

Clinical assessment

On clinical examination it is important to decide whether or not active inflammation is present and to look for a mechanism for IOP elevation. The cause may be obvious, e.g. PAS or secluded pupil, but in many cases of uveitis presenting with raised IOP the angle will be open on gonioscopy and there will be no visible obstruction to outflow. In these eyes it is important to gauge if IOP elevation is likely to be temporary, manageable with a short course of hypotensive medication, or whether long-term treatment will be required. It may be possible from the history to determine whether IOP elevation predated the use of corticosteroids or vice versa. A patient who is a steroid responder and who requires a short course of corticosteroids for a brief episode of uveitis, is better

managed medically than surgically for the acute episode. On the other hand, a patient with chronic IOP elevation between uveitic episodes, or who is a corticosteroid responder but requires chronic corticosteroid medication, is more likely to require chronic hypotensive medication and possibly filtration surgery.

The degree of glaucomatous optic neuropathy will also give an impression of the severity of the problem. The symptomatic nature of uveitis ensures that glaucoma is usually detected before the presence of visible optic nerve damage. There may only be early cupping and a normal visual field. An important early sign of significant damage is optic disc asymmetry, especially in unilateral uveitis. It is worth noting when the IOP is very high, compression of the optic nerve head increases the apparent cup size, which may be partially reversible on restoring the normal IOP.

Management

Medical The first principle of management of uveitic glaucoma is to treat active intraocular inflammation appropriately with corticosteroid therapy in order to limit long-term damage to the outflow pathways. Restricting corticosteroid use in the hope of avoiding an IOP response may result in further inflammatory damage, and glaucoma which is more difficult to control than might otherwise be the case. This is especially important in conditions such as Posner–Schlossman syndrome in which recurrent episodes of very high IOP may occur in the presence of limited inflammation of the anterior segment.[37] Posterior synechiae are rare in this condition and the angle is usually normal on gonioscopy. The episodes of raised IOP are believed to be secondary to trabeculitis which profoundly reduces conventional outflow. In patients without established glaucoma, and who do not require chronic medical topical glaucoma medication, Posner–Schlossman syndrome may sometimes be exquisitely sensitive to corticosteroid treatment, presumably by reducing trabecular inflammation and hence improving outflow. While aqueous suppressants are required in the acute phase to protect the optic nerve, it is sometimes judicious use of topical corticosteroid which will terminate the episode and prevent recurrence rather than ocular hypotensive medication. The same is generally true of elevated IOP in association with herpes simplex keratouveitis, in which case topical corticosteriods may be required in conjunction with anti-viral therapy (Figure 21.3). On the other hand, the use of corticosteroids in these conditions may have to be tempered in patients with established glaucoma, or a clear corticosteroid IOP response. Similarly corticosteroid use may be inappropriate in some types of uvietis which do not respond e.g. Fuchs' heterochromic cyclitis (Figure 21.3).

Uveitic glaucoma should be managed medically where possible. Some episodes of raised IOP may be self-limiting due to the episodic nature of the condition and intermittent use of corticosteroids. Additionally, the recurrent nature of uveitis prejudices the long-term success of surgery. Non-selective β-blockers are the first line of therapy in patients with no contraindications. Second line treatment may be an α-agonist such as brimonidine or a topical carbonic anhydrase inhibitor such as dorzolamide. In a significant proportion of cases, systemic carbonic anhydrase inhibitors will be required. Prostaglandin agonists are better avoided in uveitic patients because of a possible uveitogenic effect in some individuals[38] and a reported association with cystoid macular oedema.[39,40] Similarly cholinomimetics such as pilocarpine may potentially cause iris vasodilation, further breakdown of the blood-aqueous barrier, and posterior synechiae. In some cases, the IOP will be resistant to maximum-tolerated

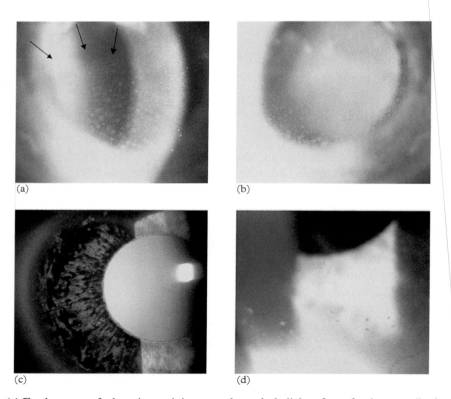

(a)

(b)

(c)

(d)

Figure 21.3   (a) Fresh mutton-fat keratic precipitates on the endothelial surface of a circumscribed area of cornea, (b) secondary cataract in herpes simplex keratouveitis. Fuchs Heterochromic cyclitis, (c) iris transillumination in Fuchs Heterochromic Cyclitis, (d) long-standing keratic precipitates in Fuchs Heterochromic Cyclitis.

medical therapy and surgical management will be necessary.

Surgical Initial surgical management of uveitis is usually trabeculectomy. The long-term success rate of filtration surgery of any type is likely to be compromised in inflammatory glaucomas by the episodic nature of the primary disease.[41] While reasonable survival has been described for both antiproliferative trabeculectomy[42,43] and seton implantation, both in the anterior chamber[17] and via the pars plana,[44] there is little long-term prospective comparative evidence on which to base management decisions. There is a theoretical basis for avoiding CPC where possible in patients with active ciliary body inflammatory disease, but again there is as yet little published evidence on which to estimate the potential risk of hypotony or phthisis.

There is a general consensus that trabeculectomy without the use of adjunctive antiproliferatives has a poor long-term chance of survival in uveitics.[35,41] But while the use of mitomycin in preference to 5-fluorouracil in uveitic trabeculectomy is widely advocated, the long-term benefits are not clearly established. A few *common sense* principles can be applied. It is unwise to perform a trabeculectomy in an eye with active inflammation, and therefore the IOP should be controlled medically as best as possible while inflammation is treated aggressively. If surgery is required in an actively inflamed eye, even mitomycin usage may not guarantee success. Other established risk factors for trabeculectomy failure should be taken into consideration, especially previous conjunctival surgery, but also race, age, and diabetes mellitus.

The risk of hypotony in the early postoperative period is greater in uveitic patients, even in the absence of overdrainage. In addition uveitic patients are often young, and consequently are more prone to the sequelae of hypotony. It is therefore desirable to suture the trabeculectomy flap securely in order to prevent drainage in the early postoperative period. Viscoelastic may also be left in the anterior chamber to help avoid early hypotony. Aqueous flow can then be established in the first one to two postoperative weeks by selective suture removal, either by using releasable/adjustable scleral sutures or argon laser suturelysis.

Patients with heavy aqueous flare from chronic breakdown of the blood aqueous barrier, even in the absence of active inflammation, may benefit from treatment with topical or even systemic corticosteroids prior to surgery.

Traumatic glaucoma

IOP elevation after trauma may occur early as a consequence of direct trauma to angle structures, angle recession, and iridodialysis. Erythrocytes in the aqueous (hyphaema) or ghost cells (erythroclasts) may obstruct the TM contributing to the IOP rise.

Hyphaema

Normal red cells in the anterior chamber can deform sufficiently to pass through the TM. Meshwork function therefore only becomes compromised in very large hyphaemas (involving more than half of the anterior chamber) or in the presence of abnormal red cells that do not deform appropriately, e.g. sickle cells or ghost cells. In the case of patients with sickle cell trait, systemic carbonic anhydrase inhibitors should be avoided as the resultant reduction in aqueous pH may precipitate sickling and exacerbate the situation. Sickled erythrocytes may produce a profound elevation in IOP in the presence of only a small hyphaema.[45]

Trauma to outflow structures

Angle recession results from a tear in the anterior face of the ciliary body with resultant posterior displacement of the iris root and a clinical appearance of broadening of the ciliary band on gonioscopy.[46] Recession is seen in up to 94% of patients after traumatic hyphaema (Figure 21.4),[47] and is of use in identifying patients at long-term risk of glaucoma. The

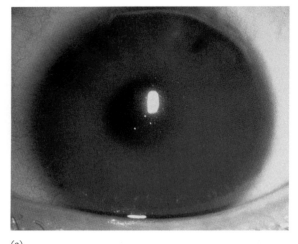

(a)

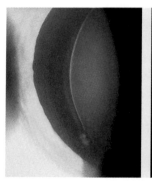

(b)

Figure 21.4 (a) Anterior chamber obscured by circulating hyphaema. Up to 94% of patients with traumatic hyphaema will demonstrate angle recession on gonioscopy afterwards and (b) the angle recession on gonioscopy

incidence of glaucoma is related to the extent of angle involvement.[48] It is useful to compare each quadrant of the angle with the corresponding quadrant in the uninjured eye when assessing the extent of involvement.

Approximately 10% of patients with angle recession will develop post-traumatic glaucoma, though up to two thirds may occur late. It has been suggested that a second peak in the incidence of glaucoma may occur more than 10 years after the initial insult,[49] hence the requirement for long-term follow-up.

Ghost cell glaucoma

Following vitreous haemorrhage (traumatic or otherwise), erythrocytes may pass into anterior chamber. The red cell life span is approximately 120 days, at which point, the cells lose haemoglobin. The biconcave shape is lost as is deformability and the resultant ghost erythrocytes in the anterior chamber may obstruct aqueous outflow. Occasionally a *tan hypopyon* forms (sometimes mistaken for endophthalmitis). Diagnosis can be confirmed by paracentesis and cytological examination of the aspirate.

Lens-related glaucoma

Lens-induced glaucoma may occur as a result of subluxation, change in lens shape (phacomorphic), leakage of lens proteins (phacolytic) or an immunological reaction to lens material (phacoanaphylactic).

Subluxed lens

Most commonly lens subluxation occurs with blunt trauma and may result in pupil-block glaucoma or occasionally vitreous pupil-block if there is marked dislocation. However, patients with lens subluxation may develop open angle glaucoma in the absence of obvious trauma to the angle structures (Figure 21.5). In cases of pupil-block surgical removal of the lens

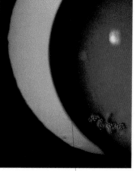

Figure 21.5 Traumatic lens subluxation in a patient with secondary open angle glaucoma

with vitrectomy may be performed via either an anterior or pars plana approach. In the case of open angle glaucoma, appropriate medical or surgical glaucoma management may be required before considering lens extraction.

Phacomorphic

In phacomorphic glaucoma an intumescent cataractous lens results in secondary angle closure. Initial medical management is similar to primary angle closure glaucoma. By definition, surgical removal of the cataractous lens rather than an iridotomy, will be required to correct the anatomical abnormality. The requirement for long-term glaucoma medication or surgical trabeculectomy will depend on the relative degree of synechial versus appositional angle closure and pressure damage to the TM.

Phacolytic

Phacolytic (lens particle) glaucoma is classically described as occurs when high molecular weight proteins become soluble as liquefaction of the lens cortex occurring in the hypermature cataract. Diffusion of these proteins through the intact capsule into the anterior chamber and to the TM results in obstruction of aqueous outflow, both by lens proteins themselves and also by engorged macrophages containing engulfed lens material. A much more common cause of glaucoma by this mechanism in clinical practice today is the presence of retained lens cortex after cataract surgery. In the postoperative cataract surgery patient, it is important to look for retained cortex, especially by gonioscopy of the inferior angle where it may be missed. While initial medical therapy should include topical corticosteroids to suppress associated inflammation, and aqueous suppressants to control the IOP, the pathogenesis of this condition is essentially mechanical and removal of retained lens cortex or the lens itself in the phakic patient, is indicated to correct the primary problem.

Phacoanaphylactic

Phacoanaphylactic glaucoma is considerably less common than phacolytic and caused by an immunological reaction to lens material in the anterior chamber or retained nuclear fragments. Classically, phacoanaphylactic uveitis occurs 14 days after cataract surgery or lens trauma, although much longer latent periods have been described. Clinically, the typical appearance is of a chronic granulomatous anterior uveitis with mutton-fat keratic precipitates and synechiae. A sympathetic inflammatory response may develop in the fellow eye. Secondary open or closed angle glaucoma may develop if treatment is not prompt. Unlike phacolytic glaucoma, IOP elevation is the result of chronic inflammation, rather than obstruction of the TM with lens material. In addition, glaucoma does not usually present in phacoanaphylactic glaucoma until some time after the onset.

Aqueous suppressants and topical corticosteroids are used in the medical management, but definitive management is to remove any retained lens material.

Pseudophakic/aphakic glaucoma

Aphakic

Aphakic glaucoma may be multifactorial, e.g. vitreous pupil-block, open angle, or synechial. The anterior chamber is usually deep. Vitreous may be visible in the anterior chamber and may adhere to the pupil margin inducing pupil-block with iris bombé and shallowing of the anterior chamber. However, in aphakic glaucoma the angle is often open. Typically the IOP rise is resistant to medical therapy and trabeculectomy survival in the pre-antiproliferative era was poor. Previously seton implantation offered the best chance of achieving long-term IOP control in cases of aphakic glaucoma, although in many practices this has been supplanted by trabeculectomy with mitomycin C in combination with anterior vitrectomy as the first surgical glaucoma procedure in aphakic patients. Diode laser CPC also offers a useful alternative.

Pseudophakic

The intraocular lens (IOL) may induce open angle glaucoma because of associated inflammation, or from pigment release from haptics chaffing on the iris. Glaucoma *de novo* in the presence of an anterior chamber IOL may be caused by iris tuck around the haptics obstructing the TM, PAS, vitreous or IOL pupil-block if no iridotomy is present, or secondary open angle glaucoma. Management of pupil-block is to perform an iridotomy if not already present, and anterior vitrectomy if appropriate. Open angle glaucoma is managed initially with aqueous suppressants and subsequently mitomycin C trabeculectomy if required.

Post-keratoplasty glaucoma

Glaucoma has been reported in up to 31% of eyes after keratoplasty. Apart from pre-existing glaucoma and aphakia,[50] glaucoma is more common in patients after multiple keratoplasties and possibly also if donor buttons are not oversized. Early IOP spikes after surgery may be the result of retained viscoelastic, blood, vitreous, uveitis, pupil-block or corticosteroid response. Although not predictive of future glaucoma, there is a higher incidence in those who have postoperative IOP spikes.

The influence of angle compression on post-keratoplasty glaucoma has received extensive theoretical attention. Olson *et al* have demonstrated mathematically how the relationship of donor to recipient diameter can influence the degree of angle compression and hence glaucoma.[51,52] The clinical evidence is less clear. Bourne reported a significantly lower mean IOP postoperatively in a study of 41 consecutive transplants, half of which were oversized,[53] whereas Perl found no difference when comparing 61 same sized to 119 oversized grafts.[54]

Post-keratoplasty glaucoma can be intractable and is a significant adverse prognostic factor for graft survival. Medical treatment often fails, ALT is inappropriate and trabeculectomy may not be feasible. For a considerable period of time cyclocryotherapy (CCT) was the mainstay of treatment,[55] despite the uncontrolled nature of the procedure and possible severe complications.

Trabeculectomy has not generally found favour with a reported high incidence of complications.[50] One would expect the success rate to be higher with adjunctive antiproliferative agents but limited clinical outcome data have been published.[56,57] Additionally, setons have been associated with an increased risk of keratoplasty failure.[58,59] Tube-endothelial contact has been implicated as a cause of chronic non-immune graft failure,[60] but a higher rate of acute allograft rejection has also been noted more commonly in tube patients.[58] Kirkness has suggested that as the tube allows direct contact with fibrovascular tissue, the blood-aqueous barrier is eliminated, thereby increasing the possibility of allograft rejection.[61] However it might also be the case that the blood-aqueous barrier is already compromised from chronic anterior segment disease and previous surgical intervention. Alternative tube entry sites have been suggested as a means of avoiding corneal touch, such as pars plana[13] and more recently, ciliary sulcus positioning.[62]

There are little comparative data regarding the relative efficacy of trabeculectomy, seton implantation and CPC. One small retrospective study has recently reported little difference in efficacy, complication rate and graft survival.[63]

Iridocorneal endothelial syndrome

Iridocorneal endothelial syndrome (ICE) is usually unilateral and, presents with iris abnormalities or visual symptoms from corneal oedema, most commonly in young women (third to fifth decade). The syndrome is caused by abnormal proliferation of altered corneal endothelium. Contact inhibition between cell types appears to be lost, and the abnormal endothelium shows an ability to spread over neighbouring structures, including the TM and iris surface. Subsequent contraction of this tissue lining the meshwork produces PAS, while contraction of the tissue over the iris causes distortion and pseudopolycoria. Glaucoma appears to be more common in cases where the posterior corneal surface is entirely replaced by iridocorneal endothelium.[64]

Clinically, the iris may demonstrate pupillary distortion, loss of crypts and ectropion uveae due to traction from the abnormal membrane on the anterior iris surface. Nodules of hypertrophic or normal iris may protrude through the ICE membrane, and atrophic full-thickness iris holes are seen in the quadrant opposite to the direction of pupillary distortion. The cornea may demonstrate a demarcation line between normal and abnormal endothelium. In more advanced cases these may not be seen if endothelium is completely replaced. Abnormal endothelium takes on a "hammered silver" appearance. The diagnosis can usually be confirmed by specular microscopy (Figure 21.6), which also permits differentiation from posterior polymorphous dystrophy, a possible differential diagnosis.[65] In advanced cases the cornea may become oedematous in the presence of only mildly raised IOP.

On gonioscopy, broad-based PAS may be seen which extend beyond Schwalbe's line. These synechiae typically progress around the circumference of the angle. The degree of glaucoma does not necessarily correlate with degree of synechial closure because clinically open angle may be covered by ICE membrane histologically.

Although the pathogenesis is identical, three major clinical patterns are recognised according to the effects of the proliferating cellular membrane within the anterior segment. In *progressive iris atrophy*, iris stromal thinning progresses to produce full-thickness iris "stretch" holes typically in the quadrant diametrically opposite the site of PAS. PAS develop early and pupillary distortion with ectropion uveae most typically points in the direction of the most prominent PAS. *Chandler's syndrome* usually manifests with corneal oedema as the dominant feature, often at normal or only moderately elevated levels of IOP. Iris atrophy is less prominent. In *Cogan–Reese (Iris Naevus) syndrome*, multiple pigmented iris lesions are seen which actually represent areas of normal iris protruding through defects in an ICE membrane which covers the anterior iris surface.

Medical management is appropriate initially, though the glaucoma in ICE syndrome is often resistant. While trabeculectomy survival at one year has been reported to compare favourably with that in primary open angle glaucoma,[66] survival at five years appears to be poor.[64] This is presumably due to endothelialisation of the filtration site which has been demonstrated histologically.[67] Similarly poor filtration survival has been reported with 5-fluorouracil trabeculectomy, and seton implantation currently may offer the best prospect for longer term IOP control.[12]

Epithelial downgrowth

Epithelial downgrowth in the anterior chamber may manifest as a limited inclusion cyst close to a previous penetrating wound, or as sheet-like downgrowth which progressively envelopes all anterior segment structures, lens, vitreous and even retina in vitrectomised eyes. Epithelial cysts typically do not progress, but

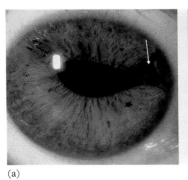
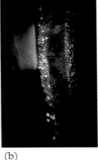

(a)   (b)

Figure 21.6 Iridocorneal endothelial syndrome (ICE): (a) pupil distortion towards contracting ICE membrane, (b) normal and abnormal endothelium on specular microscopy

may be converted to sheet-like downgrowth if incompletely excised. The natural history of sheet-like downgrowth is inexorable progression resulting in intractable glaucoma.

While fortunately rare, downgrowth typically occurs after complicated surgery involving the limbus, e.g. cataract, trabeculectomy, usually in eyes which have undergone multiple surgical procedures and in which a persistent postoperative wound leak has occurred. The leak may be as small as a full-thickness suture track (Figure 21.7).

Epithelium within the eye usually proliferates most aggressively in the vicinity of vascularised tissue, e.g. peripheral cornea and iris, and exhibits some degree of contact inhibition when it meets healthy endothelium. Downgrowth usually presents as a progressive retrocorneal membrane usually encircling most of the peripheral cornea prior to reaching the visual axis (Figure 21.7). The cornea usually remains clear until the later stages. Anterior iris membrane may be more difficult to visualise but classically blanches on argon laser photocoagulation. A mild chronic anterior uveitis is often seen.

Glaucoma develops when the leaking fistula eventually seals. Management of downgrowth is primarily to control the IOP, for which seton implantation offers the only realistic prospect.[16,68] Trabeculectomies become internally closed by proliferating epithelium and do not usually function for long. Radical surgical excision and extensive cryotherapy have been used in the past in an attempt to control epithelial proliferation, but reported long-term successes are rare. Penetrating keratoplasty may restore visual loss due to corneal decompensation.

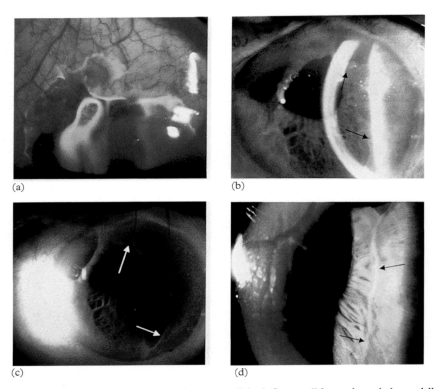

(a) (b)

(c) (d)

Figure 21.7   Epithelial downgrowth: (a) a persistent small leak from a "through and through" suture track is often responsible, (b) and (c) the retrocorneal membrane often progresses circumferentially, replacing central corneal endothelium late, (d) the sharply demarcated epithelial membrane on anterior iris surface

Post-trabecular glaucomas

Raised episcleral venous pressure may be suspected from the presence of dilated episcleral veins (Figure 21.8) or characteristic features of a predisposing cause such as a Sturge–Weber syndrome or dysthyroid ophthalmopathy.

The cause of venous obstruction should be treated where possible. In some conditions, e.g. raised IOP associated with dysthyroid ophthalmopathy, orbital decompression or inferior rectus recession may be valuable.[69] Medical treatment is the initial mainstay of glaucoma management and, in the long-term, filtration surgery may be required. Filtration surgery should be approached with caution in eyes with raised episcleral venous pressure as there is a significant risk of uveal effusion. Steps should be taken to avoid prolonged intraoperative or early postoperative hypotony by tight wound suturing and viscoelastic injection. In the aphakic patient intraocular gas injection may also be appropriate.

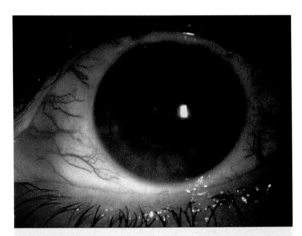

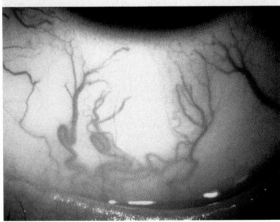

Figure 21.8 Dilated episcleral veins may raise the suspicion of elevated episcleral venous pressure in cases where regional (superior vena caval) or orbital venous drainage is obstructed

References

1 Burn RA. Intraocular pressure during haemodialysis. *Br J Ophthalmol* 1973; **57**: 511–3.

2 Sitprija V, Holmes JH, Ellis PP. Intraocular pressure changes during artificial kidney therapy. *Arch Ophthalmol* 1964; **72**: 626–31.

3 Hoskins HD Jr. Secondary Glaucomas. In: Heilmann K, Richardson K (eds). *Glaucoma Conceptions of a disease* Philadelphia: WB Saunders Co, 1978.

4 Williams RD, Hoskins HD Jr, Shaffer RN. Trabeculodialysis for inflammatory glaucoma: a review of 25 cases. *Ophthalmic Surg* 1992; **23**: 36–7.

5 Demeler U. Ciliary body excision in secondary glaucoma: a 15 year follow-up. *Dev Ophthalmol* 1991; **22**: 138–139.

6 The Fluorouracil Filtering Surgery Study Group. Five-year follow-up of the fluorouracil filtering surgery study group. *Am J Ophthalmol* 1996; **121**: 349–66.

7 Lambrou FH, Burke JM, Aaberg TM. Effect of silicone oil on experimental traction retinal detachment. *Arch Ophthalmol* 1987; **105**: 1269–72.

8 Joseph JP, Grierson I, Hitchings RA. Chemotactic activity of aqueous humor. A cause of failure of trabeculectomies? *Arch Ophthalmol* 1989; **107**: 69–74.

9 Krupin T, Mitchell KB, Becker B. Cyclocryotherapy in neovascular glaucoma. *Am J Ophthalmol* 1978; **86**: 24–6.

10 Bloom PA, Tsai JC, Sharma K, *et al.* "Cyclodiode": trans-scleral diode laser cyclophotocoagulation in the treatment of advanced refractory glaucoma. *Ophthalmology* 1997; **104**: 1508–20.

11 Spencer AF, Vernon SA. "Cyclodiode": results of a standard protocol. *Br J Ophthalmol* 1999; **83**: 311–6.

12 Wright MM, Grajewski AL, Cristol SM, Parrish RK. 5-Fluorouracil after trabeculectomy and the iridocorneal endothelial syndrome. *Ophthalmology* 1991; **98**: 314–6.

13 Lloyd MA, Heuer DK, Baerveldt G, *et al.* Combined Molteno implantation and pars plana vitrectomy for neovascular glaucomas. *Ophthalmology* 1991; **98**: 1401–5.

14 Mermoud A, Salmon JF, Alexander P, Straker C, Murray ADN. Molteno tube implantation for neovascular glaucoma. *Ophthalmology* 1993; **100**: 897–902.

15 Eid TE, Katz LJ, Spaeth GL, Augsburger JJ. Tube-shunt surgery versus neodymium: YAG cyclophotocoagulation in the management of neovascular glaucoma. *Ophthalmology* 1997; **104**: 1692–700.

16 Costa VP, Katz LJ. Glaucoma associated with epithelial downgrowth controlled with Molteno tube shunts. *Ophthalmic Surg* 1992; **23**: 797–800.

17 Hill RA, Nguyen QH, Baerveldt G, *et al.* Trabeculectomy and Molteno implantation for glaucoma associated with uveitis. *Ophthalmology* 1993; **100**: 903–8.

18 Naumann GOH, Schlötzer-Schrehardt U, Küchle M.

Pseudoexfoliation syndrome for the comprehensive ophthalmologist. *Ophthalmology* 1998; **105**: 951–68.

19 Kivelä T, Hietanen J, Uusitalo M. Autopsy analysis of clinically unilateral exfoliation syndrome. *Invest Ophthalmol Vis Sci* 1997; **38**: 2008–15.

20 Popovic V, Sjöstrand J. Course of exfoliation and simplex glaucoma after primary trabeculectomy. *Br J Ophthalmol* 1998; **83**: 305–10.

21 Farrar SM, Shields MB. Current concepts in pigmentary glaucoma. *Surv Ophthalmol* 1993; **37**: 233–52.

22 Campbell DG. Pigmentary dispersion and glaucoma: a new theory. *Arch Ophthalmol* 1979; **97**: 1667–72.

23 Richter CU, Richardson TM, Grant WM. Pigmentary dispersion syndrome and pigmentary glaucoma. *Arch Ophthalmol* 1986; **104**: 211–5.

24 Richardson TM, Hutchinson BT, Grant WM. The outflow tract in pigmentary glaucoma: a light and electron microscopic study. *Arch Ophthalmol* 1977; **95**: 1015–25.

25 Ritch R, Liebmann J, Robin A, *et al.* Argon laser trabeculoplasty in pigmentary glaucoma. *Ophthalmology* 1993; **100**: 909–13.

26 Lehto I. Long-term follow-up of Argon laser trabeculoplasty in pigmentary glaucoma. *Ophthalmic Surg* 1992; **23**: 614–7.

27 Breingan PJ, Esaki K, Ishikawa H, Liebmanm JM, Greenfield DS, Ritch R. Iridolenticular contact decreases following laser iridotomy for pigment dispersion syndrome. *Arch Ophthalmol* 1999; **117**: 325–8.

28 Gartner S, Taffet S, Friedman AH. The association of rubeosis iridis with endothelialisation of the anterior chamber: report of a clinical case with histopathological review of 16 additional cases. *Br J Ophthalmol* 1977; **61**: 267–71.

29 Tsai JC, Feuer WJ, Parrish RK II, Grajewski AL. 5-Fluorouracil filtering surgery and neovascular glaucoma. Long-term follow-up of the original pilot study. *Ophthalmology* 1995; **102**: 887–93.

30 Krupin T, Kaufman P, Mandell AI, *et al.* Long-term results of valve implants in filtering surgery for eyes with neovascular glaucoma. *Am J Ophthalmol* 1983; **95**: 775–82.

31 Armaly MF. Statistical attributes of the steroid hypertensive response in the clinically normal eye: I. the demonstration of three levels of response. *Invest Ophthalmol Vis Sci* 1965; **4**: 187–97.

32 Armaly MF. The heritable nature of dexamethasone-induced ocular hypertension. *Arch Ophthalmol* 1966; **75**: 32–5.

33 Becker B. Intraocular pressure response to topical steroids. *Invest Ophthalmol Vis Sci* 1965; **4**: 198–205.

34 Dreyer EB. Inhaled steroid use and glaucoma. *N Engl J Med* 1993; **329**: 1822.

35 Panek WC, Holland GN, Lee DA, Christensen RE. Glaucoma in patients with uveitis. *Br J Ophthalmol* 1990; **74**: 223–7.

36 Toris CB, Pederson JE. Aqueous humor dynamics in experimental iridocyclitis. *Invest Ophthalmol Vis Sci* 1987; **28**: 477–81.

37 Posner A, Schlossman A. Syndrome of recurrent attacks of glaucoma with cyclitic symptoms. *Arch Ophthalmol* 1948; **39**: 517–33.

38 Fechtner RD, Khouri AS, Zimmerman TJ, *et al.* Anterior uveitis associated with Latanoprost. *Am J Ophthalmol* 1998; **126**: 37–41.

39 Colonna D, Fellowman RL, Savage JA. Latanoprost-associated cystoid macular edema. *Am J Ophthalmol* 1998; **126**: 134–5.

40 Miyake K, Ota I, Maekubo K, Ichihashi S, Miyake S. Latanoprost accelerates disruption of the blood-aqueous barrier and the incidence of angiographic cystoid macular edema in early postoperative pseudophakics. *Arch Ophthalmol* 1999; **117**: 34–40.

41 Towler HMA, Bates AK, Broadway DC, Lightman S. Primary trabeculectomy with 5-fluorouracil for glaucoma secondary to uveitis. *Ocular Immunol Inflamm* 1995; **3**: 163–70.

42 Patitsas CJ, Rockwood EJ, Meisler DM, Lowder CY. Glaucoma filtering surgery with postoperative 5-Fluorouracil in patients with intraocular inflammatory disease. *Ophthalmology* 1992; **99**: 594–9.

43 Prata JA, Neves RA, Minckler DS, Mermoud A, Heuer DK. Trabeculectomy with Mitomycin C in glaucoma associated with uveitis. *Ophthalmic Surg* 1994; **25**: 616–20.

44 Sheppard JD, Shrum KR. Pars plana Molteno implantation in complicated inflammatory glaucoma. *Ophthalmic Surg* 1995; **26**: 218–22.

45 Goldberg MF. The diagnosis and treatment of secondary glaucoma after hyphema in sickle cell patients. *Am J Ophthalmol* 1979; **87**: 43–9.

46 Treacher Collins E. On the pathological examination of three eyes lost from concussion. *Trans Ophthalmol Soc UK* 1892; **12**: 180–6.

47 Tönjum AM. Gonioscopy in traumatic hyphaema. *Acta Ophthalmol* 1966; **44**: 650–64.

48 Kaufman JH, Tolpin DW. Glaucoma after traumatic angle recession. *Am J Ophthalmol* 1974; **78**: 648–53.

49 Blanton FM. Anterior chamber angle recession and secondary glaucoma. *Arch Ophthalmol* 1964; **72**: 39–43.

50 Foulks GN. Glaucoma associated with penetrating keratoplasty. *Ophthalmology* 1987; **94**: 871–4.

51 Olson RJ, Kaufman HE. A mathematical description of causative factors and prevention of elevated intraocular pressure after keratoplasty. *Invest Ophthalmol Vis Sci* 1977; **16**: 1085–92.

52 Olson RJ. Aphakic keratoplasty. Determining donor tissue size to avoid elevated intraocular pressure. *Arch Ophthalmol* 1978; **96**: 2274–6.

53 Bourne WM, Davison JA, O'Fallon WM. The effects of oversize donor buttons on postoperative intraocular pressure and corneal curvature in aphakic penetrating keratoplasty. *Ophthalmology* 1982; **89**: 242–6.

54 Perl T, Charlton KH, Binder PS. Disparate diameter grafting. Astigmatism, intraocular pressure, and visual acuity. *Ophthalmology* 1981; **88**: 774–81.

55 Binder PS, Abel R, Kaufman HE. Cyclocryotherapy for glaucoma after penetrating keratoplasty. *Am J Ophthalmol* 1975; **79**: 489–92.

56 Figueiredo RS, Araujo SV, Cohen EJ, Rapuano CJ, Katz LJ, Wilson RP. Management of coexisting corneal disease and glaucoma by combined penetrating keratoplasty and trabeculectomy with Mitomycin-C. *Ophthalmic Surg Lasers* 1996; **27**: 903–9.

57 Sharma A, Kumar S, Ram J, Gupta A. Trabeculectomy with Mitomycin-C for postkeratoplasty glaucoma: a preliminary study. *Ophthalmic Surg Lasers* 1997; **28**: 891–5.

58 McDonnell PJ, Robin JB, Schanzlin DJ, *et al.* Molteno implant for control of glaucoma in eyes after penetrating keratoplasty. *Ophthalmology* 1988; **95**: 364–69.

59 Price FW Jr, Wellemeyer M. Long-term results of Molteno implants. *Ophthalmic Surg* 1995; **26**: 130–5.

60 Sherwood MB, Smith MF, Driebe WT, Stern GA,

Beneke JA, Zam ZS. Drainage tube implants in the treatment of glaucoma following penetrating keratoplasty. *Ophthalmic Surg* 1993; **24**: 185–9.

61 Kirkness CM, Moshegov C. Post-keratoplasty glaucoma. *Eye* 1988; **2 Suppl**: S19–S26

62 Rumelt S, Rehany U. Implantation of glaucoma drainage implant tube into the ciliary sulcus in patients with corneal transplants. *Arch Ophthalmol* 1998; **116**: 685–7.

63 Ayyala RS, Pieroth L, Vinals AF, *et al*. Comparison of Mitomycin C trabeculectomy, glaucoma drainage device implantation, and laser Neodymium: YAG cyclophotocoagulation in the management of intractable glaucoma after penetrating keratoplasty. *Ophthalmology* 1998; **105**: 1550–6.

64 Laganowski HC, Kerr-Muir MG, Hitchings RA. Glaucoma and the iridocorneal endothelial syndrome. *Arch Ophthalmol* 1992; **110**: 346–50.

65 Laganowski HC, Sherrard ES, Muir MG, Buckley RJ. Distinguishing features of the iridocorneal endothelial syndrome and posterior polymorphous dystrophy: value of endothelial specular microscopy (see comments). *Br J Ophthalmol* 1991; **75**: 212–6.

66 Kidd M, Hetherington J, Magee S. Surgical results in iridocorneal endothelial syndrome. *Arch Ophthalmol* 1988; **106**: 199–201.

67 Eagle RC Jr, Font RL, Yanoff M, Fine BS. Proliferative endotheliopathy with iris abnormalities. The iridocorneal endothelial syndrome. *Arch Ophthalmol* 1979; **97**: 2104–11.

68 Fish LA, Heuer DK, Baerveldt G, Minckler DS, McDonnell PJ. Molteno implantation for secondary glaucomas associated with advanced epithelial ingrowth. *Ophthalmology* 1990; **97**: 557–61.

69 Kalmann R, Mourtis MP. Prevalence and management of elevated IOP in patients with Graves' orbitopathy. *Br J Ophthalmol* 1998; **82**: 754–7.

Acknowledgements

The author would like to thank the following for kindly granting permission to use certain photographs as illustrations; Riaz Asaria FRCOphth of Moorfields Eye Hospital, London for Figure 1, Richard K. Forster M.D. and William W. Culbertson M.D., both of Bascom Palmer Eye Institute, University of Miami School of Medicine, Miami for Figures 6 and 7 respectively.

Index